"What a treasure trove we have in this book. It exemplifies my belief that psychoanalysis should be viewed as the natural history approach to psychology much as Darwin's study of the natural world opened up biology. This method of work requires sustained observation and builds theory from the observed data as the writers in this volume have done, across a wide range of topics of clinical interest. I recommend it most warmly."

Ronald Britton, psychoanalyst and author,
past President of the British Psychoanalytic Society

"At a time when the need for novel interdisciplinary approaches to mental health research is increasingly recognised, this excellent book provides a compelling account of the distinctive tradition of qualitative child psychotherapy research. It is a fascinating read, offering rich insights from the frontline of children's services."

Eilis Kennedy, Director of Research, Tavistock
and Portman NHS Foundation Trust

"This impressive collection of papers is testimony to the rich tradition of research into child psychotherapy undertaken at the Tavistock Clinic over the last 20 years. It will be of great interest to those working therapeutically with children, as well as those seeking inspiration regarding psychoanalytic research methods."

Nick Midgley, Associate Professor, UCL, and the
Anna Freud National Centre for Children and Families

NEW DISCOVERIES IN CHILD PSYCHOTHERAPY

New Discoveries in Child Psychotherapy presents eleven new contributions to child psychoanalytic research, most of them based on the experience of the clinical consulting room. Each chapter is the work of an experienced child psychotherapist or child analyst, vivid in their description of the children and families they encountered. Their understanding of the "inner worlds" of patients and the clinical consulting room is clearly evidenced in their analysis of clinical presentations.

The chapters are the result of the psychoanalytic clinical and observational practices of their authors, allied to their use of rigorous qualitative research methods, in particular Grounded Theory and interpretative phenomenological analysis (IPA). They describe developments of child psychoanalytic knowledge in several fields, including autism, psychotherapy with severely deprived children, and the study of early infancy. They demonstrate advances in child psychoanalytic theories and methods and the development of new forms of clinical service provision. Contested issues in psychoanalytic research are thoroughly evaluated, showing how it can be made more accountable and rigorous through the adaptation of established qualitative research methods to the study of unconscious mental phenomena.

New Discoveries in Child Psychotherapy will be an essential text in the field of child psychoanalysis and will be highly useful in psychotherapy and psychoanalysis training courses and for psychoanalytic researchers, as well as for practitioners.

Margaret Rustin is a prominent child psychotherapist and child psychoanalyst. She was Head of Child Psychotherapy at the Tavistock Clinic for many years and continues to teach and supervise there. She contributed significantly to the IMPACT research study on adolescent depression. She is the author and editor of many books, including, most recently, with colleagues, *Short-Term Psychoanalytic Psychotherapy for Adolescents with Depression,* and, with Michael Rustin, *Reading Klein.*

Michael Rustin is Professor of Sociology at the University of East London and a Visiting Professor at the Tavistock Clinic where he has taught for many years. He has written widely on psychoanalysis and its applications. His book *Researching the Unconscious: Principles of Psychoanalytic Method* has also recently been published by Routledge in the Tavistock Clinic Series.

Tavistock Clinic Series

Margot Waddell, Jocelyn Catty, & Kate Stratton (Series Editors)

Recent titles in the Tavistock Clinic Series

Childhood Depression: A Place for Psychotherapy, *edited by Judith Trowell, with Gillian Miles*
Conjunctions: Social Work, Psychoanalysis, and Society, *by Andrew Cooper*
Consultations in Psychoanalytic Psychotherapy, *edited by R. Peter Hobson*
Contemporary Developments in Adult and Young Adult Therapy. The Work of the Tavistock and Portman Clinics, Vol. 1, *edited by Alessandra Lemma*
Couple Dynamics: Psychoanalytic Perspectives in Work with the Individual, the Couple, and the Group, *edited by Aleksandra Novakovic*
Doing Things Differently: The Influence of Donald Meltzer on Psychoanalytic Theory and Practice, *edited by Margaret Cohen & Alberto Hahn*
Inside Lives: Psychoanalysis and the Growth of the Personality, *by Margot Waddell*
Internal Landscapes and Foreign Bodies: Eating Disorders and Other Pathologies, *by Gianna Williams*
Living on the Border: Psychotic Processes in the Individual, the Couple, and the Group, *edited by David Bell & Aleksandra Novakovic*
Making Room for Madness in Mental Health: The Psychoanalytic Understanding of Psychotic Communication, *by Marcus Evans*
Melanie Klein Revisited: Pioneer and Revolutionary in the Psychoanalysis of Young Children, *by Susan Sherwin-White*
New Discoveries in Child Psychotherapy: Findings from Qualitative Research, *edited by Margaret Rustin & Michael Rustin*
Oedipus and the Couple, *edited by Francis Grier*
On Adolescence: Inside Stories, *by Margot Waddell*
Organization in the Mind: Psychoanalysis, Group Relations, and Organizational Consultancy, *by David Armstrong, edited by Robert French*
Psychoanalysis and Culture: A Kleinian Perspective, *edited by David Bell*
Researching the Unconscious: Principles of Psychoanalytic Method, *by Michael Rustin*
Reason and Passion: A Celebration of the Work of Hanna Segal, *edited by David Bell*
Short-Term Psychoanalytic Psychotherapy for Adolescents with Depression: A Treatment Manual, *edited by Jocelyn Catty*
Sibling Matters: A Psychoanalytic, Developmental, and Systemic Approach, *edited by Debbie Hindle & Susan Sherwin-White*
Social Defences against Anxiety: Explorations in a Paradigm, *edited by David Armstrong & Michael Rustin*
Surviving Space: Papers on Infant Observation, *edited by Andrew Briggs*
Talking Cure: Mind and Method of the Tavistock Clinic, *edited by David Taylor*
The Anorexic Mind, *by Marilyn Lawrence*
The Groups Book. Psychoanalytic Group Therapy: Principles and Practice, *edited by Caroline Garland*
Therapeutic Care for Refugees: No Place Like Home, *edited by Renos Papadopoulos*
Thinking Space: Promoting Thinking about Race, Culture, and Diversity in Psychotherapy and Beyond, *edited by Frank Lowe*
Towards Belonging: Negotiating New Relationships for Adopted Children and Those in Care, *edited by Andrew Briggs*
Turning the Tide: A Psychoanalytic Approach to Mental Illness. The Work of the Fitzjohn's Unit, *edited by Rael Meyerowitz & David Bell*
Understanding Trauma: A Psychoanalytic Approach, *edited by Caroline Garland*
Waiting to Be Found: Papers on Children in Care, *edited by Andrew Briggs*
"What Can the Matter Be?": Therapeutic Interventions with Parents, Infants, and Young Children, *edited by Louise Emanuel & Elizabeth Bradley*
Young Child Observation: A Development in the Theory and Method of Infant Observation, *edited by Simonetta M. G. Adamo & Margaret Rustin*

NEW DISCOVERIES IN CHILD PSYCHOTHERAPY

Findings from Qualitative Research

Edited by Margaret Rustin & Michael Rustin

Routledge
Taylor & Francis Group
LONDON AND NEW YORK

First published 2019
by Routledge
2 Park Square, Milton Park, Abingdon, Oxon OX14 4RN

and by Routledge
52 Vanderbilt Avenue, New York, NY 10017

Routledge is an imprint of the Taylor & Francis Group, an informa business

British Library Cataloguing-in-Publication Data
A catalogue record for this book is available from the British Library

Library of Congress Cataloging-in-Publication Data
Names: Rustin, Margaret, editor. | Rustin, Michael, editor.
Title: New discoveries in child psychotherapy : findings from qualitative research / edited by Margaret Rustin and Michael Rustin.
Description: Abingdon, Oxon ; New York, NY : Routledge, 2019. |
Series: Tavistock clinic series | Includes bibliographical references and index.
Identifiers: LCCN 2019004247 (print) | LCCN 2019005419 (ebook) | ISBN 9780429282294 (Master) | ISBN 9781000001297 (Adobe) | ISBN 9781000014655 (Mobipocket) | ISBN 9781000008135 (ePub3) | ISBN 9780367244101 (hardback : alk. paper) | ISBN 9780367244071 (pbk. : alk. paper) | ISBN 9780429282294 (ebk)
Subjects: | MESH: Psychotherapy—methods | Child | Qualitative Research
Classification: LCC RC480.5 (ebook) | LCC RC480.5 (print) | NLM WS 350.2 | DDC 616.89/14—dc23
LC record available at https://lccn.loc.gov/2019004247

ISBN: 978-0-367-24407-1 (hbk)
ISBN: 978-0-367-24410-1 (pbk)
ISBN: 978-0-429-28229-4 (ebk)

Typeset in Palatino
by Swales & Willis, Exeter, Devon, UK

CONTENTS

SERIES EDITORS' PREFACE

Since it was founded in 1920, the Tavistock Clinic—now the Tavistock and Portman NHS Foundation Trust—has developed a wide range of developmental approaches to mental health which have been strongly influenced by the ideas of psychoanalysis. It has also adopted systemic family therapy as a theoretical model and a clinical approach to family problems. The Tavistock is now one of the largest mental health training institutions in Britain. It teaches up to 600 students a year on postgraduate, doctoral, and qualifying courses in social work, systemic psychotherapy, psychology, psychiatry, nursing, and child, adolescent, and adult psychotherapy, along with 2,000 multidisciplinary clinicians, social workers, and teachers attending Continuing Professional Development courses and conferences on psychoanalytic observation, psychoanalytic thinking, and management and leadership in a range of clinical and community settings.

The Tavistock's philosophy aims at promoting therapeutic methods in mental health. Its work is based on the clinical expertise that is also the basis of its consultancy and research activities. The aim of this Series is to make available to the reading public the clinical, theoretical, and research work that is most influential at the Tavistock. The Series sets out new approaches in the understanding and treatment of psychological disturbance in children, adolescents, and adults, both as individuals and in families.

In *New Discoveries in Child Psychotherapy: Findings from Qualitative Research*, Margaret Rustin and Michael Rustin bring together a diverse range of studies, united by the common endeavour of using systematic research methods to explore the practice of psychoanalytic child and adolescent psychotherapy. All the research presented in this innovative and engaging book originally comprised, or was a key element in, the doctoral research of the authors, conducted as part of the Tavistock's doctoral programme in child psychotherapy.

Dividing the book into "Mainly Theory and Clinical Method" and "Mainly Practice", the editors situate the book within a distinguished tradition of studying the "phenomena of the unconscious" in the clinical consulting room. They observe: "Most psychoanalytic concepts have as their principal empirical reference phenomena that have first become known in clinical settings . . . The links between psychoanalytic discourse and clinical practice are particularly marked in the British psychoanalytic tradition." As they explain, the authors bring alive the interplay between theory and practice, concept and patient, by "engag [ing] with the psychoanalytic ideas that give meaning and explanation to these 'individualized' phenomena . . . , seeking in many instances to show how an explanatory idea actually applies, or needs to be amended or even challenged, in the light of the evidence of 'clinical facts' that authors have encountered in their work." They also draw attention to the secondary purpose of the book: to demonstrate the methodological interest and innovation of the studies, which represent an adaption of the methods of social science and psychology in the psychoanalytic context. Their Introduction lays out, with exceptional clarity, the history, development, and implications of these methods—principally Grounded Theory, thematic analysis, and interpretative phenomenological analysis —for both the initiated and the uninitiated alike.

Part I, "Mainly Theory and Clinical Method", displays a range of ways in which the authors and researchers have integrated clinical and research practice, many of them using Grounded Theory. Wendy Shallcross describes the use of the method to explore and understand her observation with a mother and baby where there was a significant trauma and disruption during the early months. In Louise Allnutt's study, it is used to examine the impact of the researcher's clinical work with a looked-after 2-year-old on the child's development. Carlos Tamm and Emily Ryan each use this method to illuminate and explore theoretical and clinical ideas: respectively, "the K link" and "aspects of autistic functioning and language development". Miriam Creaser's chapter, the final one of the section, shows the author taking up a different position in relation to the data: that of researcher utilizing data collected as part of a larger study, the IMPACT study of adolescent depression. Yet here, too, the interplay between clinical and systematic "research" thinking is vividly illustrated, as Creaser immerses herself in the clinical process by exploring and interpreting the divergences between process and audio recordings of child psychotherapy sessions, leading to conclusions with significant implications for training.

Part II, "Mainly Practice", presents the reader with a range of clinical situations and research methodologies. Ferelyth Watt and (in the penultimate chapter) Rajni Sharma both use interview methods informed by their clinical insight to study the impact on their clinical work of the experience of pregnancy in, respectively, Bangladeshi mothers and child psychotherapists. Both chapters demonstrate the clinical relevance and immediacy of this method, which is more commonly associated with other disciplines, and they provide an eloquent counterpart to the chapters in this section focusing on child psychotherapy practice in diverse forms: intensive work (in Liselotte Grünbaum's study of breaks and siblings), assessment (in Marie Bradley's study), and short-term psychoanalytic parent work (in Kristine Tiltina's study). In the final chapter, Jenifer Wakelyn makes a particular case for the clinical relevance of research, in showing the work that developed from her original doctoral research on therapeutic infant observation: her intervention developed from the insights gained from this research, "Watch Me Play!", is described here, along with her ongoing research into its utility for looked-after infants and young children.

As Wakelyn remarks, "The dialogue between clinical research and practice is a fruitful one". This illuminating and rewarding book brings that dialogue alive for a wider audience.

ACKNOWLEDGEMENTS

We are grateful to the many child psychotherapists who have played a part in supporting the research work described in these pages, as clinical colleagues and supervisors. In particular, Catrin Bradley and her course team, together with their academic administrative colleagues, have been a much-valued resource for this doctoral programme of whose outcomes this book represents only a part.

We would like to thank Margot Waddell, Kate Stratton, and Jocelyn Catty for their encouragement and help in the production of this book. Particular thanks are also due to Eric and Klara King of Communication Crafts and to Natalie Clark of Swales & Willis for their meticulous editing of its final text, and to Algy Craig Hall for the cover image.

ABOUT THE CONTRIBUTORS

Louise Allnutt is a child and adolescent psychotherapist in a specialist team at the Tavistock working with traumatized families. She has an interest in early development and the developmental impact of psychoanalytic psychotherapy on parents and children. She also teaches and supervises on the child psychotherapy training at the Tavistock.

Marie Bradley is a child and adolescent psychotherapist now in private practice after working in mainstream and adolescent specialist NHS services for many years. She has a special interest in working with children who are fostered or adopted, with their families, and with the professional networks around them. She also works independently with children from age 4 years through to early adulthood, with an emphasis on work with adolescents and including work with young adults who have been adopted. She undertakes the assessment of young people facing serious criminal charges. As an adult psychotherapist her work includes psychotherapy and clinical supervision with child and adult psychotherapy trainees.

Miriam Creaser is a senior child and adolescent psychotherapist at Oxleas NHS Foundation Trust with a specialism in working with looked-after child and their networks. She trained at the Tavistock and Portman NHS Foundation Trust and has taught extensively on

Tavistock courses. She would like to explore further the implications of her research for the training of child and adolescent psychotherapists.

Liselotte Grünbaum, a psychologist, is a specialist practitioner and supervisor of clinical child psychology and psychotherapy, currently in private practice in Copenhagen. She is a collaboration partner and part-time associate professor at Aalborg University, teacher and supervisor at the Danish training programme for psychoanalytic child and adolescent psychotherapists, and former Child & Adolescent Section and Research Coordinator of the European Federation of Psychoanalytic Psychotherapy. Her doctoral work, which concluded with the dissertation *Breaks as a Window to Core Object Relationship Themes* (2014), was carried out at the University of East London and the Tavistock and Portman NHS Foundation Trust.

Emily Ryan is a child and adolescent psychotherapist who trained at the Tavistock Clinic. She is based in Bristol where she leads Bridge in Schools, a programme of the Bridge Foundation which provides a specialist mental health service to schools in the Bristol area. She teaches on the Wessex-Bridge PG Diploma on Psychodynamic Approaches to Counselling Children and Young People in Community and Educational Settings. She is also a clinical supervisor on the Sino–British programme, coordinated through the National Psychoanalysis Demonstration Unit, P.R. China.

Wendy Shallcross is a child and adolescent psychotherapist working in the child and adolescent mental health service for Cornwall Foundation NHS Trust. She has had a major role in promoting infant mental health in the county and has developed an ongoing child psychotherapy trainee programme within the Trust. She was the course organizer for the Devon Psychoanalytic Observational Studies course and has taught and supervised infant observation both in Britain and abroad.

Rajni Sharma is the professional lead for child and adolescent psychotherapy in Manchester and Salford Child and Adolescent Mental Health Service. She has extensive clinical experience of working in community outpatient and inpatient settings. Rajni also heads the Psychoanalytic Observational Studies postgraduate programme at the Northern School of Child and Adolescent Psychotherapy (NSCAP) and teaches on the Child Psychotherapy Clinical Training.

Carlos Tamm is a child, adolescent, and adult psychoanalyst and psychotherapist. Before he came to London, he was a psychiatrist and psychoanalyst in Brazil. He has a PhD in the field of child psychoanalytic psychotherapy, based on his research at the Tavistock on autistic functioning and language development. He is a supervisor, tutor, and lecturer at the Tavistock and Portman NHS Foundation Trust, and a training analyst for the Association of Child Psychotherapists. He is a Fellow of the British Psychoanalytical Society, where he is a member of the Child Analytic Training Committee. He has been teaching Infant Observation as well as the Emotional Development of Children and Adolescents for over fifteen years and has published and lectured on autism, language development, psychoanalysis, and literature, and the works of W. R. Bion.

Kristine Tiltina is a child and adolescent psychoanalytic psychotherapist in the Belfast Trust. Her current research interests include the impact of early trauma, especially on fostered and adopted children, their carers and adoptive parents, and the wider Social Services system. She is currently an International Psychoanalytical Association candidate of the Northern Ireland Association for the Study of Psychoanalysis (NIASP).

Jenifer Wakelyn is a child and adolescent psychotherapist working in a specialist outreach service of the Tavistock Centre. She has a special interest in therapeutic work with babies and young children in transition. She is a teacher and supervisor in the Tavistock Child Psychotherapy training, clinical research coordinator, and co-chair of the Tavistock Fostering, Adoption and Kinship Care Workshop. She has published articles on psychoanalysis and visual art, sibling assessment for the family courts, psychotherapy with children in transition, and therapeutic applications of infant observation.

Ferelyth Watt is lead Child and Adolescent Psychotherapist in Haringey CAMHS and Haringey CAMHS lead for the Child Sexual Abuse Hub. Prior to this she worked in Tower Hamlets CAMHS (East) where she set up Help at Hand, an outreach project in a children's centre. She is also working at the Baobab Centre for Young Survivors in Exile. She is a member of the Board of Trustees at the British Psychotherapy Foundation (BPF) and Chair of the Independent Psychoanalytic Child & Adolescent Psychotherapy Association at the BPF.

Introduction

Michael Rustin & Margaret Rustin

Origins

Since 1995, many child psychotherapists who trained at the Tavistock Clinic (now the Tavistock and Portman NHS Trust) have undertaken research as part of a professional doctorate programme,[1] accredited for many years through the Tavistock's partnership with the University of East London, and in particular its (then) Faculty of Social Sciences.[2] In the first years, these researchers were already qualified child psychotherapists, who were able to prepare for doctoral study through a supplementary programme concerned with research methods.[3] But, at the same time, this professional doctorate was incorporated as an option into the child psychotherapy curriculum, and many trainees have chosen to pursue research projects during or soon after the completion of their clinical training. To date, over 80 child psychotherapy doctoral theses have been completed within this framework (their authors and titles to date are listed in the Appendix at the end of the book).[4] This volume presents accounts of research findings from nine of these completed projects, together with two chapters written from PhD theses that were supported by parallel supervision arrangements at the Tavistock.

This doctoral programme was based on a distinctive approach to research in psychoanalysis and child psychotherapy. Its assumption was that psychoanalysis, since Freud, has *always* been a research programme, located at first, and principally thereafter, in the context of its clinical practice, and that it was upon such research that the substantial knowledge base of psychoanalysis, encompassing both its theories and practices, has been based. This programme disputed an idea that has become fashionable: that a lasting and critical failing of psychoanalysis has been its indifference to scientific principles and the research methods consistent with them. This view was in defiance of Freud's own commitment to the conception of psychoanalysis as a new and revolutionary form of science, comparable in its potential, as he claimed (Freud, 1917a), to the scientific revolutions (and the injuries to "the universal narcissism of men") that had been brought about by Copernicus and Darwin.

A further assumption of this programme was that the most substantial development of knowledge in psychoanalysis had been achieved by clinical practitioners. This was not only by psychoanalysts, working mainly with adult patients, but also in the post-war period by the new profession of psychoanalytic child psychotherapists.[5] While this development had been founded on the pioneering work of psychoanalysts of children such as Anna Freud, Melanie Klein, and Donald Winnicott, and continued to draw on theoretical advances in mainstream psychoanalysis (by such figures as Wilfred Bion, Donald Meltzer, Hanna Segal, Betty Joseph, Edna O'Shaughnessy, Ronald Britton, and John Steiner), child psychotherapy has, nevertheless, for many years been the principal location in Britain of psychoanalytic work with children and adolescents. We argue that it has generated its own substantial knowledge base, in regard to both psychoanalytic theory and therapeutic technique. Among the sub-fields in which it has advanced psychoanalytic understanding are the autistic spectrum of disabilities, the treatment of severely deprived children, and problems of eating disorders and of adolescent development. It has been a principal aim of the Tavistock's child psychotherapy doctoral programme to add to this body of knowledge, and this book offers examples of new discoveries in the wide range of work undertaken by child psychotherapists.

Since psychoanalysis was first established as a scientific and therapeutic practice, there have always been criticisms of its claims and status as a form of knowledge. Polemics against it, by philosophers and psychologists committed to various kinds of scientific empiricism, have provided a persistently hostile context for psychoanalytic work (Cioffi, 1970, 1998; Crews, 2017; Crews & Crews, 1997; Eysenck, 1973, 2002; Popper, 1963). However, the area of critique that we have found most challenging and stimulating has come from those who are close to psychoanalysis and are essentially in sympathy with its achievements and purposes. Psychoanalysts such as Robert Wallerstein (Wallerstein, 1988, 2005; Wallerstein & Fonagy, 1999; Wallerstein & Sampson, 1971) and Peter Fonagy (1993, 2003) have argued not against psychoanalysis and its value, but for its defence and enhancement through a closer engagement with "mainstream" scientific methods, especially those of its competitors in the field of mental health services. One facet of this argument has focused on the deficient quality of the evidence usually offered in support of psychoanalytic theories. Writers such as Donald Spence (1984, 1994, 1998, 2000, 2002, 2007) have noted the excessive reliance by psychoanalytic writers on brief clinical examples and vignettes, rather than on a systemic analysis of rigorously sampled segments of clinical material. "Internal critics" of psychoanalysis who are themselves analysts, such as Peter Fonagy, have given much attention to the issue of the measurable effectiveness of treatments.[6] How can we show that it "works", that it actually achieves clinical improvement, has been the main emphasis of the research programme that has followed from this critique of traditional psychoanalytic practice. This is a critique that has had considerable resonance in child psychotherapy, since in the current era of "evidence-based medicine" the absence of empirical research of treatment outcomes threatens the position of psychoanalytic therapies within public mental health services, and their relevance to those who suffer mental illness. It has often seemed that the recent demand for "more research" in psychoanalysis and child psychotherapy has been essentially a demand for evidence only of treatment outcomes, disregarding any other research aims.

Psychoanalytic psychotherapies have found themselves facing severe competition in the mental health field (or quasi-market, as it has become) from therapies such as Cognitive Behaviour Therapy (CBT) which allegedly have a stronger evidence base than psychoanalytic treatments (Layard & Clarke, 2015). The theory of "mentalisation" (Fonagy, Gergely, Jurist, & Target, 2004) and treatments based on this theory developed by Anthony Bateman and Peter Fonagy (2010, 2016) has been one project to develop measurable and cost-effective therapies in this market-sensitive environment. This approach draws not on the core ideas of cognitive psychology, as CBT does, but, rather, brings together those of attachment theory (its idea of "internal working models" and its focus on empirical measurement) and of psychoanalysis (in particular, Bion's theory of thinking: Bion, 1962b; O'Shaughnessy, 1981).

Psychoanalysts and psychotherapists have in recent years taken a significant role in outcome studies and fully recognized their value and importance. These studies have included, in Britain, the Child Depression

Study (Trowell, 2011), the TADS Study (Fonagy et al., 2015), and the IMPACT Study (Goodyer et al., 2017), each of them highly significant examples of their kind. However, it has been a central feature of our research programme that it has been focused on central goals of psychoanalytic research broader than that of treatment effects. Its research interests have included the development of personality, the phenomena of the transference and the countertransference, the development of new forms of treatment and intervention, and other issues fundamental to psychoanalytic understanding. There is a risk that such "fundamental" research questions are being relegated to insignificance by the insistent demand to measure treatment efficacy, above all else. Yet if there had never been fundamental research of the kinds this collection of theses demonstrates, no treatments in psychoanalysis or child psychotherapy would exist.

Another line of relevant "internal critique" of psychoanalysis has called for a closer engagement between psychoanalysis and adjacent fields of research into the mind. Such convergences—with the developmental psychological study of infancy by researchers such as Daniel Stern (1985) and Colwyn Trevarthen (2010), or in a renewed rapprochement with attachment theory (Fonagy, 2001), or with neuroscience, in the work of Mark Solms (2015) and Jim Hopkins (2004)—are necessary and beneficial. Indeed, they offer the possibility of setting psychoanalysis on a broader base of scientific evidence. However, although references to such convergences are to be found in the chapters of this book, they are not its main topic.

Principles and methods of research

A central assumption of the Tavistock's child psychotherapy doctoral research programme was that clinical practice has always been the principal source of knowledge in psychoanalysis and child psychotherapy. Psychoanalytic theories and clinical techniques have evolved primarily through the treatment of patients, allied with the theoretical creativity of the major figures of psychoanalysis, Freud foremost among them. It is the clinical consulting room that has provided the principal context for the discovery and validation of psychoanalytic ideas. This has been the "laboratory" (M. J. Rustin, 2001a, 2019) where the phenomena of the unconscious have been most clearly identified. This has taken place in particular through the study of the transference–countertransference relationship, in clinical settings that are purposefully protected from external disturbance and "noise". Most psychoanalytic concepts have as their principal empirical reference phenomena that have first become known in clinical settings. Psychoanalytic ideas become more difficult to use reliably and consistently the greater the distance of their application from clinical contexts and from those, such as exercises in group relations, with similar boundaries. The links between psychoanalytic discourse and clinical practice are particularly marked in the British psychoanalytic tradition. In its literature, psychoanalytic concepts and ideas are almost invariably exemplified and illustrated through clinical descriptions.

The embedding of this doctoral research programme within or closely following a clinical training followed from the understanding of psychoanalytic knowledge summarized above. The theories and techniques underpinning child psychotherapy have largely emerged from clinical work with patients. Klein's discovery of "play therapy" (Klein, 1932; Rustin & Rustin, 2017, chap. 4) and her understanding of the vicissitudes of early infant development are examples of such discoveries. The therapeutic struggles with at first almost unmanageable child patients, which are reported in the literature on psychotherapy with severely deprived children (Boston & Szur, 1983) and in early work with children with autism (Tustin, 1972), are later instances of this kind of learning. Child psychotherapists have drawn substantially on ideas that emerged in the analysis of adults to inform their understanding of their child patients. Hanna Segal's (1957) theory of the development of symbol formation, and Betty Joseph's (1985) understanding of the "total transference situation", have, for example, deeply influenced recent psychotherapy with children and adolescents. So has Winnicott's understanding of the maternal environment (1990) and of the phenomenon of "hate in the countertransference" (1949b). The links made in Bion's work between the psychotic states of mind he observed in adult patients, and the functions of projective processes and the "container–contained" relationship, have become crucial to child psychotherapists' understandings of infancy and the early development of mind, and they were also formative in the development of the practice of psychoanalytic infant observation.

Given this assumption of the centrality of clinical experience, the understanding of every clinical case embodies an element of discovery (and thus research) in its own right, since psychoanalytic patients are of interest and value in their particularity and individuality, and not only as instances of "kinds" of pathology or symptom. Normal clinical practice in psychoanalysis involves trying to bring an understanding of the particulars of individual personalities and their experiences within a therapeutic relationship, while drawing upon psychoanalytic theories that are found to be useful as explanatory resources.

Bion (1962b) described the experience of infant development as one in which a conception (for example, of the breast) has to become conjoined with a "realization"—the actual presence of the breast or maternal object—for development to take place. The psychoanalytic process has some similarities with this relation between idea and experience, insofar as the observation and experience of a particular patient or episode in a therapy may be understood as the realization of a concept. Perhaps a better way of understanding a psychoanalytic perception is as an experience of "seeing as", in which a phenomenon becomes recognized as being of a given kind, and as thus having meaning. Psychoanalytic research is, however, not only devoted to the understanding of the particularities of individual patients. While psychoanalytic concepts and theories are often primarily a resource for enabling meaning to be assigned to clinical phenomena, they also sometimes become a topic in themselves, an object of research in their own right. This happens when it is found that innovations in concepts and theories have been needed in order to give meaning to a phenomenon that may resist understanding through familiar categories. Sometimes a hitherto unknown or unrecognized phenomenon calls for a new idea. Freud's writing was full of such new ideas, which became the foundation of psychoanalysis, and many of these arose from his encounters with his clinical cases. The evolution of psychoanalytic theory, most visibly in "the British School", can be understood as the history of a research programme the main stimulus for which has been the need to describe, explain, and account for hitherto unseen or unrecognized clinical phenomena.

The chapters in this book should, we hope, enable readers to come to "know" many actual persons (seen as patients, observed or talked with) and to recognize their living qualities. But the chapters also engage with the psychoanalytic ideas that give meaning and explanation to these "individualized" phenomena. They explore these ideas as having their own significance, seeking in many instances to show how an explanatory idea actually applies, or needs to be amended or even challenged, in the light of the evidence of "clinical facts"[7] that authors have encountered in their work. The "New Discoveries in Child Psychotherapy" of our title each have a conceptual and theoretical aspect, as well as aiming to give a "lived reality" to the individuals through which these are realized.

The specific kinds of meaning with which psychoanalysts are most concerned are those that have an unconscious dimension. To understand the force of phantasy in shaping a patient's or an analyst's own perceptions or behaviours requires an understanding of the unconscious structures and patterns of mind in which phantasies have their valency. Almost by definition of the nature of unconscious mental life, such understandings are elusive. It is because assigning conceptual meanings to the phenomena of the transference and countertransference is an uncertain and difficult task that psychoanalysts and psychotherapists have to undergo, a prolonged and patient kind of learning. Theories in themselves can be learned in more or less didactic ways and merely illustrated with clinical or other examples. But the therapeutic or observational use or application of theories has to be learned by practice and example, through engagements with particulars, and especially emotional particulars. It is for this reason that psychoanalytic training is so iterative in its nature. A two-year weekly infant observation may well involve the need to experience and reflect on 80 or more separate observational hours. An intensive clinical training case seen three times per week for two years will consist of around 240 clinical sessions. (Child psychotherapy trainees will have three of these cases.) If an analysis is more intensive in frequency, or of longer duration, as it may be, this number may be considerably greater. In the background is also the trainee's own personal analysis of many years' duration. The matching of experiences against theoretical understandings in this work is only accomplished by means of learning from a multitude of learning experiences, many of them occasions for supervisory or subsequent reflection. This is as much an experience of learning a craft as of learning a science, although, of course, the practices of the sciences also involve craft-like skills, such as those required to undertake laboratory work (Knorr-Cetina, 1999; Latour & Woolgar, 1979).

It is for this reason that many of the understandings shared between analytic practitioners are what the school of sociology known as "ethnomethodology" defines as "indexical" in their nature (Garfinkel, 1967; Heritage, 1984). An indexical understanding is one that depends on shared implicit assumptions about the meaning of elements in a communicative exchange which do not normally require or obtain explicit clarification or definition. (These sociological ideas were greatly influenced by Husserl's phenomenology.) Most communications in everyday language are of this kind. For example, most of the time we understand the meaning and performative import of a phrase such as "good morning", when it is said to us, without our needing to ask in what respect it is good, or what leads the speaker to believe that it is morning, or indeed that mornings exist. The ethnomethodologists at one period demonstrated the degree to which everyday life was based on such implicit understandings by staging unsettling human "experiments" in which these were put in question. For example, students visiting with their parents would ask them about the rent they owed, even though they were staying in what everyone had recognized to be their family home.

Psychoanalytic literature has long depended for its effective communication among analysts on the sharing of "indexical" or implicit mutually held assumptions. A brief clinical vignette in a psychoanalytic paper can be held to provide telling evidence for, or at least an illustration of, a theoretical contention, because its readers can recognize from their own similar experience its veracity (the probable truthfulness and accuracy of its descriptions), as well as understand the meanings and implications of the ideas that inform it. Sociologists of science have, however, pointed out that this property of "indexicality", of implicit assumptions and beliefs shared among practitioners, is common to most scientific communities.[8] It is thus not unique to psychoanalysis. Indeed, this quality of shared implicit understanding is the precondition for the pursuit of what T. S. Kuhn described as "normal science" (1962), the everyday practices of laboratory life, which do not afford time to explain ideas fundamental to an investigation at its every step. However, what people may be prepared to accept as unavoidable where arcane topics of natural science are concerned, and where one has usually to leave matters to the experts, becomes contentious with theories that purport to interpret the phenomena of everyday mental life. Psychoanalysts are understandably expected to be able to make clear, and justifiable, exactly what they mean in every respect, since what they have to say may refer directly to you and me. Arguments about psychoanalysis—for example, in professional mental health settings—often turn out to be not about the relevance or truthfulness of a specific psychoanalytic hypothesis, but, rather, about whether the core assumptions of psychoanalysis are valid or not.

This element of the implicit or "taken for granted" in much psychoanalytic writing, and in the justifications analysts offer for their theoretical assertions, has given rise to much internal criticism of psychoanalytic methodology. One of the challenges that the academic accreditation of a doctoral programme has presented for child psychotherapists is how to overcome these seeming—but also, to a degree, real—deficiencies of method. It is a requirement of an academic research thesis that its topic is situated in a specified disciplinary context, that its investigations are located within a published literature, that it can specify a definite and acceptable method of study, and that its findings are validated by the method it has set out. It has turned out that these academic challenges were sometimes helpful in enabling psychoanalytic psychotherapists to respond to the methodological criticisms to which their field has long been subjected.

Significant for the development of our programme was an earlier battle that raged in the broader field of the human and social sciences, which concerned the justification for qualitative as distinct from quantitative research methods. An orthodoxy, derived from a conception of the hierarchy of credibility of the natural sciences that placed physics at its summit, held that what could not be measured in quantitative terms had only an inferior scientific status. Much of biology, which had been long concerned with the description and classification of "kinds" of organism, conformed poorly to this model. But for the human and social sciences, where differences of cultural and subjective meaning were fundamental to most forms of useful understanding, this insistence on quantitative measurement as the sole criterion of scientific validity was potentially catastrophic, excluding from view many "qualitative" aspects of phenomena which are of the greatest significance. The necessity for recognizing the significance of qualitative differences was recognized since the inception of sociology and anthropology as social sciences, but it has nevertheless remained contentious.

In fact, the development of systematic methods of qualitative analysis in the social sciences (including some sub-fields of psychology) was the precondition for the emergence of qualitative research methods for investigating psychoanalytic phenomena. Indeed, it has been possible to transpose, as several chapters in this book demonstrate, methods such as grounded theory, thematic analysis, and interpretative phenomenological analysis (IPA) from their original fields of sociology and psychology, while adapting them to the study of the phenomena of unconscious mental life which are distinctive in psychoanalytic inquiry.

Thus, a second purpose of this book, complementary to its dimension of "discovery" and innovation in the domains of concepts, theories, clinical techniques, and interventions, lies in the field of research methods. We aim to show that the discoveries described are of both substantive and methodological interest. This will be through demonstrating that they have been achieved through the use of more systematic and rigorous qualitative research methods than are customarily displayed in clinical psychoanalytic writing.[9] It is nevertheless the case, of course, that such clinical writing has often conveyed great depths of theoretical understanding. Our purpose is to show how the procedures of psychoanalytic discovery can be enhanced, not to devalue or discredit the established body of knowledge of psychoanalysis. We do not subscribe to the view that research in psychoanalysis has now to begin from a point somewhere near zero.

Qualitative methods of research in psychoanalysis

Systematic qualitative research methods, such as grounded theory and IPA, were initially developed in fields of study in the social and human sciences which were not psychoanalytic in their orientation.[10] In sociology, the pioneering text was *Discovering Grounded Theory*, by Glaser and Strauss (1967). This represented a challenge to the dominant orthodoxy of sociology as it then was. This prior hegemonic model was committed to the development of a "general theory" of the social system, and to the idea that research should be focused on the empirical testing of specific hypotheses derived from such a general theory, or its subordinate theories. In parallel with this, although distinct from it, was an equally strong mainstream commitment to quantitative research methods, on the grounds that numerical measures permitted the most rigorous empirical testing of theoretical hypotheses. This emphasis on the quantitative was particularly important in the policy and practical applications of social scientific ideas, where, for example, it might be desired to establish the causes of a social problem or the effectiveness of a social policy. Such practical and policy concerns by authorities have a considerable and understandable influence on social scientific practices, as the current vogue for "outcome measures" in mental health reminds us.

Glaser and Strauss (1967) instead argued for a form of investigation in which theoretical ideas should not define *a priori* the agendas for empirical investigations, but, on the contrary, for one in which theories would emerge from such investigations as their "inductive" outcomes. Encounters with facts, evidence, and experiences should come first, and theories be their eventual product, emerging as the means of finding meaning in them. Theories would thus, in Glaser and Strauss's terms, be "grounded" in observed data, in the lived realities of the social worlds in which sociologists chose to investigate. There was an assumption in this perspective that social environments are particular and diverse in their nature, and that the differences between them are of consequence. There was also a commitment to understanding the ways in which the actual subjects of research experienced their own life-worlds, in preference to "imposing" the theoretical categories of researchers upon them, as if from above. Contemporary with the development of grounded theory, the perspective of "symbolic interactionism" (Blumer, 1992) proposed that the social world be understood as a product of the definitions given to it by its participants.

In these ways, *The Discovery of Grounded Theory*, written at a point of considerable cultural turbulence in the 1960s, was part of a larger reaction against hierarchy. Grounded theory has a long-standing affinity with the idea of a "social science from below", receptive to the perspective of ordinary social subjects, even though its founders did not approach these issues in an especially political way. Several kinds of sociology were at this time challenging the received representations of social reality. It was argued that what were often represented as "social facts", objective reflections of reality, were in fact the outcome of categorizing procedures imposed by the powerful upon the weak. Rationalization and self-justification was rife, as the ethnomethodologists showed, in the ways that institutions maintained their credibility, both to themselves and others. Goffman's *Asylums* (1968) described the procedures by which mental hospitals sought to manage the identities of their inmates, and forms of resistance to these practices. Sociologists of education in Britain provided an account of social interactions of classrooms from the point of view of students, especially of conventionally less successful students, quite different from that of their teachers or the governments who set the educational agendas.

Glaser and Strauss, and their collaborators and successors in the development of grounded theory (e.g., Charmaz, 2006; Corbin & Strauss, 2008), took an inclusive and eclectic view of the kinds of data through which understanding of society could and should be obtained. Although they did not reject the relevance of quantitative data, their approach was primarily sensitive to the many qualitative dimensions of social phenomena, and was therefore open-minded and inventive about the methods through which these might be captured. In their own empirical investigations of experiences of dying in hospital, Glaser and Strauss (1965) made use of observations and of the content and meaning of communications of staff and patients. Their research had a quantitative dimension, insofar as the frequency and intensity of attention to patients in different social circumstances were relevant to the theoretical understanding of "status passage" they developed. Indeed, most "qualitative research" involves very basic kinds of quantitative assessment, concerning the presence or absence of phenomena, or their frequency or intensity, even if these are not measured in precise numbers.

The essence of the method of grounded theory lies in its procedures of "coding". Investigations based on grounded theory are often those that are likely of their nature to generate large amounts of data, shaped in one way of another by the human or social subjects of research, rather than according to the prior categories of researchers. Interviews conducted within this methodological framework are likely to be open-ended and, at most, "semi-structured". Criticisms of forms of interview or questionnaire that only aim to test predetermined hypotheses are that they generate no information that is not already defined by an interview schedule. "Box-ticking", as a means of assessing the quality of a social performance, is an extreme version of this limited kind of data gathering. Media outputs or fictions have the characteristics given to them by their producers, not by those who are researching them. The critical problems in researching such relatively unstructured data-sets are therefore (1) how to be sure they are representative of any phenomenon broader than their own particularity, and (2) how to identify what is significant and recurrent in the phenomena they report, and to grasp what attributes most fully explain their shape and character. The first problem is related to the issue of "sampling", even though, with a qualitative method, criteria of representativity cannot usually be established through statistical procedures. The second is the problem of generalizing from particular findings, of ensuring that research findings are more than a description of an entirely unique and particular phenomenon. Indeed, without some procedure that enables "kinds" and "types" to be recognized, it is not even possible to identify that a phenomenon is indeed one of its kind.

All qualitative research thus involves a procedure of "coding" of some sort. Coding is a method of generalizing, of identifying definite attributes of a phenomenon, through the sequential study of its particular manifestations. This may, in the first instance, be a matter of counting the incidence of such attributes. For example, in an interview transcript the frequency of occurrence of a word or phrase may be a measure of its causal or conceptual significance. Or, in an observation of a social setting, how often an individual of one social status communicates with another of similar, superior, or inferior status may draw our attention to the existence of hierarchical social relations. But informative kinds of "coding" usually go well beyond measures of frequency. What may be recognized is a pattern, a recurrent moment of intensity or conflict, whose significance does not rest on the number of times it occurs, but on its consequences or causes when it does.

Grounded theorists describe a desirable progression from a particular datum or fact to a code, to a concept, and lastly to a theoretical category, each representing a higher or more generalized level of abstraction.

They at first believed in the "discovery" of new theories from the examination of primary empirical data. In those circumstances, therefore, the final representation of a phenomenon in terms of its essential "categories" was the point at which its "grounded theory" had been "discovered." This was, in their initial view, an "inductive" approach, according to which theories would be inferred essentially from the inspection and accumulation of instances—that is, from their "constant correlation", by using what Glaser and Strauss (1967) referred to as the "constant comparative method".

Later exponents of grounded theory, such as Kathy Charmaz (2006), came to recognize that the idea of an entirely theory-free approach to data, which Glaser and Strauss had first advocated, did not reflect the way in which social researchers usually approached any field of study. Indeed, it is doubtful if a field could even be identified without reference to some implicit or explicit conceptual categorization. This follows the idea that all facts are perceptions that are "theory loaded" in some way. Thus, for example, the farmer's perception of a field is different from that of the botanist, the impressionist painter, or the ornithologist, though there will often be links between their ways of seeing and understanding. Thus, all researchers will necessarily bring some frame of reference to their topic. Indeed, without such a frame of reference, a "topic" could hardly be identified. Even the initial advocates of a "tabula rasa" or clean-slate approach to a research topic, such as Glaser and Strauss originally were, can be shown to have held in mind core ideas—such as social role, the constructed meaning of a situation, and social status—as presuppositions of their own investigations, although they filled out these core concepts to encompass the qualities of the phenomena they observed.

C. S. Peirce [1839–1914] was an American pragmatist philosopher whose concept of "abduction" has proved to be an invaluable addition to the interpretive methods of grounded theory (Gallie, 1952, chap. 4; Reicherz, 2007). It allows that the meanings that investigators may find in a phenomenon are most likely to involve its relation to or correspondence with some existing frame of reference and do not necessarily, or even usually, involve the discovery or invention (by "induction" from numbers of cases) of an entirely new concept or category. "What is this an example of, what typical pattern does it represent?" is the question one asks of data when working abductively. Charmaz (2006, p. 186) summarizes this procedure as:

> A type of reading that begins by examining data and after scrutiny of all these data, entertains all possible explanations for the observed

> data, and then forms hypotheses to confirm or disconfirm, until the researcher arrives at the most plausible interpretation of the observed data.[11]

Peirce's formulation enables one to understand that "normal science", in Kuhn's terms, usually involves the locating of specific phenomena within an existing conceptual field. Which fields may have explanatory relevance, whether there might be more than one that is relevant, and what interpretive problems are posed if a location or "fit" within a field proves to be anomalous, are problems that may well be faced by researchers.

The adaptation of grounded theory methods to psychoanalytic research

A strong affinity between the clinical method of psychoanalysis and child psychotherapy and grounded theory methods was recognized by the first researchers in the Tavistock's doctoral research programme (Anderson, 2003, 2006; Hindle, 2007; Reid, 2007). This arose from similarities between the procedure of "coding" recommended by grounded theorists and the methods of analysing and interpreting clinical data followed by psychoanalysts. Indeed, it became recognized that the procedures of "line-by-line" supervision of clinical (and infant-observation) session material essentially prefigured, for these researchers, the grounded theory procedure of coding. The discovery of meaning and coherence in a single clinical session, and subsequently in sequences of sessions, and indeed in an entire case history, were close, it was realized, to the procedures by which grounded theorists identified meaning and developed theories from their data sets. It appeared that just as Molière's M. Jourdain in *The Middle Class Gentleman* had been speaking prose all along, without knowing it, so child psychotherapists had been implicitly "doing grounded theory".

The grounded theorists recommended a procedure of "theoretical sampling" of data, in contrast to the random and representative sampling methods proposed according to the standard hypothetico-deductive approach to scientific research. This followed from the priority given to theory generation in the grounded theory approach and, one might also say, to the priority it has tended to give to the "context of discovery" over the "context of verification" (Hoyningen-Huene, 1987; Swedberg, 2012). That is to say, grounded theory methods are better adapted to the discovery or development of theories in a specific context than to testing out their empirical scope or incidence of application. The representation by a sample of the attributes of a larger population is the province of sampling theory, with the randomized controlled trial as its so-called gold standard. It is reasonable, in pursuing an investigation of phenomena whose nature and development is partly unknown, to attend to the phenomena that seem most anomalous or interesting, and to go in search of extreme or "ideal types" to investigate in depth, rather than determine what is average for the sample.

Theoretical sampling is relevant to the psychoanalytic use of grounded theory, at the stages of both data collection and data analysis. Something like theoretical sampling is, in a sense, what takes place during the therapeutic process itself, within the interactions between patient and analyst. Although a patient will bring to the session whatever he or she wishes, analysts will choose to take up some aspects of this material in preference to others. Patients too may come to recognize what is analytically most significant—to themselves or their analyst—and give more attention to that. For example, patients may come to recognize that dreams have a particular relevance in the analytic setting and report them more than they would be likely to do in any other context. Thus, although from one point of view a record of sessions will represent everything that occurs in them, what has taken place may already be structured by considerations of clinical relevance. In other words, psychoanalytic clinical material has already been subject to a degree of theoretical sampling, even before selections from the clinical data for subsequent analysis are made.

At the stage of data analysis of a clinical or other psychoanalytic record, a form of theoretical sampling may well be preferred to random sampling. Carlberg's (2007) concept of "turning points" in therapy provides one criterion for the selection of data for examination that a researcher may have good reason to follow. Another might be of interactions that demonstrate the existence of a negative transference. As we have noted, psychoanalysts also have reason to attend to the representativeness of the data samples they choose. This is necessary in order to avoid an imputation that they are selectively drawing attention only to data samples that give support to their own theoretical point of view. Thus, in practice, researchers need to have both theoretical and representative grounds for sample selection in mind, and to maintain some balance between them. To ignore theoretical criteria for selection may give rise to analysis that omits what is of most substantive interest in case material, while to neglect issues of typicality may risk producing findings that are theoretically interesting, but whose scope of application cannot be assessed, even in relation to the body of material from which they are chosen. Of course, the relevance and scope of application of a finding can also be assessed by reference to the published literature on the topic in question.

As several chapters in this book demonstrate, the child psychotherapists discovered, that the retrospective analysis of their own clinical notes could be a productive step in the generation of meaning from case material. This, of course, was already a familiar procedure with respect to clinical case studies that were written up for qualification. Such analysis could often be deeper and more complex than had been possible during the original conduct of a case, even taking account of its concurrent clinical supervision. Outside the conduct of academically accredited research projects, psychoanalytic writers had often engaged in such a process of retrospective reflection upon their case material—and, indeed, many if not most influential clinical papers in the psychoanalytic literature have come about through such a method, informal as it has for the most part been. Within this doctoral programme, however, the use of grounded theory and other forms of systematic qualitative analysis has often been the means by which new discoveries have emerged.

Significant adaptions to the methods of qualitative analysis described above had to be made to make them useful in psychoanalytic research. In the first place, it was essential that the "abductive" as well as "inductive" nature of this form of analysis was recognized. No understanding of psychoanalytic research is possible without recognition of the indispensability of the psychoanalytic frame of reference and at least some of its core theoretical assumptions. Although Bion at one point recommended that psychoanalysts approach clinical phenomena "without memory and desire", he was recommending openness to emotional experience within each particular clinical setting, in its immediate present, not that analysts should banish all that they know of psychoanalysis when they later come to reflect on the meaning of their clinical experiences. At least it is certain, from the theoretically rich and deeply sourced nature of Bion's writing, that he himself paid close attention to the psychoanalytic tradition in formulating his own ideas. Indeed, it seems that one can best account for theoretical discovery in psychoanalysis as a process by which anomalies between new clinical findings and existing conceptualizations are identified, and not as a pure invention of ideas, *ab initio*, that lie outside any existing conceptual field (Hughes, 2004; M. J. Rustin, 2001a).[12]

A second critical adaption of grounded theory for psychoanalytic use required the inclusion of the domain of *unconscious* phenomena within the domain of investigation. This focus has been a significant departure from the common uses of grounded theory methods in social science. Although grounded theory has been earlier advocated as an appropriate method in the psychoanalytic literature (Tuckett, 1994), the Tavistock's doctoral programmes (not only in child psychotherapy, but also in other disciplines such as social work and organizational consultancy) have been probably so far the largest embodiment in practice of this approach. There is a theoretical departure from conventional social science and psychology inherent in the idea that phenomena may have, and may convey, unconscious as well as consciously recognized meanings. However, this theoretical acknowledgment seems to involve no specific challenge to investigation at the level of method. To demonstrate the existence and causal potency of an unconscious level of meaning, it is necessary merely to identify and specify its presence within a sequence or field of data (i.e., to "code" for its existence), and to clarify when, in what conditions, and with what other correlates this occurs. One can give as an example patients' responses to impending or actual separations from their analysts (holiday breaks, or unintended breaks in treatment occurring for other reasons). One may expect to see responses to such situations in "excess"[13] of what might have been anticipated in the absence of an unconscious transference relationship between patient and analyst. These responses might take many forms, in words and actions. The "coding" of psychoanalytic phenomena involves the identification and exploration of many phenomena of unconscious significance, extending all the way to the understanding of an entire personality configuration as being to some degree shaped by unconscious structures of mind.

A third specific adaptation of grounded theory methods to psychoanalysis is parallel to what is also required of them in other fields of inquiry. This concerns the issues of sampling and its representative status. When one is dealing with large volumes of relatively unstructured data, in which meaning is found through its ongoing or retrospective analysis, it is necessary to demonstrate that samples of data that are selected for detailed analysis are indeed adequate representations of the whole, and are not biased by the researcher's preconceptions. It has been a frequent criticism of the psychoanalytic literature that it offers mere "vignettes" of material as evidence in support of its theories, with little explanation of how and why such vignettes have been selected. They may thus be seen to be merely persuasive illustrations of a prior theoretical argument, rather than as evidence or proof of its validity. But where the data-set for a grounded theory analysis consists, as it often does, of large numbers (perhaps even hundreds) of detailed session records, it is feasible and necessary to select samples from these by reference to explicit criteria. These may be of a randomized kind (every *n*th session, or from beginning, middle, and end of a case), or chosen, as discussed above, by theoretical criteria (e.g., the idea of "turning points"), whose attributes may additionally be validated by the blind-rating of the sessions concerned.[14]

These are among the adaptations to grounded theory procedures which have been evolved to enable them to be employed in the analysis of psychoanalytic data.

Interpretative phenomenological analysis

Parallel to the development of grounded theory methods in the field of sociology, an equivalently rigorous approach to the analysis of qualitative data emerged in the field of psychology. Its central text has become *Interpretative Phenomenological Analysis: Theory, Method and Research* (2009) by Jonathan A. Smith, Paul Flowers, and Michael Larkin, but its origins lay in papers published in the 1990s (Smith, 1996; also two collections edited by Smith, Harré, & Van Langenhove, 1995a, 1995b). This work represented a departure from the orthodoxy of "positivistic" or "nomothetic" research methods that at that time dominated the field of psychology, consistent with its aspirations to the credentials of a natural science. Smith's 1996 paper argued for an approach to psychology which was able to capture the experiential and qualitative. But the aim of this approach was to remain in dialogue with mainstream psychology, and to stake a claim for a qualitative approach centred in psychology, rather than importing one from different disciplines. The purpose was to return psychology to its more pluralist origins in the work of William James (Smith, Flowers, & Larkin, 2009, p. 4).

The resources on which the IPA theorists drew to bring greater experiential depth to psychological study were largely philosophical, among them the phenomenological writings of Edmund Husserl, Martin Heidegger, Hans-Georg Gadamer, and Maurice Merleau-Ponty. Phenomenology provided ways of thinking in which the complexities of consciousness and subjective meaning could be explored in their various dimensions. These included the relations between individual consciousness and received ways of thinking, issues of bodily embodiment, the time-boundedness of experience, and the reflexive and self-creating nature of human identities. Different sub-fields of qualitative research methodology (e.g., narrative analysis, conversation analysis, and discourse analysis) developed from this philosophical matrix, as well as the IPA method which has been taken up in some child psychotherapy studies.

There are many similarities between the methods of IPA and grounded theory in their application to clinical psychoanalytic research, as essays in this volume show. Both are highly attentive to the particularities of experience, of personal interactions, and of cases seen as integral wholes. Both recognize subjective experience to be complex and hold that its layers of meaning need to be investigated in depth and in detail, usually with small data samples. Each recommend that researchers immerse themselves in their material and investigate it slowly and meticulously. To this end, they have both developed procedures of "coding", of line-by-line or segment-by-segment analysis of "material", anticipating that superordinate "themes" will emerge as iterations proceed. The main data source for IPA research are interviews of a semi-structured or open-ended kind, but in its application to psychotherapy this may be clinical sessions or group discussions. IPA practitioners seek to identify, through their procedures of coding, recurrent patterns of subjective meaning and connections between "parts and wholes". Such links make up what Smith and his co-authors refer to as the "hermeneutic circle". The coding practices of grounded theory are more oriented to the identification of explanatory concepts and categories, in a hoped-for development of a theoretical explanation of the phenomena in question.

There are both significant similarities and differences between these approaches in their original locations in psychology and sociology, respectively. The "negative similarity", of omission, lies in the fact that neither grounded theory nor IPA, in the work of its mainstream practitioners, has previously given much attention to unconscious mental phenomena. But it has been essential for psychoanalytic researchers using grounded theory methods that they do investigate this additional dimension of unconscious meaning and causal effectivity. By extending the scope of its coding procedures, they have sought to make transparent the significance of "unconscious scripts" (McDougall, 1986)—that is, disavowed and unrecognized but nevertheless potent beliefs and desires—in the minds of the subjects they study, for the most part in clinical settings. The methodological success of this work depends on how far this demonstration has been accomplished.

A significant difference between these methods lies in their disciplinary origins. Although the grounded theorists were rebelling against the dominant "general theories" of their sociological field, they were, all the same, committed to the intrinsic value of theoretical explanation. They sought to develop new, "grounded", experience-based theories, but these were explanatory theories nevertheless. We have seen how, as grounded theory evolved, its earlier "ground-zero" approach to pre-existing theories diminished. It came to be recognized, through, for example, the idea of "abduction", that theoretical presuppositions are inherent in *any* investigation. Its method came to be seen as a way of exploring new phenomena in the light of existing theories, and challenging them in the light of experience. One could not always expect to be discovering new "Grounded Theories" *ab initio*. This dialogic conception of the links between empirical investigation and an evolving body of ideas is consistent with the pattern of most psychoanalytic investigation. Psychoanalysis as a field is similar to sociology and anthropology in its fundamentally "theoretical" nature. Just as sociology can trace the origins of its paradigms back to its founding figures, so there is a continuing line of filiation between contemporary psychoanalytic theory and its classic early formulations.

Psychology, the parent discipline of IPA, is much less "theoretical" and more "empiricist" in its mainstream orientation. IPA has a correspondingly different emphasis from grounded theory. Its purpose has been to capture the experience of subjects, in all their complexity, rather than to develop generalizing theories about them. Its interest is in explicating patterns of meaning, rather than determining structures of cause and effect. The substantive focus of the central IPA text (Smith, Flowers and Larkin 2009) is on changing patterns of identity, as these are formed within such life contingencies as those of motherhood or illness. By giving expression and articulation to these, this perspective aims to facilitate the choices. adaptation, and well-being of its subjects. But the main idea is that is from the subject him/herself that such understandings will emerge, not from any theory "external" to that person's situation. Even in descriptions of research, in this text, into conditions such as psychosis and addiction, there is a marked reluctance to enter the territory of unconscious meanings.

In practice, some IPA research has been theoretically generative. (This is the case for studies reported in this book.) One influential figure in the "critical psychology" movement to which IPA is linked, Rom Harré, has been a leading advocate of the theoretical nature of scientific understanding (Harré & Madden, 1975). Conversely, psychoanalytic grounded theory research is usually as concerned to capture the individual experience of patients and their clinical interactions as with theoretical issues. Nevertheless, we believe that grounded theory's commitment to the discovery and development of theories gives it a particular relevance to psychoanalytic research.

The use of systematic qualitative methods in this research has two principal purposes. The first has been to facilitate clinical and theoretical discovery by child psychotherapist researchers, beyond what might have otherwise been likely. We believe that this volume gives evidence of the productive use of methods of systematic qualitative analysis. A second purpose has been to enhance the transparency and accountability of psychoanalytic findings, through showing that its understandings can be grounded in empirical evidence. The specification of definite methods of research (this sometimes involves changes in the ways in which data is collected as well as analysed) may make it easier for psychotherapists and analysts to undertake research at earlier stages in their careers than usually happens. Such approaches may enable recently qualified clinicians not only to learn about their individual patients, but also contribute to the larger field of psychoanalytic knowledge.

An outline of the book

The substance of this book is arranged in two sections. The first of these, "Mainly Theory and Clinical Method", clusters chapters whose main contribution is to offer some development of the conceptual and theoretical ideas that shape the contemporary field of child psychotherapy and child analysis. The second, "Mainly Practice: Contributions to Service Development",[15] groups chapters that describe innovations in the interventions and techniques available to child psychotherapists in the response they and their services offer to the needs of their patients and their networks and communities. Both of these dimensions are crucial to the modern profession and practice of child psychotherapy. While one important outcome study (IMPACT) has been the context of research for one chapter of this book (chapter 5), for the most part the aims of the research reported are different from that of measured treatment outcome. Without research into individual (or small numbers) of cases, and into specific innovations in clinical technique and practice, there would be few treatments in existence whose effects would be worth measuring. Such "fundamental" kinds of research are therefore crucial to the development of the field, as we argued earlier.

The book does, we think, convey something of the experience of the clinician researchers who came to feel that their research was adding something important to their clinical skill and understanding. At times, the excitement of discovery was palpable; at others, the careful interrogation of material led to a greater clarity or depth and to great satisfaction in the growth of conviction. All seem to have noted and valued the slowing-down of coming to conclusions inherent in the further level of scrutiny involved in the research process, and all enjoyed the realization that their work meant that they had something of interest to communicate to colleagues, whether informally, in conference presentations, or in publications, as in these chapters and in the doctoral theses themselves.

In inviting colleagues to contribute to this book, we hoped to demonstrate the range of clinical work done by child psychotherapists—individual psychotherapy, both intensive and on a weekly basis; parent work; work based in multidisciplinary teams; and work involving wider professional collaboration—and also to represent other research dimensions of child psychotherapy activity. The data presented is, therefore, quite varied, and the methods of data gathering are also varied, as, of course, is the method chosen by the individual researchers to analyse their data.

Our first section, "Mainly Theory", begins at the beginning of life, with a chapter by Wendy Shallcross in which she revisits her experience of an infant observation that she undertook many years previously. Her retrospective analysis of this observation, making use of a grounded theory method, proposes a revised view of the earliest development of mind. Her data links with W. R. Bion's, Esther Bick's, and Donald Meltzer's theorizations and is an important extension of Melanie Klein's earlier account. Louise Allnutt (chapter 2) describes psychoanalytic therapy with a very young child in which the different theories of Melanie Klein, Donald Winnicott, and Frances Tustin with respect to autistic phenomena are seen to represent different aspects and moments of development. She also explores the question of how to work with a small child's carer when the child cannot yet manage separation. The next two chapters are both explorations of the relevance of Bion's theory of thinking to the practice of child psychoanalysis. Carlos Tamm (chapter 3), in comparing weekly work with two children on the autistic spectrum, uses Bion's Grid alongside a grounded theory analysis of the clinical data. This reveals significant patterns of mental organization shared by his two patients, despite important differences between them, and describes their atypical language development. Emily Ryan (chapter 4) describes intensive work with a fostered boy with a very painful history and enormous problems in learning and relating, in which her focus on the "K" link elucidated by Bion proved to be the convincing centre of her patient's capacity to change. O'Shaughnessy's paper, "A Commemorative Essay on W. R. Bion's Theory of Thinking" (1981) has been widely read, but Ryan's work is one of the first to apply its argument so rigorously to clinical practice. Looking in a quite different direction, Miriam Creaser (chapter 5) reports on her research into the nature of the differences between the traditional process notes of psychotherapy sessions and their audio-recording and transcription. The IMPACT study provided an opportunity to compare these two forms of clinical record. Creaser's compelling account not only lays out the kinds of difference to be observed but proposes a theoretical understanding of the origins of these differences. Process notes, she suggests, understandably and rightly, focus on "clinical facts"—namely, the evolution of transference and countertransference relationships. This means that they are highly susceptible to distortions arising from countertransference dynamics. This important discovery lends additional weight to the emphasis given within psychoanalytic practice to the centrality of ongoing supervision and opens up questions about the value of studying audio-records, hitherto somewhat disregarded as a source of valuable data, alongside process records.

In our second section, "Mainly Practice", the involvement of child psychotherapists in work with under-fives and its background in infant observation, highlighted above in Wendy Shallcross's and Louise Allnutt's chapters, are further developed with respect to service provision. Ferelyth Watt (chapter 6) describes her investigation of the understandings among Bangladeshi mothers of the minds of babies and young children, and their attitudes to the supportive services in the community. Her use of observation and her own emotional reactions are of particular interest in her method of analysing material gathered in focus groups. Her attention to the experience of an ethnic group poorly represented in child and adult mental health services (CAMHS) work is exemplary. Liselotte Grunbaum's (chapter 7) meticulous case-study of a child in long-term foster care is focused on the significance of temporal breaks, planned and unplanned, in the therapeutic process. This revealed, additionally and unexpectedly, the particular significance of sibling relationships for this child—both the birth siblings from which she was separated and the foster siblings she encountered in her foster family. This work expands our capacity to understand the complex interaction between the internal and external situation of a child, which is typical of so many patients seen by child psychotherapists. It brings together in an original way two areas of current thinking: the treatment of children in care, and the significance of sibling relationships. It has important relevance for decisions made about placements and contact with birth families.

Marie Bradley (chapter 8) and Kristine Tiltina (chapter 9) both write about new models of brief work in a CAMHS context. Bradley describes her model of a child psychotherapy assessment provided as part of the wider assessment of children in care, with respect to their placement and their emotional and potential therapeutic needs. Her practice was fully integrated with the work of social work colleagues and is one of a number of current models of child psychotherapy contributions in such settings. This particular model combines, in a highly convincing way, a role in assessment with a potentially more long-term involvement in these children's lives, as therapists or as consultants to the network, thus establishing the continuity of care so often lacking for children in the care system. Bradley's chapter, like many others in this collection, describes the additional insight obtained from the meticulous use of a method of qualitative analysis of her clinical data. Tiltina's focus is on the problematic experience of foster-carers, both investigating their psychological-mindedness and also attempting to expand their capacity to relate emotionally to the troubled children placed with them. Her modest four-session intervention is a model that surely has wide relevance. Rajni Sharma (chapter 10) describes her study of the impact of pregnancy on child psychotherapy practice, using both a detailed case study from her own work and interviews with a number of other child psychotherapists. For a largely female profession, pregnancy is a significant fact of life, and Sharma's work raises thought-provoking questions. Both case management and therapeutic technique are often challenged when a therapist become pregnant, and this chapter can help us begin to think more deeply about both these elements.

Finally, Jenifer Wakelyn (chapter 11) describes the development of a borough-based service for babies and young children in care which arose from her doctoral research, in which she had reported her "therapeutic observation" of a baby who was in foster-care from birth until his adoption a year later. She describes ongoing clinical and training work in partnership with many professional groups with responsibility for this highly vulnerable group of children. This chapter provides an example of the potential wider impact of research rooted in the child psychotherapy clinical context, and the value of the psychoanalytic observation stance when it is translated into quite everyday contexts.

As will be evident, our two sections overlap in many ways, and other potential groupings of chapters are implicit—for example, work with under-fives, work with children in care, work with carers and networks. Readers will find all sorts of evocative echoes across the various chapters. We think, however, that this book is making a contribution in both theoretical and clinical directions. The work presented has relevance to the shape of CAMHS provision, to the specification of NICE guidelines, to the lives of children in care, and to child psychotherapy training, as well as to its central focus on child psychotherapy theory and practice. Our contributors have made use of the qualitative research methods outlined earlier to demonstrate that psychoanalytic researchers can draw on their core psychoanalytic thinking to pursue the topics they address, and thus exemplify the research potential of psychoanalytic clinical work.

There is one further aspect of this research to note. It is consistent with classical psychoanalytic practice that most of the work described in this book began from the experiences and ideas of clinical practitioners. These doctoral theses were the initiatives of their authors and were not the outcome of any larger schemes of research. This is, in part, in the nature of psychoanalysis—an aspect, perhaps, of its belonging to the humanities as well as to the sciences. But it is also the consequence of the exclusion of psychoanalysis, until recently, from the academy and its structures of funded research. We should point out that virtually all of the work on this and other doctoral research programmes at the Tavistock has been undertaken by students without the support of research grants, and in their own time.

There are limitations to such an approach to research, from the point of view of the accumulation and systematization of knowledge. The problem arises of how the findings of researches like these can be verified and generalized. In principle, it is not difficult to envisage how studies like these could be scaled up, and their findings tested more broadly, although in present circumstances this seems unlikely to happen any time soon. Now that research in child psychotherapy has reached its present level, there is the need at least for a greater degree of mapping, consolidating, and even planning in these fields of research. We hope that this book might encourage such a development.

Notes

1. The first research degree proposals were registered by already-qualified child psychotherapists with the university in 1995. Regulations for the professional doctorate were approved in 1994.

2. Parallel professional doctorates were developed during these years in other Tavistock disciplines, including social work, systemic family therapy, and psychoanalytic consultation to organizations.

3. The first child psychotherapists to be awarded doctorates in this programme were Debby Hindle, Marguerite Reid, Janet Philps, and Janet Anderson. Their doctoral work has had a continuing influence on child psychotherapy practice and research.

4. In addition, Doctorates by Published Work have been awarded through the Tavistock to 17 child psychotherapists in recognition of research and publication by them achieved before doctoral study was readily accessible to their profession.

5. Child psychotherapy was initiated as a professional training at the Tavistock Clinic in 1948 by Esther Bick and John Bowlby. Its professional association, the Association of Child Psychotherapists (ACP), was established in 1949, and it became recognized as a mental health profession within Britain's NHS in the 1970s. There are now approximately 900 qualified child psychotherapists accredited by the ACP, a number considerably in excess of the British Psychoanalytical Society's current membership. Professional qualification now requires members to have undertaken a two-year pre-clinical course in Psychoanalytic Observational Studies, followed by a four-year clinical training, which includes a personal analysis, education in psychoanalytic theory, and the undertaking of three intensive clinical cases, six or more once-weekly cases, a manualized treatment model such as short-term psychoanalytic psychotherapy (STPP), and a variety of the modalities of clinical and consultative work required of child psychotherapists in public CAMHS. This model of professional education has been adopted internationally in several countries, including Italy, France, and India, with a less direct influence in many other places.

6. Fonagy has been centrally involved in several major outcome studies, including IMPACT and TADS. He is co-author of *What Works for Whom? A Critical Review of Psychotherapy Research* (Roth & Fonagy, 1998) among his many other writings.

7. The idea of "clinical facts" as essentially arising in a transference relationship is developed in several papers in the Special Issue of the *International Journal of Psychoanalysis* in 1994 devoted to clinical facts. See also M. J. Rustin (2019, chap. 10).

8. Indexical or implicit meanings are significant in the analysis of qualitative data, as pointed out by Bryant and Charmaz (2007, chap. 1) in their useful introduction to the grounded theory method.

9. Two earlier volumes (Midgley, Anderson, Grainger, Nesic-Vuckovic, & Urwin, 2009; Urwin & Sternberg, 2012) originating within child psychotherapy, in which the late Cathy Urwin had a significant role, had a purpose related to this one.

10. The most substantial anthology devoted to grounded theory (Bryant & Charmaz, 2007) contains virtually no reference to psychoanalysis as a field of study.

11. It should be noted that this concept is far from unambiguously defined in Peirce's writing. Peirce's approach is delightfully compared by Eco and Seboek (1988) to Sherlock Holmes's.

12. There are moments in the sciences when an entire theoretical field is challenged and brought into question, perhaps leading to a radical departure. These are the moments of "revolutionary science" defined by Kuhn. But these are distinct from the moments of less discontinuous theoretical discovery that have taken place throughout the history of psychoanalysis, and indeed of all other sciences.

13. The term "excess" has been usefully deployed by Slavoj Žižek (1990, 1993) to note the presence of unconscious dimensions of meaning in a situation, beyond what might otherwise be expected.

14. An earlier doctoral thesis by Janet Philps (2009) made influential use of a blind-rating procedure to demonstrate that her assessment of the meaning of a patient's state of mind in certain sessions had validity, or "inter-rater reliability".

15. Many readers will recognize that these titles echo those of the two volumes of Elizabeth Spillius's *Melanie Klein Today* (1988a, 1988b).

PART I

MAINLY THEORY AND CLINICAL METHOD

CHAPTER ONE

A single case of psychoanalytic infant observation and what it reveals about loss and recovery in infancy

Wendy Shallcross

> Why didst thou promise such a beauteous day,
> And make me travel forth without my cloak,
> To let base clouds o'ertake me on my way,
> Hiding thy bravery in their rotten smoke?
> 'Tis not enough that through the cloud thou break,
> To dry the rain on my storm-beaten face,
> For no man well of such salve can speak
> That heals the wound and cures not the disgrace:
> Nor can thy shame give physic to my grief;
> Though thou repent, yet I have still the loss:
> The offender's sorrow lends but weak relief
> To him that bears the strong offence's [cross].
> Ah! But those tears are pearl which thy love sheds,
> And they are rich and ransom all ill deeds.
>
> [Shakespeare, Sonnet 34]

When encountering new findings, it is expected that one would experience a capacity within oneself to imagine and wonder: opening the mind to elements of experience that are preverbal and deeply important to understanding the developing mind of the infant. This chapter illustrates this potential, by presenting research findings from infant observation records made two decades ago. I aim to demonstrate how, by looking closely at the infant's lived experience, we can learn something about loss and recovery in very young babies. These findings arose from a research project in which observational transcripts were reviewed and coded, starting from when the baby was 4 days old until after his second birthday. The whole experience sensitized me to the earliest relationship between parent(s) and infant, and, in so doing, it brought meaning to the struggles associated with life-long fluctuations in states of mind. Just how the baby begins this journey of knowing their own and others' minds was at the heart of this study.

Two principal aims emerged from the evolving investigation. The first concerned the methodology involved in examining observational data using psychoanalytic methods, and the second was the exploration of what can be learned from the systematic study of a single recorded case of infant observation using grounded theory. The use of line-by-line coding, abductive reasoning, and the formation of categories led to a focus on the following details: the first month of life; exploration of the period in this baby's life when mother was traumatically absent; her eventual return; and selected observations that revealed parent–infant recovery.

An earlier chapter published in *Infant Observation and Research: Emotional Processes in Everyday Lives* (Urwin & Sternberg, 2012) concentrated on the first four weeks following birth. There I described how coding revealed how defences at 3 months of age, constructed as a result of trauma, had in fact been preconfigured as proto-defences in the earliest weeks. Several conclusions were reached regarding the observed infant. The first concerned the identification of synchronous rhythms or patterns in the mother–infant relationship where they were found to form a backdrop to aesthetic reciprocity. Rupture in aesthetic attunement was instrumental in activating a cascade of early proto-defensive organization into later development. This took the form of oral preoccupation—namely, regurgitation, rumination, and choking (Shallcross, 2012). While this defensive organization may have been specific to the observed infant, the study draws attention to developmental processes that may be relevant to infants in general. Evidence to support Bick's (1968) idea that babies are more integrated than first thought and are "open" to triangular relating from the beginning was also revealed.

The first weeks post-birth were full of promise—a "beauteous day"—yet within a short time the baby at the heart of this investigation experienced the sudden loss of close intimacy. This chapter details this period, which can be likened metaphorically to the infant travelling forth without the cloak of maternal warmth and security. As Shakespeare's sonnet suggests, the struggle towards recovery was a complex task. This involved the infant managing feelings associated with ambivalence, betrayal, and a lack of trust in order to establish the recovery of the lost good object.

Infant observation and research

There still exists a significant amount of debate as to whether the unconscious as inferred in the infant observation setting can be reliably examined in a research context (see, e.g., Groarke, 2008). The consulting room has been the long-held research preserve for the study of unconscious phenomena. Yet M. J. Rustin (2012), in furthering the analytic connection between the unconscious as perceived in the consulting room and how it is encountered in the observational setting, writes:

> It came to be realized that observers, and even the seminar groups who discussed their observation reports, were being exposed to a field of unconscious feelings, both between mother and baby but also often including the observer herself. . . . If one wants to "see" the unconscious, one can find it in the setting of infant observation as well as in the consulting room. [pp. 14–15]

The major debate centres on the reliability of such observations, given that in the clinical setting analytic formulation can be tested through interpretation. It could be argued that "testing" in this context still remains open to distortion, given the power imbalance in the therapeutic relationship. The supervisory "corrective" is as relevant to the clinical setting as it is to the practice of infant observation.

The existence of unconscious mental states within individuals is a fundamental premise in psychoanalytic enquiry. However, unconscious states are, by definition, not readily transparent and only come to be "known" from the detailed observation of self and other in relation to their effects. Concisely examining such phenomena outside the confines of analysis is a methodological challenge. However, the conjunction of facts arising from psychoanalytic thought, line-by-line, *in-vivo*, and focused selective coding established the meaning and cause of such effects.

In the consulting room, the focus of study centres on individual difficulties, interpersonally and intrapsychically, whereas infant observation, importantly, allows for the study of both risk and difficulty (see, e.g., Briggs, 1997), as well as factors associated with growth, resilience, and development. It could be argued that infant observation offers a distinctive opportunity to research the border area between health and factors associated with anti-development. Significantly, as a research method it is well positioned to study emotional truths relevant to the emotional experience and development of the infant's personality and, in the mother's case, her developing identity as a parent.[1] Wendy Hollway (2012), in reviewing the Tower Hamlets study (Hollway, Phoenix, Elliott, Urwin, & Gunaratnam, 2008), writes of how the infant observation method was able to "access what could not be verbally expressed by research participants; it could go beyond the intentional account and beyond narrative coherence" (p. 27).

Through the course of the study, Hollway, in the tradition of qualitative research practice, reflected upon the methodological implications of infant observation. Specifically, she addressed how emotional responsiveness in the observers was an essential element of the research study. Yet, how to make sure that this subjective element reflected the emotional tone of the observational setting rather than the observers' own biases and preferred views of the infant's world was an important methodological consideration. Traditionally, in the field of research, significant emphasis had been placed upon "objectivity" as a way of managing these dilemmas. The supposed neutrality of the researcher has, however, been criticized, and Hollway, in recognition of the technical challenges associated with drawing on emotional inference, suggests that "keeping an open mind, so central to training in infant observation, provides an alternative epistemological basis for the practice of objectivity" (p. 29). Drawing on the work of Judith Edwards (2008), she outlines three distinct periods of time and process, where the observer/researcher can draw meaning from what is or has been observed: in the actual observational setting, during the course of writing up the observational notes, and in the later seminar presentation and discussion. At each of these stages, an "open-minded corrective" to possible preconceptions entering the field of study can be made.

M. J. Rustin (2012) writes of the advantages of infant observation, in that the method remains close to the experience of the "lived lives" (p. 17) of infants and families. It can provide a complementary addition to quantitative laboratory forms of investigation, and, importantly, the method has the means of identifying distinctive patterns in "being" and relating, which may, over the course of time, influence and direct development. The normal two-year infant observation allows for the close study of inter-personal and intra-personal factors as they develop. Although the duration exposes the observer/researcher to ever-increasing complexity, the lengthy observational period allows for the most prominent features of the observation to surface, often with distinctive clarity.

The infant observation presented here concerns aspects of developmental continuity/discontinuity, with reference to how significant environmental change impacted upon the infant's developing psyche. Earlier, healthy developmental processes were increasingly overshadowed by protective and defensive structures as the infant struggled to relate to a substitute carer who took on the characteristics of a bad object. Paradoxically, these defensive constructions became more entrenched when the infant's mother returned after a period of hospitalization, suggesting that phantasy and the reorganization of memory can and does influence new stages in development and maturation. The challenge was how to concentrate the research enquiry without predetermined "overvalued ideas" (Britton & Steiner, 1994) determining the focus of enquiry.

In researching the observational material, two forms of data examination have been referred to. The first concerns the narrative account, the analysis of which offered a framework for the contextualization of the infant's development. This method is akin to the way in which observation transcripts are approached in the infant observation seminar. The second form of data analysis was approached more systematically, using grounded theory methods. The application of line-by-line coding, clustering, and categorization were processes that, by their very nature, took segments of observational material apart, creating a more abstract view. These two research methods were inextricably linked together throughout the research process, and the binocular account they provided led to the eventual grounded theoretical formulation presented here.

Infant development

The first years of life and their relevance to later personality development first found clinical and theoretical exploration in the work of Freud (1905d). His views about the child's strongly felt emotions of love, hate, and jealousy and the struggle associated with life as a sexual being from birth were revolutionary (Diem-Wille, 2011, p. xix). The idea that early childhood phases and influences could persist into later development, influencing both normative and pathological[2] processes, has received significant attention, expanding beyond the original confines of psychoanalysis. Developmental theorists, neuroscientists, and attachment researchers have latterly contributed towards this exploration. This has created a rich opportunity to triangulate learning from psychoanalytic practice, laboratory-based experimentation, and infant observation. Psychoanalytic infant observation holds a unique position in relation to this ongoing theoretical interplay, as it both continues the psychoanalytic tradition and establishes the technique as a valid method of studying babies in a naturalistic setting.

Internal objects are in live dynamic interplay with external object(s); this is most noticeable when considering how the infant's most primitive fears and anxieties are managed. The carer's ability to contain the infant's emotional states and the internalization of this function by the infant creates a sense of interiority—a space inside (Bion, 1962a). The infant who experiences carers/parents who consider and hold in mind their experience while at the same time relating to each other opens up a "triangular space" (Britton, 1989, p. 86). This model of being thought about is internalized and creates the basis for self-reflection, security, and learning from experience.

Findings from this study reveal how the infant was subject to a triangular presentation from the beginning. Accommodating, tolerating, and imagining external reality as represented by the presence of the third, together with the baby's capacity to endure depressive anxiety, has been thought psychoanalytically to occur at around 5 or 6 months of age. The case cited here would question this assertion and would suggest that the infant was able to tolerate and manage depressive thought from a much earlier age (Shallcross, 2012). Although defensively preoccupied when experiencing the sudden temporary loss of his mother, the baby was able to adjust to the changed environmental circumstances and retain a level of integration necessary for object seeking and relating. The following account details the infant's experience during his mother's absence and his presentation on her return. I begin with a short introduction to Kieran and his family.

Baby Kieran and his family

Kieran, a fair-haired, sturdy infant, was the second child born to Susan and Mark; they had been together for some time, appearing emotionally secure and living comfortably. They lived some considerable distance from immediate family. The home was warm and welcoming, and it was with relative ease that I was able to remain in the observer role. Kieran's piercing blue eyes held a steady, enquiring gaze; this was noticeable during breast-feeding, which was usually calm and relaxed. At this stage he was able to hold his head unsupported and had a real interest in the world around him. He signalled his distress with confidence, and his frustrated cries were full of protest. However, by the thirteenth week, Susan held the expectation that Kieran could begin to rely upon an internal container to manage short periods of frustration. All observations had taken place without hindrance, until I received a telephone call from Mark to say that his wife was in hospital, having sustained serious injuries.

The elaboration of defences: Observation 14

The following account details the first observation of baby Kieran in the care of the young nanny (Mary). Kieran had initially greeted me with animated cooh's and ahh's, perhaps in anticipation that my presence would reinstate that of his mother's. Distress soon followed; it was the beginning of the third day without his mother.

> Pulling away from the nanny, with eyes averted, Kieran tensed his body, and his crying intensified. Gone were the soft smiles of a few minutes ago, to be replaced now with a taut, determined, angry cry. Kieran started to chew on his fist; Mary went to collect the juice bottle, telling Kieran that he might be thirsty. Returning with the bottle, Kieran let out a scream as Mary tipped him backwards on her lap to insert the teat into his mouth. He fought with the bottle, and Mary appeared to fight back; however, Kieran managed to push the bottle away, and Mary placed it back on the table.
>
> ... Mary took a bottle of milk from the fridge; taking a teat from the sterilizer, she returned to her chair with both items. While she fixed the teat to the bottle, Kieran began to cry; he let out a loud, long yell as Mary tipped him backwards, his head lower than his feet, the teat placed straight into his O-shaped mouth. Kieran continued to scream. Mary jiggled the bottle in his mouth, his cries now muffled by gargled milk; eventually, Kieran took the teat between his lips, and he began to suck. Kieran strained his head away from Mary in such a way that he was determined not to look at her or the bottle as he fed. He focused instead on the light streaming through the door into the shaded kitchen. Both looked uncomfortable; Mary's arm was bent back, now feeding Kieran at rights angles to her body, Kieran still straining away from Mary. I felt a sense of shock at the thought of the (cold?) pre-prepared milk hitting his stomach.
>
> ... Kieran became limp and motionless; his sucking decreased. Mary pulled the bottle from his mouth and watched as the air bubbles noisily reached the surface of the remaining milk. Then, swiftly, the teat was re-inserted.

> This pattern was repeated several times; at one point Mary exerted quite a lot of pressure removing the teat, and it came away with a pop not unlike the cork from a bottle.
>
> ... As she moved around the kitchen, Mary began to jig Kieran up and down. His eyes averted, they closed and widened open with each up-and-down motion. I began to feel nauseous, and with each downward movement I felt as though I were falling. Kieran started with hiccups. His face screwed in distaste as he brought up a small quantity of milk into his mouth. Kieran's eyes closed, and his lips curled as the milk and saliva started to dribble down his chin. With clenched fists and through the hiccups, Kieran began to cry.
>
> *Observation 14: Kieran (3 months, 2 weeks)*

Kieran's distress is clearly evident. He is unable to sustain eye contact with Mary, and her ministrations are clearly out of tune with the baby. Their struggle to establish reciprocal, meaningful contact is demonstrated in the conflicted exchange over the feeding bottle. It appears to represent in a concrete manner the agent of intrusion. The eyes and mouth as portals of entry are barred to Mary's endeavours to feed him, and she, in turn, enters into a battle of forced access. It is a challenging situation; the responsibility for the survival of such a young, distressed, hungry infant who refused all feeds was clearly a strain.

In this observation we see the first instance of regurgitation: the bringing up of small amounts of milk and saliva, in this instance as a passive consequence of his helplessness when faced with the force-feeding consequent on Mary's anxiety. She grew increasingly persistent that Kieran should take the bottle; his diagonal positioning on her lap appeared to be the final act in his submission. Seeking an alternative to Mary's face—one that we imagine being a source of persecution for him—Kieran glues himself to the light source streaming through the open kitchen door and, later in the observation, to the family dog. This *second-skin formation* (Bick, 1968) serves as a defence against catastrophic anxiety.[3]

What followed was a repeated exchange between Kieran and Mary characterized by avoidance, intense distress, and mounting hostility. Baby and nanny were clearly mis-attuned; Kieran was held visually too close to Mary's face, her movements with him lacked fluidity, and his communications were constantly misread. Mary, in turn, spoke about her feelings of persecution: Kieran had scratched her skin, and he cried each time she sat down with him. As a consequence her arms ached from holding him upright as Mary paced the kitchen floor. It was clear that the baby was projecting his significant distress into the nanny, and she, in turn, was trying her best to ameliorate his mounting sorrow by giving recognition to how Kieran needed to be continuously held and kept on the move. This was in sharp and stark contrast to the way in which Susan, with her graceful and fluent movements, tended to her baby. Mary was desperate to soothe Kieran in his grief; in ordinary circumstances her ministrations would have been enough to calm him. However, Kieran's state of mind in these unusual conditions seemed to communicate an intense split between an idealized object and one that, by replacement, was experienced as persecutory or bad.

Ambivalence and development: Observation 15

The following week I was welcomed into a small room opposite the kitchen. Kieran was lying on a play mat in front of the television; the nanny, Mary, was sitting on the sofa, with Kieran at her feet.

> Mary turned to look at Kieran and smiled, saying "you want a drink now, Kieran, you want a drink now, I think it is time that you had a bottle, you would like a bottle would you." Mary stood up and again offered Kieran one of the small toys. He almost went to take it with his hand, and instead of reaching forward, he opened his mouth. Mary moved the toy towards his fingers and turned and left the room to make his bottle. Kieran watched Mary as she disappeared and then started to make small noises of discontentment, of "ah ah" and "mmm, mmm". He looked at me with expectation, and I gave him what I thought was an empathic facial acknowledgement of how difficult it was to wait. Turning towards the doorway, Kieran kicked his legs vigorously and again let out a squeal. He began to suck with his lips before again letting out a further squeal and a cry. Turning his attention towards the television, he again appeared to be watching the mouth of the presenter before scanning and examining the faces on the screen. This momentarily held his attention, until he once again began to kick his legs and let out a small cry. In the doorway, Mary said, "the bottle is being warmed, Kieran, it won't be a moment". Kieran looked at her and started to make mouthing movements.
>
> *Observation 15: Kieran (3 months, 3 weeks)*

The observational extract records how Kieran's urgent vocalization (proto-communication) was responded to in a manner that made it meaningful. The sense Mary makes of these utterances scaffolds[4] (Bruner, 1978) a development in thinking, demonstrated by how Mary communicates back to the infant her understanding of his hunger. The synchronicity between Kieran's integration of the face on the television screen and that of Mary's reappearance serves to highlight how both nanny and infant were prepared to struggle for contact, to find a fit, however briefly. This could be understood as an innate search for a K link (Bion, 1992) as a representation of growth and transformation.

As the observation progressed, Kieran's agitation intensified, escalating in tone and pitch, accompanied now by his knees drawn into his chest as though in pain. His cries became staccato, ending with a long, high-pitched squeal that sounded as though he were cross. At the time I found myself wanting to use my own voice to soothe,[5] wishing to de-escalate the rising pitch of his cry. The intensity of the experience, coupled with the powerful nature of the projective identification, created the illusion in the mind of the observer and later the researcher that there was a complete absence of a regulatory capacity in the form of *"parentese"*[6] (*"Motherese"*: Bateson, 1971; Fernald, 1985) and containment.

Bion's description of the absent breast (no breast) creating a negative realization[7] is particularly pertinent here. This was especially noteworthy because Kieran was expelling the frustration associated with the absence of his mother's breast and the presence of the bottle (substitute carer) in such a forceful manner (which came to be categorized as: –orientation/ –transformation/ –expansive). It gave every indication that he was defending against such a realization. The urgency of his need seemed to communicate the phantasy that he might not survive the experience. Yet in order to do so, he needed to find a way to tolerate his frustration as a means of commencing the important task of thinking about and perhaps grieving for the absent breast.

Just how Kieran adapts to this change is quite remarkable: there is a tangible diminution of affect-attunement, parentese, and containment, yet against this backdrop there appears to be a surge in vocal development. It could be speculated that in the absence of refined object sensitivity, the baby seeks the means by which interactive connection can be further elaborated. In effect, the infant is spurred on to make a more robust communicative link with others, thereby promoting vocal development in a similar way to that which Bion (1962b) describes: the absent breast in ordinary good-enough circumstances provoking thought and the means to think.[8] In order to do this, the infant requires an internal resilience that can withstand the uncertainty and doubt created by broken contact and to find the means by which new links can be sustained and nourished.

Kieran's glance towards the doorway where Mary had made her exit would seem to suggest that he could, at age 3 months, not only track the movements of the individual but also begin to anticipate her return. This, over time, promotes a capacity to hold in mind the absent object and to perhaps self-regulate the impact of the non-appearance. Yet despite his developing capacities of three-dimensional triangularity, internal object regulation, and increased vocal communication, Kieran still struggled with the rapid change from breast to bottle and the altered intimacy in the feeding encounter. The following extract details the adjustments that both Kieran and Mary made in order to sustain feeding contact.

> Mary sat down, with Kieran on her knee. She reached backwards for the bottle and tipped Kieran's upper body below the horizontal position in order to insert the bottle straight into his mouth. He let out a small cry at the sudden and unexpected tipping backwards. Mary then lifted him higher, with the bottle firmly held in his mouth, until he reached a completely horizontal position. Instead of cradling Kieran in her arms, she rested his head on a cushion, and Mary sank back into the sofa to watch television. Kieran watched her intently as he sucked on the bottle. Occasionally, as he fed, Mary smiled at him and held his hand. Kieran grasped the bottle to him with his right hand as he began to suck rhythmically. Suddenly, without warning, the bottle was removed from Kieran's mouth by Mary; air bubbles rose to the surface. The surprise on Kieran's face appeared "frozen". Quickly, again without any signal, the teat was reinserted. This pattern continued throughout the feed. The removal of the bottle while Kieran sucked rhythmically was very difficult to observe. It made no sense to me whatsoever. I noted how still and composed my body became, as though suspended.
>
> *Observation 15: Kieran (3 months, 3 weeks)*

The unusual style in which Mary fed Kieran meant that it was very difficult for him to refuse the teat; there was no alternative but to take the bottle. It precluded the earlier struggle of the desire and need for nourishment followed by rejection because it was not his mother's breast. Whether Mary's style was influenced by Kieran's ambivalence was hard to tell. What is clear, however, was how determined Mary was in controlling the timing and positioning of Kieran for the feed.

The cushion as an alternative to Mary's embrace appears to be a thoughtful compromise, one that allowed Kieran to once again make eye contact. The hand-holding and occasional smile from Mary offered reassurance and the opportunity of skin-to-skin contact. It seemed to promote and support Kieran's grasp of the bottle, giving the illusion, perhaps, that he had regained some omnipotent control over the feeding experience, thereby avoiding a state of helplessness and uncertainty associated with the breast's disappearance.

There was a functional and somewhat mechanical quality to the sudden and unexpected removal of the teat from Kieran's mouth, as if Mary's attention was taken up entirely by the removal of air from the bottle. The erratic nature of the withdrawal bore no relation to Kieran's rhythm of feeding or any observable cue that the baby had slowed or stopped. Kieran's "frozen response" would seem to indicate a protective function, as though he is highly alert to the threat of total withdrawal. Mary's actions and Kieran's reply seemed to capture the traumatic moment of loss—one that is replayed over again with each abrupt removal of the teat from Kieran's mouth. This occurred frequently during this and every observed feed with the nanny thereafter.

The observer's feeling of body suspension (an indication, perhaps, of a strong identification with the infant's experience of frozenness) draws attention to how time is perhaps distorted by traumatic events, supporting the idea of continual replay. The surprise of Susan's sudden and abrupt absence appears to be captured in this moment—as if Mary and Kieran had come together as a nursing dyad in a somewhat startling, incoherent manner. Yet, in other aspects, Kieran and Mary were forging a relationship that conveyed intimacy and receptivity.

The expression of ambivalence was further elaborated upon when the nanny spoke directly to the observer about the previous night's feed. It was reported how grandmother had given Kieran his bottle of milk, which he had "guzzled down" with vigour, only for the entire bottle to be regurgitated shortly afterwards. This turned out to be the beginning of a regular pattern[9] that saw Kieran returning the milk in this manner. It drew attention to how trauma associated with the loss of the breast and the change in aesthetic from breast to bottle found expression in an oral display of regurgitation. Vividly it drew attention to how many feeding styles Kieran had to manage and adapt to.

Mother's return—pleasure and pain: Observation 17

On entering the playroom at the family home the following week, I was surprised to see Susan reclining on the sofa, with Kieran sitting beside her. The surprise changed to a dawning sense of shock as I noticed how pale and ill Susan looked. Slumped against his mother's body, Kieran stared out into the room. It was a sorrowful sight. I greeted them both;

Kieran smiled in response, but it faded quickly before he intently looked into my eyes. He held a steady, penetrating, solemn gaze as his mother told me that she was having a "difficult day" and that she "wasn't used to her mood being so low". As though trying to enliven the serious tone, Kieran smiled once again, followed by an intense stare. His smile did little to punctuate Susan's reflection on her mental state. She described how she was normally "emotionally even-keeled" and that her "mood naturally was quite a buoyant one". However, she now "felt detached" ... "I just feel switched off", she concluded. Susan's capacity to reflect on her own state of mind suggests that she recognized how the impact of trauma had altered her. She noted how her responses to Kieran were now incongruent to his communicated affect. Susan noticed, too, how aversive and reticent she was in responding to her baby's cries, and how reliant she was upon others to care for her son. In the following extract, mother and baby are physically close yet remain psychically estranged. While Kieran was able to appreciate a spatial awareness beyond the organizing principles associated with his mother's face, his positioning, facing into the room and away from her, was not accidental, for he was reluctant to engage in sustained eye contact.

> Susan turned her attention to Kieran, who had started to grizzle and complain. She showed him the toys that she had on the seat beside her. Kieran in response stared at them intently. One squeaked, and Susan danced the toy up and down in front of Kieran. However, Kieran began to slump forward, and Susan gently coaxed him back up into a sitting position. It looked uncomfortable for the both of them to play, since Kieran could not see her face.
>
> *Observation 17: Kieran (4 months, 1 week)*

In this episode, Kieran's mood seemed to match that of his mother: even the squeaking, dancing toy did little to enliven him. Visually, his slumped "C" position seemed to capture an impression that an internal collapse was taking place, appearing to symbolically represent his mother's voiceless presence and her physical difficulty in caring for her son. There appeared to be little in the way of a psycho-skeletal structure that would offer support and containment.

A short time later Mary resumed the care of Kieran; he received the bottle in the now familiar horizontal position, and once again the teat was removed several times. Kieran, in response, sucked vigorously, and the feed concluded with milk seeping from the corners of his mouth. Kieran's defensive strategies became increasingly revealed by the line-by

-line coding: sucking vigorously as a way of regulating intimacy and perhaps his aggression; staring out into the room as an alternative to the face, and finding organization from a replacement source; and, finally, the expression of indifference related to seeping and leaking milk as it dribbles from his mouth. As the coding frequency of these defensive responses was traced through the observational transcripts, a clustering of them into a definition or categorization of aesthetic conflict gained credibility.

Mother's first feed: Observation 18

This was the first observed account of mother and son holding sustained eye contact following her accident. It undoubtedly contributed to the bringing together of eye, mouth, and sound. However, in the following extract we see just how fragile the object–infant union actually was.

> Turning his attention back to the bottle, Kieran continued fingering and holding it with both hands. It was surprising to see how widely stretched his fingers were and how he used his thumb hooked underneath the bottle and around the teat area to explore, while his fingers rested on the top of the bottle. At one point, Susan moved her hand away, and Kieran alone momentarily supported the bottle.
>
> Milk started to dribble from the corners of Kieran's mouth. Susan removed the bottle and reached for a cloth to wipe him. She held the bottle in front of Kieran, and he watched it intently. He started to murmur and then to cry, his fists clenched as he looked at the bottle. Susan offered it to him again, and Kieran began to suck. Susan smilingly called him "a little guzzler".
>
> *Observation 18: Kieran (4 months, 1 week, 3 days)*

The inevitable break in intensity between mother and son caused by Susan momentarily removing her hand from the bottle was enough to break Kieran's good relationship with it. This small, barely discernible event was only recognized through the close analysis of the observational data.[10] It revealed how sensitively related current events were to the loss of the breast. Susan's removal of her hand perhaps reawakened the absence of the object, and, as milk seeped from the infant's mouth, it is feasible to consider how Kieran experienced it anew as a faulty fit between teat and mouth. The bottle so tenderly explored earlier in the observation was now looked at as though something persecutory had taken its place. This would suggest that while an aesthetic quality is linked to the restoration of a good object, alone it lacks the robustness of depressive thought encountered in more integrated states.

In the following extract, Kieran had returned once more to feeding on the bottle, the teat filling his mouth and securely held in place by his tighter lips. This comfortable alliance was to be short-lived.

> Susan once again offered Kieran the bottle. He was immediately content, as soon as the teat was in his mouth. However, Susan had left the muslin cloth underneath the bottle. She realized this immediately and said, "I'm sorry Kieran, I know you like to hold the bottle." Susan briefly removed the teat from Kieran's mouth and removed the cloth. Kieran watched the bottle intently and began to make mouthing movements as Susan once again placed the bottle into his mouth. Kieran resumed feeding, sucking quietly, his eyes fluttering shut into a milky sleep.
>
> The dog jumped up and started to bark in a high-pitched, frenzied manner, making Susan and myself jump in fright. Kieran opened his eyes momentarily, then closed them again and sucked unconcernedly on the teat. After a while he stopped sucking, and Susan removed the bottle. There was a small amount of milk left in it, and Susan placed it beside her on the bed. She moved tentatively to wipe some milk that had started to dribble from Kieran's mouth. He suddenly opened his mouth, and a small amount of milk came back. Susan instinctively moved Kieran to a higher position when suddenly he opened his eyes wide and was sick in a projectile manner. The whole contents of a full bottle of milk came pouring out of Kieran's mouth.
>
> *Observation 18: Kieran (4 months, 1 week, 3 days)*

In this observation, mother and son were once again enveloped in intimacy, one that is delicate and sensorial—for example, the way in which Kieran fingers the teat. Despite the changes associated with the bottle and his positioning next to his mother rather than held on her lap, there was a return of sensorial integration, eye, and touch. It is perhaps the very return of the integrating object that left Kieran vulnerable to "aesthetic conflict", as first described by Donald Meltzer (Meltzer & Harris Williams, 1988). Meltzer relates how conflict within the infant arises when the truth of an experience is unbearably beautiful. In this instance, the return of the feeding, nurturing mother perhaps evokes conflict associated with the unknowable aspects of her near-death experience or, as Kieran felt it, the object's absence. Was this an aspect related to the violent expulsion of milk—that something within, despite the environmental security, was impacting on the container–contained (Bion, 1959) function.[11]

After enduring such a traumatic separation, to encounter the vulnerability of the object seems to me to be a supremely conflicted experience for Kieran. For he was, once more, looking towards his mother, drinking her in, along with the milk. The resulting conflict is quite different from that experienced with the substitute object/nanny. For example, as the baby by sight and touch infuses the image of the bottle with meaning, a sequence of events appears to be set in motion that culminates in the expulsion of milk. There is both a re-enactment of the trauma associated with mother's accident—the forceful loss of the milk/breast—and a suggestive purging that may conceivably relate to the presence of something indigestible.

Restoration of the object: Observation 19

Seven weeks after Susan's accident and three weeks into the shared care arrangement with the nanny, Susan began to reflect in my presence upon her mental state. She spoke of how she had "woken up" and now felt "switched on again" after several weeks of feeling "switched off, lacking in energy or thought for anything". As though to confirm her increasing restored mental availability, Susan in this observation began to read and voice her baby's cues, and as the observational hour progressed, these observations were shared with the nanny, thereby creating a link comparable to that of a parental couple. In response, Kieran was more playful, which Susan noted as she commented upon her son's restored "animation".

> Kieran appeared to get excited by the coffee cups; he made mouthing movements as he carefully observed them on the table. He turned his attention to his left hand and watched his hand for a moment as he lightly touched the pram cover, moving his hand closer to the toy worm. After a moment or two of considering the worm, he used his right hand to grasp it, pulling it forward towards him and then pushing it away. At one point the worm tippled over, and again he repeated pushing away and pulling forward the toy. One of his movements was vigorous, and the worm fell to the floor. In response Kieran looked very serious, and he immediately took his right hand to his mouth, chewing on his thumb and fist for the briefest of moments. He removed his thumb and continued with mouthing movements, his lips coming together in rhythm. Mary spotted that Kieran had dropped his worm, and she picked it up, using it to play peek-a-boo,

bopping Kieran on the head with a "boo" after the worm had been out of sight.

Observation 19: Kieran (4 months, 2 weeks, 3 days)

Kieran's activity with the toy worm would seem to capture, in a symbolic manner, his preoccupation with the closeness of the object and then its distance—recreating perhaps the to-and-fro in the feeding relationship. The associative mouthing that occurred at the start differed significantly from that of Kieran's state of mind displayed at the end. For then, Kieran's look conveyed anxiety when the worm dropped from view, indicating concern for the object. Kieran may well have experienced a sense of persecutory guilt, signified by how his fist went into his mouth, and he began to gnaw on his thumb and knuckles. However, something of a transformation followed when Kieran began his rhythmic sucking. It might convey how at this point the infant had a more benign phantasy in his mind, conceivably of a good object. There was, perhaps, "the desire to restore" (Klein, 1936b, p. 294) a good object presence, especially after the aggressive pushing away that had caused the fall of the worm. Mary understood the nature of Kieran's play, and she elaborated it into a full disappearance of the object. The worm's sudden return as a "boo", once again capturing the rather startling and sudden reappearance of the object for Kieran, reinforced for the infant that the restoration of the object is dependent upon the management of his own ambivalence.

Alongside these developmental opportunities, Kieran still struggled to remain in contact. He would demand once more to be held upright, with some distance between his body and that of the other. Eye contact although present was not sustained, and commonly *while seated on the lap, he turned away from the gaze of the carer.* Most frequently his distress was noted in the feeding relationship. Susan reported how Kieran occasionally regurgitated his feed; not knowing what the trigger was, she believed it to be somewhat idiosyncratic. By way of explanation, the family and nanny continued to refer to him "as a little guzzler". The term may well capture a particular internal significance for Kieran: a defensive aspect, which, while satisfying the immediate need for "good" sustenance, fails to "paralyse the action of the 'bad' objects and substances inside the body" (Klein, 1931, p. 247).

At this stage in the data analysis, codes, as previously mentioned, began to coalesce and cluster into emerging categorization (see Appendix 1.1). The next stage in the narrative analysis was, therefore, to select individual observations that explored these themes and emerging categories in greater depth. Before returning to the observational narrative, however, I pause in order to explore the findings from Phases 2 and 3[12] of the observational narrative.

The legacy of mother's accident

The observations in this section record the care the infant received from the nanny during mother's absence. They capture the baby's adjustment to his changed circumstances and record defensive preoccupations, which characterize so many of his interactions with the mother substitute.

It would appear that the trauma associated with mother's accident had coalesced with an already existing developmental task associated with weaning from the breast. Managing these first separations was a delicate and necessary undertaking for both mother and baby. Mother's abrupt hospitalization occurred at an important point for the infant, since he had begun an evening bottle just one week prior to the accident.

Throughout Observations 14–16 there is a continual movement between ambivalence and a more depressive position. Linked to this oscillation, we see fluctuations between unintegrated and integrated states. In the former, we see how the baby struggles to maintain a coordinated body rhythm as he writhes and flails in the nanny's arms. His unintegration is also noted in his visual part-object fixation.

Observations 14–16 in summary

- » A process of forced entry enters the feeding relationship. Control and authority were asserted as a way of managing the baby's conflicted state.
- » Early proto-defensive strategies first noted in Observations 1–4 become habituated as protective measures.
- » The baby becomes the recipient of the nanny's anxious projections.
- » By Observation 16, Kieran was at times resistant to the soothing approaches of the nanny—a further blockade—and his prolonged grievance delayed amelioration of his distress.
- » In Observation 17, a mixture of ambivalence and blocked access manifests itself as indifference when his mother returns home from hospital. This continues for some time, and although first noted in

Observation 14, the infant's turning away from the carer persists into Observation 20.

» Passive leaking of milk was related to a faulty fit in the container/contained relationship.
» There is a surge in vocal development, possibly related to the toleration of frustration and developing communicative repertoire.

Mother's return

The observations prior to the accident detailed many examples of how capable mother was at assessing her baby's state of mind, and likewise how capable the infant was in evaluating the mother's.[13] This facilitated joyous reciprocal exchanges at times, and in a rarefied manner, was evident when mother and son presented a unified depressed state when mother returned in her altered state. Regurgitation began at this point and coincided with mother's temporary mental unavailability, indicating perhaps the indigestible nature of the infant's psychic pain.

When the infant does allow himself to be "gathered together" into reciprocal exchanges, his body movements return once again to a more discernible rhythm, and he enters a more integrated state. There is a return to coherent synchronized emotional patterns, and these have some bearing on how a process of mentalization becomes established following mother's accident.

Observations 17–20 in summary

» Analysis of later observations detailed how important synchronized emotional patterns were both to the establishment of a contingent adaptation as seen in Observations 15, 18, 19, 20, as well as to the later recovery of mother/infant attunement.
» The infant attunes himself to mother's state of mind.
» Rumination was defined by the urgent taking in of milk, followed by forceful projection outwards.
» Painful pleasure characterized playful interactions.
» Aesthetic conflict was activated by mother's return in her altered state.
» There was a continuation in defensive preoccupation characterized by gaze avoidance, blockading, and second-skin adaptation.
» The infant uses triangular referencing as a way of bringing nanny, mother, and observer together.

Reparation and a loss realized: Observations 22, 38, 46

Having identified selected themes from Observations 1–19, examined in three distinct time frames,[14] I then turned to reviewing the categories of *synchronous patterns, defensive strategies, aesthetic conflict, the progress of rumination as a defensive strategy, indifference to mother's presence* and *the demonstration of painful pleasure* in the remaining observations. Observations were selected from when the infant was 4 months, 3 weeks old (Observation 20) to just past his first birthday. It was hoped that this selective process would help to check, qualify, and elaborate on the already identified themes.

From Observation 22, there was further amplification of the infant's oral preoccupation; a choking response was noted, as was further reference to the regurgitation of milk. Kieran took to placing a teething ring so far into his mouth that he started to retch. However, these defensive preoccupations were interspersed with intimate and joyous exchanges with his mother. In the following account Susan had left the room.

> Kieran watched as his mother slowly stood up and made her way to the door. He then turned to glance up at himself in the mirror, turned away, and glanced towards the doorway, where his mother now was. Kieran then turned to look in the mirror and caught sight of himself again. A serious expression passed across his face, his eyes intently focused in an inwardly thoughtful manner. Kieran returned to playing with the toys and let out well-formed "mmn, mmn" and "ahh ahh" sounds. He found the teething ring and started to chew on it vigorously. Once again he pushed it so far back into his mouth that he started to choke. He removed it as I moved forward to check on his safety. Kieran slumped forward and using the firmness of the play frame he pushed the ring further back into his mouth. He started to choke and gag. Kieran collapsed further against the ring, the teething ring firmly lodged into his mouth. He was choking excessively now; I quickly looked towards the door for the arrival of mother. Seeing that she was not there and thinking about the time involved in collecting her (especially because of her slow movement on crutches), I moved forward to lift Kieran into an upright position. There was an urgency I felt to take action, as if his choking was a fight for survival.
>
> *Observation 22: Kieran (5 months, 2 weeks)*

The sequence begins with Kieran's anticipation of his mother's imminent departure. The play ring and, especially, the mirror are taken as substitute objects in mother's absence. Looking towards his departing mother and then turning back to the mirror would seem to suggest that his reflection[15] was invested with mental processes associated with managing his mother's absence. He seems to give vocalization to these ideas, but something more orally urgent takes precedence. We might imagine how at this point his mother's absence is felt on an oral level; the teething ring consequently is inserted forcefully, and choking begins. At this point the teething ring appears to take on sadomasochistic qualities, for it is inserted so far into the mouth as to cause considerable distress. The earlier satisfying feed with his mother is replaced by something more painful in her absence.

The activity of choking and regurgitation would seem to be a very apt representation of being intruded upon by an attacked object. Repeating the activity over again was an important element in overcoming or mastering the experience. Kieran may also have imagined that his mother's absence, and later return in a damaged state, was related to him, as though he had contributed to it. This is a different explanation of regurgitation and choking from that made by Gaddini and Gaddini (1959), who understood the process as a denial of dependence and, as they called it, "the first perversion".

When Kieran was 6 months, 2 weeks old, his mother returned to work; this change was responded to by increased physical development: Kieran was attempting to crawl, rolling with ease onto his stomach and pushing up through his arms. I learned that there were occasions when he regurgitated his milk, and choking on objects continued. Yet despite these defensive pre-occupations, Kieran communicated in a lively, engaging manner; there was evidence of knowing others' minds and teasing. By 7 months, 2 weeks (Observation 28), he practised standing, could clearly say "mum, mum, mum", and was able to coordinate objects with both hands fluently. He was studious and observant of his surroundings, and it was clear that he was thriving with his greater sense of physical independence. With the cutting of his first tooth at age 7 months, 2 weeks (Observation 30), and coinciding with Susan reconsidering her professional role in light of her parenting commitments, she finally decided to leave work. Kieran's regurgitation at this point came to an end. At 8 months, Kieran was able to read my emotional engagement in his activity of dropping a spoon over the side of his chair and, I believe, infer my next action—whether I would pick up the spoon or not. This is not usually seen in infants until they are 1 year old (Phillips, Wellman, & Spelke, 2002) and serves as an example of his precocious physical and mental development.

Despite these developments in Kieran's capacity to theorize the intentions of others, a week later he began what was to become, over time, a familiar action. He accompanied eating and drinking with the vocalization of "mum, mum, mum", and as long as his mother was visually accessible, he continued to eat or drink. However, as soon as she moved away, Kieran began to complain, throwing his head back until he started to choke on the food that he had in his mouth. Mother spoke of Kieran's continued regurgitation of milk, especially at night. Although there was parental recognition that this was, perhaps, related to separation, there was also a growing realization in mother's mind that the infant was still feeling the impact of her accident. Symbolic resonance appeared to penetrate many aspects of their relationship, and I began to wonder whether there was an internal need for the infant to continually find ways in which loss was recreated, whether this was by the regurgitation of milk and the choking response to draw attention to the oral catastrophe, or in the creation of a barrier, one that served to keep the object at a distance. Playing games associated with absence and presence, appearance and disappearance, is not unusual in early infancy; it is, rather, the intensity and passion that gave these events such particular meaning. In the following example Kieran has been placed in his high chair awaiting his bottle.

> Susan offered Kieran a baking tin full of items, including Duplo, a small rolling pin, and a wooden spoon. Kieran, with serious intent, took each of the items from the bowl and dropped them immediately onto the floor, looking over the edge of his seat as they fell. Momentarily he waved a wooden spoon above his head; the accompanied vocalization had a scolding tone, and the spoon, too, was dropped to the floor. Picking up the now empty metal tin, he gazed at the light reflections captured on its surface from around the kitchen. Kieran pushed his head into it, feeling its smooth ridged interior. This, too, was then thrown to the floor. It made a tremendous clattering noise as it spun on the stone floor, startling Kieran. As though checking to see what had occurred, he leant over the side of his chair and began to grizzle. It felt as though he was telling them—the discarded items—off. His eyes swept across the kitchen to where his mother was measuring his milk, and he now included her into his complaint.
>
> *Observation 38: Kieran (10 months, 1 week, 2 days)*

The angry complaint from Kieran had a clear intention: to communicate his dissatisfaction and growing anger at waiting for his longed-for milk. The discarding of various items was purposeful; for he seemed to gain gratification from looking over the edge of his seat and seeing the items discarded on the floor below. It seemed to demonstrate how Kieran was able to face his negative feelings without being overwhelmed. The act appeared to capture a sense of potency, as though Kieran could remain positive about negative feelings towards the object.

Having developed the capacity to manage ambivalent feelings, Kieran welcomed others to join him in his play, as illustrated in the following example.

> Kieran held the lid from his feeding bottle firmly between his lips. The size of it obscured his face, and he looked like he had a yellow button for a nose. It looked very funny as he crawled along. Kieran snorted with laughter, as though enjoying the joke himself. He then began a game whereby he threw the lid of the bottle and then set about retrieving it. He did this all around the kitchen and dining area. At one point, Susan asked Kieran if she could join his game. Kieran offered her the yellow lid and then withdrew it while smiling at her. She returned his smile and asked again; this time he offered her the lid, and she threw it. It skimmed the kitchen and dining room floor and flew out of sight into the hallway. Susan explained to Kieran that she had not meant to throw it so far from him. Kieran looked up at his mother, and she encouraged him to look for it. In a determined manner he made his way across the kitchen and dining-room floors, and I was able to observe how he smiled when he spotted it in the hallway. Susan watched him regain the lid and commented on "how clever he was" and clapped. Kieran, with a beaming smile, resumed his game.
>
> *Observation 46: Kieran (1 year, 2 weeks)*

Kieran's playful inventiveness with the lid of the bottle captured his ongoing preoccupation with the loss and retrieval of objects. His curiosity facilitated him finding different modes of expression for restitution. Humour, whether that of self-awareness or in the act of teasing, seemed to be an important component of his play, perhaps enabling him to face his fear of loss and disappearance. Humour has been shown to "neutralize anxiety-provoking situations by somehow reappraising and looking at them from another perspective, and of course humour is very much a social, interpersonal act" (Music, 2011, pp. 217–218). The sequence began with Kieran's awareness of the funny nature of the yellow lid held between his lips. He may not have been conscious of it acting as an amusing replacement to his nose, but he certainly communicated how, even to him, the activity was unusually funny. The cognizance of self is thought to develop in infants' minds from around 2 years of age; the early self-awareness demonstrated by Kieran would suggest that, for some infants, this might occur at an earlier time. There were frequent examples of how he held in mind how others perceived his actions.

Although initially cautious to retrieve the out-of-sight lid, Kieran looked to his mother to contain his anxiety; she inspired him with confidence that it could be found, and Kieran went off in search of something temporarily lost from view. The fact that Susan wished to share in this game was particularly important and demonstrated how, for the good object to be recovered internally, both mother and son were required to once again engage in meaningful and symbolic activity, with recognition given to the loss that had been suffered and endured. All ill deeds are not necessarily cancelled, but a realistic appreciation of the object leads to a recovered optimism and the expression of shared symbolic meaning.

Conclusion

Despite significant advances in the methodological application of psychoanalytic observation (see, e.g., Bradley, Selby, & Urwin, 2012; Gretton, 2006; Wakelyn, 2012b), there are surprisingly few detailed research studies using this methodology in the field of early infancy. Psychoanalytic infant observation has not yet been primarily deployed as a research method—there is no systematic body of work derived from this source that describes what babies can do and when. To my knowledge, to date this is the first in-depth research analysis of a single case of psychoanalytic infant observation (conducted initially for educational purposes). Given that there is no baseline from which to draw, how does one know what is a theoretical advance? The field of study closest to this is child development research, yet findings from its laboratory-based methods are sometimes open to challenge from naturalistic observation. As such, there are no comparable studies from which to consider my developing hypothesis. As a result, this research investigation has relevance both to the generation of knowledge in relation to the emotional experience and sensitivities of infants and to the epistemological and methodological use of grounded theory in relation to psychoanalytic infant observation.

This research study has revealed the far-reaching aspects of aesthetic sensibility and the consequences when a breakdown in aesthetic reciprocity occurs. The findings suggest how aesthetic values govern the parent–infant relationship beyond that of early infancy and into the second year of life, thereby transcending the to-and-fro movement between the paranoid-schizoid position and the depressive position envisioned by Klein (1946) and Bion (1963). Close analysis of the observations revealed a convergence between aesthetic conflict and the trauma-driven response of regurgitation and rumination.

Meltzer considered how aesthetic conflict arose from the impact of the outside "'beautiful' mother, available to the senses, and the enigmatic inside which must be construed by creative imagination" (Meltzer & Harris Williams, 1973, p. 22). He theorized how the infant could feel overwhelmed by the experience, of the mother's breast, her touch, smell, or taste. This study makes a distinctive contribution to this discussion by considering how the shadow of the absent object disrupts and disturbs aesthetic impressions in the infant who had come to rely upon the beauty of the object. Freud originally discovered how the experience of trauma penetrated the psychic shield, disrupting the regulation between conscious and unconscious factors. For a young infant like Kieran, I propose that this protective membrane is made up of an aesthetic contribution from the mother as well as the infant's own aesthetic response. The refusal to take the teat, avoidance of eye contact, and the straining away from closeness all indicate a disturbance in aesthetic appreciation. Yet we see how the infant and nanny eventually find a way of adapting. It is with the return of the object that we see a cascade of aesthetic disturbance entering into the feeding relationship. The mouth becomes a hole from which the milk seeps out, vomiting begins, and the mouth as the original site of aesthetic appreciation becomes the scene of disturbance, as rumination continues beyond weaning. It is my contention that the aesthetic "skin" binding mother and infant is ruptured during trauma, and, from the observational evidence, this breach is not easily or quickly repaired.

Initially I observed the fierce protestations of a baby who was ready to complain about the absence of the object. As Brenman (2006) writes in "The Recovery of the Good Object Relationship": "When there is a breakdown in the good object relationship the superego holds sway" (p. 94). The nanny's feelings of inadequacy and persecution and the reproachful engagement with his mother on her return are testament to this. Given the nature of Kieran's sustained protestation, we cannot know whether there were feelings of guilt or responsibility for the return of the object.[16]

The sudden upheaval in the mother–infant relationship resulting from the accident led to a premature ending of *subject relates to object*. Furthermore, the absence of eye contact and the physical pulling away from the object and later regurgitation and rumination were suggestive of *subject destroys object*. This is usually conceived of as occurring in phantasy for the infant. Of interest is whether this phase was actually experienced by the infant as a real, rather than an imagined, experience. This question arises because of the eight-month struggle Kieran endured to recover the lost good object.

The way in which Kieran experienced rumination as something distasteful might suggest that he had an innate realistic expectation of what was meaningful for life and development. This capacity to distinguish between healthy and unhealthy aspects of self and others does not exclude the possibility that the underlying motive for ruminatory behaviour may have been fuelled by defensive preoccupation with damaged aspects of self and object.

There is a question as to whether a thorough qualitative method of data analysis such as an adapted version of grounded theory provides a satisfactory way to examine data derived from psychoanalytic infant observation. The issue is, what can be further gained from subjecting observational material to an abductive/inductive qualitative methodology? For example, are its findings any different from those emerging from psychoanalytic exploration in the seminar setting? Several decades before the modern development of qualitative research methodology and the discovery that researchers are included in, rather than outside, the body of their own research, Freud had formulated the workings of the countertransference.[17] This study has relied heavily upon the regulated manner by which the countertransference has informed theoretical enquiry and the elevation of categories from the main body of the data. Although qualitative researchers emphasize the role and importance of reflexivity in their data analysis, especially with regard to memo writing, the use of the countertransference as referred to here concerns the exploration of possible unconscious processes in the observer (subsequently the researcher) and their later theoretical formulation. This, in my opinion, is quite a different and distinct process from that of a reflexive enquiry. Not withstanding these important distinctions, there are, however, significant areas of overlap between the *ordinary* analysis that takes place in the infant observation seminar and that of qualitative analysis. The careful consideration of the recorded material, the attention to detail, the discovery of subtle meanings, and the constant questioning to discover how much of oneself is in the formulation are just a few examples.

Coding gave a structured, focused way of viewing the material. Yet I was to encounter how a code could simultaneously capture a particular aspect of the infant's experience while also revealing properties of such complexity that it was difficult to yield an analysis without oversimplification. Toleration of this uncertainty was overcome by several means; the first was related to a state of mind in the researcher where the premature quest for certainty could be held in check by observational training, clinical experience, and personal analysis, together with coding flexibility in qualitative research practice. The going forward and backward through the observational material helped to scrutinize the significance of specific codes and, importantly, captured maverick detail that halted this process. For example, the discovery of triangular thought processes occurring so early in infancy and being related to the vertical position of the baby was a revelation. This detail had not been considered in the observation seminar. Similarly, the detailed line-by-line analysis captured the frequency of the ruminatory response and elevated the importance of this defensive activity into theoretical consideration. Seminar discussion had principally focused on the infant's more general defensive preoccupation.

The qualitative research component of this study has primarily utilized the method of line-by-line coding as a means of identifying grounded categories arising from the observational data. However, it is important to refer back to the original analysis of the material undertaken at the time when the observation was conducted. As previously stated, over the course of the two years a small number of observational scripts were examined in the seminar context and led to a psychoanalytic narrative that remained relevant during the later qualitative analysis. Although the line-by-line coding tested and questioned assumptions that had been made at the earlier time—for example, the somewhat distorted time-line of the infant's recovery from trauma[18]—there were, nevertheless, aspects that confirmed the earlier formulations. I am thinking in particular about the sensitivity with which the mother approached her baby and the thoughtful containment that was so characteristic of parental involvement, which, despite the trauma, became the foundations on which the infant flourished.

Notes

1. See for example: Elliott, Gunaratnam, Hollway, and Urwin (2014), *Identities in Process: Becoming Bangladeshi, African Caribbean and White Mothers in Tower Hamlets*, which is part of the Identities and Social Action programme, Project no: RES 148-25-0058; and "Maternal Identities, Care and Intersubjectivity: A Psycho-Social Approach", RES 063-27-0118.

2. With regard to the persistence of pathological processes influencing later developmental stages, the work of Alvarez (1992, 2006), Alvarez and Reid (1999),

Bick (1968), Meltzer (1992), Tustin (1972), Williams (1997), and Winnicott (1956), among others, has contributed significantly to this discussion. By sensitizing the clinician to early infantile states, first encountered and discovered from the close observation of babies, they extended psychoanalytic understanding. This was particularly so in relation to the interpretation of defences, with Alvarez stating that deprived and abused children relied upon their defensive position in order to survive the psychological impact of abuse and neglect. Williams placed emphasis on different forms of container function and similarly focused upon technical issues in relation to the timing of interpretation.

3. Esther Bick described the second-skin formation as follows: "The need for a containing object would seem, in the infant unintegrated state, to produce a frantic search for an object—a light, a voice, a smell, or other sensual object—which can hold the attention and thereby be experienced, momentarily at least, as holding parts of the personality together. The optimal object is the nipple in the mouth, together with the holding talking smelling mother" (1968, p. 485).

4. "Scaffolding" as a term originates from child development literature and is used to describe the psychological support the parent provides for the infant, particularly in regard to stepped learning.

5. Looking back after so many years, it is noticeable how constrained I was as an observing student by the traditional non-interventionist stance of infant observation. I now wonder whether I might have taken a more helpful and participatory role, given the circumstances.

6. "Parentese" or "motherese" describes a way of talking with babies that most adults adopt. This is seen across cultures and is characterized by a higher tone and pitch in the voice when speaking directly to the infant. It is also referred to as "infant-directed speech" in child development literature.

7. For Bion and Klein, the *no breast* is thought to represent presence–absence—that is, gaining a *negative realization* of how absence of the breast provokes an emotional response, one that replaces absence with the presence of a "bad breast".

8. Løpez-Corvo (2003) writes of the infant's struggle with the "no breast' as conceived by Bion as follows: "If the capacity to tolerate *frustration* is adequate the internal 'no breast' will transform into a thought and an apparatus for thinking will be developed, which will make frustration more bearable" (p. 282).

9. I am unsure as to the frequency of whole-bottle regurgitation. It was mentioned several times to the observer over a long period of time, giving the impression that it was a regular pattern. It occurred both at night and during the day. I directly observed the regurgitation of only one whole bottle of milk; the rest of the time it was smaller, partly digested amounts.

10. Although this small detail was brought to attention by the line-by-line coding, it is important to consider whether I was "looking harder" to discover the links between things—that is, searching harder until you find what you may be (unconsciously) looking for.

11. The violent projection of milk I am equating with an "Attack on Linking".

12. Phase 1 has been discussed in Shallcross (2012).

13. Emde (1988a, 1988b) describes how mother and baby perceive each other's emotional state and describes this as "affective attunement".

14. Time frames consisted of the *first four weeks of life, the weeks following mother's hospitalization followed by her return.*

15. In the laboratory setting it has been found that infants begin to recognize their own reflection in a mirror at approximately 16–18 month of age. However, in the home this has been observed at 3–4 months of age. Its use here would suggest that the infant was transposing onto the mirror a representation of mother's return—perhaps a form of a transitional phenomenon. Freud (1920g) describes "baby gone" when a child crouches down so that his own reflection in the mirror is no longer visible.

16. Here I am referring to the return of the object that had been changed by the experience of near death and made somewhat unrecognizable to the infant as a result.

17. Laplanche and Pontalis (1973) define countertransference as "the whole of the analyst's unconscious reactions to the individual analysand—especially to the analysand's own transference" (p. 92). Freud formulated how the analyst was only able to go as far analytically as his or her own internal resistances and complexes would allow. Post-Freudian enquiry into the role and function of the countertransference, most notably by Wilfred Bion, has led to the countertransference being viewed as a communicative tool that exists in relationship to another. Work with babies, young children, and those suffering from personality disturbance, including psychosis, furthered the conceptualization and analytic employment. However, debate still surrounds its role in psychoanalysis: whether to reduce its manifestation by structuring the analytic situation to focus exclusively upon the patient's transference, or to make use of it in a more controlled fashion. There is also a third position, in which interpretation is based upon countertransference reactions. "This approach is based on the tenet that resonance 'from unconscious to unconscious' constitutes the only authentically psycho-analytic form of communication" (p. 93).

18. This refers to the infant observation paper written on completion of the observation. There was discussion of the attuned relationship, together with an account of the baby's loss and later defensive preoccupations (regurgitating whole bottles of milk, induced choking, provoked retching on solid food, and later rumination). Healthy developmental processes were over-emphasized, and the baby's internal world was superficially referred to. The paper was clearly observationally led yet did not explore in depth the observed material; rather, it was *reported upon*. In this context, the baby's recovery from trauma was perhaps overemphasized.

Appendix 1.1 Chart detailing research findings (abbreviated and shortened for publication)

Research methods	*Observational narrative Part 1 Observations 1–4*	*Observational narrative Part 2 Observations 14–16*	*Observational narrative Part 3 Observations 17–20*	*Observational narrative Part 4 Selected Observations: 21, 22, 30, 38, 46.*
Narrative analysis	coherent synchronized emotional patterns	processes that interfere with satisfaction at the breast; filling mother's absence; rumination; aesthetic conflict	gaze aversion; rigidity; leakiness between lips and teat; choking	choking; rumination; taking self as object; recovered intimacy
Line-by-line coding	visual tracing as an organizing, gathering-together principle; reverie, gaze mentally drawing the infant closer to mother; regulating gazing; mother engaged in extended periods of reverie; baby has a preference for the face; internally preoccupied; voice as an organizing principle	exploring available space; expanding and stretching, using own resources; discharge and expulsion of unwanted affect; determination an important factor in remaining positive about the infant's capacity to manage mother's absence; regurgitation	anticipation of his mother's departure; being left alone with something unmanageable	distress can be managed; active curiosity in others' minds; infant working out whether something remains in place even when it cannot be seen

Selected codes	expulsion; internal life; family; orientation; borderline between unconscious and conscious factors; agitation and expulsion; expansive/self resourcefulness; loss of integration; synchronous patterns	expansive and flexibility; agitation and expulsion; transformation/familiar sound as a reorganizing principle; protective functions; loss of integration; predicting object constancy	search for the transformation of the experience; restored hopefulness; shared symbolic meaning painful pleasure	shared symbolic meaning; predicting object constancy; recovery of the good object; combined intimate relationship of infant and mother extending to other object relationships
In-vivo coding	attributing a mind to the infant; naming mummy and daddy as a source of interest, triangularity;	naming infant's needs; physical determination to meet infant's requirements	nanny reflecting on own observations; recognition given to the infant's confusion between pleasure and pain; the infant with a mind of his own; "little guzzler"—a reference to the infant's difficulty in regulating the flow and quantity of milk consumed; mother reflecting on own state of mind	naming infant's distress and recovery from loss; recognition of infant's preferences/adjusting accordingly; family orientation

(*Continued*)

Appendix 1.1 (Cont.)

Research methods	*Observational narrative Part 1 Observations 1–4*	*Observational narrative Part 2 Observations 14–16*	*Observational narrative Part 3 Observations 17–20*	*Observational narrative Part 4 Selected Observations: 21, 22, 30, 38, 46.*
Clustering around themes	immersion orientation expulsion expansive and flexibility forging family links transformation–reorganization	–orientation + –transformation + –expansive + rumination = aesthetic conflict		–orientation + –transformation + –expansive + rumination = aesthetic conflict orientation + transformation + expansive = cogitation

CHAPTER TWO

Finding a place of one's own: a grounded theory approach to reviewing the developmental impact of child psychotherapy with a looked-after 2-year-old child

Louise Allnutt

This chapter focuses on a single-case research study in which grounded theory methodology was applied for a retrospective analysis of the clinical material from an intensive psychotherapy treatment. The child was 2 years old when he started psychotherapy, which, being quite unusual, prompted further exploration. However, it is also a case that will strike many child psychotherapists as fairly common—he was a looked-after child who had very clear indications of developmental delay. As child psychotherapy has had a long history in the field of looked-after children, it seemed important to further the understanding of the treatment of this particular population with a focus on early development. Many themes emerged during the clinical experience that one might expect from such a case, including problems with communication, anxiety, hyperactivity, disorientation, and difficulties with transitions; however, with the application of grounded theory methods, greater depth and understanding of these themes evolved, which I hope to summarize here.

In addition to this greater depth of understanding of the themes, this method also served to offer additional understanding of the developmental impact of our work with a much younger child. The early problems of looked-after children can often be overlooked and assumed to be of less importance emotionally and developmentally.

It is demanding work, where the impact of being in close proximity with disturbed and distressed states of mind needs to be experienced and digested alongside a more overarching attention given to the child's past and ongoing experiences of the external environment. Jenifer Wakelyn highlights this in "Transitional Psychotherapy for Looked-After Children in Short-Term Foster Care" (2008). Written primarily for social workers, Wakelyn's account demonstrates the important impact of a child psychotherapist's work on both an individual child and her family and, additionally, the wider professional network.

In this chapter, I illustrate this phenomenon with reference to the clinical material and its retrospective analysis. I give a brief outline of the case followed by a summary of the methodologies applied in the analysis, prior to a discussion of the material.

Referral history

Joseph was a 2-year-old boy in a short-term placement in foster care when he began intensive psychotherapy. He had come to the attention of many of the professionals whom he had met along the way as he was showing signs of significant developmental delay—including speech and communication difficulties, problems with emotional regulation, and severe behavioural problems. The referral for psychotherapy coincided with his removal from his parents' care by order of the family court. He had been neglected and emotionally abused. Prior to individual psychotherapy, both he and his foster carer were seen for parent–child therapy to support their developing relationship.

This joint work was successful, as Joseph became increasingly communicative and interested in those around him. His foster carer reported that he had become more playful and responsive in his relationship with her. From the point of view of development, Joseph was showing that the earlier attachment difficulties that had been identified were shifting towards a greater availability for positive relationships, which was in turn supporting more ordinary social behaviour and communication. However, there were some areas of Joseph's emotional life that were still concerning and apparently unpredictable. Ordinary boundaries would provoke the most overwhelming fury and violence in him. Perhaps even more distressing was his loss of orientation at times of ordinary transition, when he would suddenly appear completely lost as if navigating through a dark tunnel while blind. At these moments, Joseph would seem to lose his own bodily sense of himself and drop to the ground without warning.

While his foster carer was a very committed and supportive figure for Joseph, she understandably struggled to fully embrace some of the ways Joseph expressed his sense of loss and confusion, and some of his emotional distress and behaviour was proving too much to manage. It was at this point that we decided to offer an individual approach in order to address his emotional development in relation to his internal world. Joseph was seen three times per week by me, and his foster carer was seen by a colleague once per week. His foster carer in particular was relieved to be able to think about Joseph with someone who appreciated the impact of his confusing and unpredictable emotional distress. Joseph, on the other hand, struggled to manage the fundamental structure of psychotherapy, including the transition to the consulting room, the boundaries of the setting, including time and space, and the connection and separations from his therapist. These fundamental coordinates became the main focus of the work. There was something deeply physical and unmentalized about the work that reflected that there were aspects of his early development that had not evolved in a way that could help him at times of anxiety to retain inner security. I noted this as a need to find a "greater sense of his own place in relation to others and himself." This was the starting point of the analysis, the focus of which can be identified through a statement of three basic premises:

1. In a good-enough environment a child develops a sense of spatial orientation. This development is both an internal and an external process.
2. With inadequate early relationships and a lack of a stable environment, the development of the capacity to perceive and secure a sense of one's own place within space is sometimes impaired or lost. This has a subsequent impact on social and emotional development.
3. A psychotherapeutic relationship is capable of good outcomes in helping a child orientate him/herself in space and time and subsequently establish a place of his or her own, which underpins a secure sense of self. Child psychotherapists can therefore potentially support the external transitions between birth parents and care environments as well as support a child with his or her development.

Methodology

Given that a psychotherapist's work is so often focused on the slow and intimate development of a relationship, it is difficult to imagine what kind of research method could effectively clarify or accurately follow its finer contours. However, qualitative research methods have been developed in the human sciences as an attempt to reflect the emotional experiences and complexities that are part and parcel of human relationships and thus offer a form of research relevant to psychoanalytic practice. This is subjective research, recognized over many years as the only methodological process that can accurately account for the individual and unique formations of human interaction and social behaviour. Anthropological observation, which tries to account for the cultural formations of human behaviour, communication, and relationships through ethnography, participant observation, and broader fieldwork, is one neighbouring form of inquiry. While psychotherapeutic work is not the same as work in the anthropological field, it is nevertheless the setting for a unique and individual human relationship. The agency of change and development in psychotherapy, whatever one's school of thought, is the therapeutic relationship; therefore, if one would like to trace its impact, I believe it is imperative that there are some areas of research that focus on the intimate and micro-analysis of this. I think it is fair to say that most child psychotherapy trainees and qualified clinicians are applying an unusually high level of rigorous investigation to the process of making relationships with their patients. Detailed notes are commonly made following patient contact, reflective practice is an integrated and expected experience, and wider professional discussion is an important additional forum for re-examination of clinical data. The important backdrop to this is, of course, one's own personal analysis.

The research discussed in this chapter can thus be said to be rooted in two levels of enquiry. The first level consisted of those processes that are part of the child psychotherapist's everyday clinical practice and includes the work that took place in the consulting room, the recollection of the experience afterwards, the reflective processes that occurred in between the sessions, and the supervision process that took place alongside the treatment. This level was primarily required by the treatment but also had a research dimension. As Michael Rustin argues, research has always been inherent within the psychoanalytic clinical process (M. J. Rustin, 1997). The second level of enquiry was a research-motivated task, in that the primary aim of this secondary analysis was to seek out and explore differing and new ways of thinking about the clinical work, without an immediate therapeutic aim. This does not exclude, however, the high likelihood that such an analysis of one case has clinical implications for other cases in the future. This level of analysis is retrospective and, in this, instance took place after the treatment had ended. The analysis relied almost exclusively on the written recollections of the sessions that were produced during the first level of enquiry. This retrospective analysis not only brought about new ways of understanding the clinical material, but also opened up new lines of enquiry. While I began with one set of ideas that emerged from the first level of enquiry, further ideas and questions emerged from the second level in the analysis. The use of grounded theory as a research method, therefore, is a tool that was utilized to deepen this exploration. The process of such exploratory research is not radically different from the processes used in the day-to-day clinical encounter with our patients, save for the benefit of time for greater reflection and consideration of one case. The main task in this type of research can be described as a systematic exploration and reflection on the clinical experience and what it can contribute to our understanding of a particular case in relation to cases with similar attributes. It is, to all intents and purposes, a contribution to an accumulative case-study research base (Midgley, 2006).

While the field of looked-after children and child psychotherapy inevitably needs to take account of a broad landscape, the main focus here is on the experiences that emerge in therapy through a therapist's relationship with the child's internal world. In line with a Kleinian and post-Kleinian model of psychoanalysis, this work was approached by me with a close eye on the link between internal processes and external experience. The emphasis, therefore, in the title on finding a "place" is a signpost to the idea that having a sense of place within oneself is borne out of early experience of the place one has inside the mind of another, and that the growth of the infant's mind is acutely subject to the relationship he has with his caregivers' emotional world. Or, as Klein puts it, "and thus from the beginning object-relations are moulded by an interaction between introjection and projection, between internal and external objects and situations" (1946, p. 2).

It goes without saying within this theoretical model that any kind of disturbance in the early relationship between infant and caregiver is likely to impact upon the growth of the infant's mind and to affect how able a child is to use his mind to experience, perceive, and respond to external relationships. Klein describes this memorably in relation to her schizophrenic adult patient who still experienced the bodily symptoms of the sudden weaning and loss of his mother he experienced as an infant. "Much light was thrown in the analysis on the influence these experiences had on his whole development. His outlook and attitudes in adult life were based on the patterns established in this early stage" (Klein, 1946, pp. 15–16).

Previous research in the field

Since the early years of child analysis and child psychotherapy, our understanding of the profound impact of early disturbance in the primary infant–caregiver relationship has grown substantially. Work with traumatized, deprived, and neglected populations of children is commonplace for psychotherapists. There is a wealth of literature and research that demonstrates the development and growth of such work in our profession over the years, including Boston and Szur's *Psychotherapy with Severely Deprived Children* (1983) and several publications with regard to the Tavistock's study of children in the care system (Boston & Lush, 1994; Lush, Boston, Morgan, & Kolvin, 1998; Midgley, 2009).

As is noted in the recent critical review by Nick Midgley and Eilis Kennedy (2011) of the profession's evidence base, the outcome of one of the earliest Tavistock studies of children in the care system showed that "The majority of children in the study had improved by the end of treatment" (p. 241). In recent years the UK government has called for children in care to be prioritized within CAMHS, as highlighted in the *Care Matters* paper (Department of Education and Skills, 2006). Underlying these developments is the awareness and understanding that deprivation, abuse, and neglect are factors that contribute to ongoing educational underachievement as well as mental instability and disturbance, which have a pervading influence on a child's and adult's capacity to negotiate relationships and maintain emotional equilibrium throughout life. For example, "consistent evidence suggests that both physical abuse and sexual abuse are associated with a doubling of the risk of attempted suicide for young people who are followed up into their late 20's" (Gilbert et al., 2009, p. 75). We also know from research that children who are looked after suffer elevated rates of mental health problems (Ford, Vastanis, Meltzer, & Goodman, 2007). In this study comparisons were made between children who were looked after by the local authority and those who were raised in private households. In those children who were looked after by the local authority, there is a higher incidence of psychiatric disorder across all areas—even in comparison with those children who were socially and economically deprived yet living in private households. The figures are cited as follows: behavioural disorders (39% vs. 4%), ADHD (9% vs. 1%), anxiety disorders (11% vs. 4%, especially PTSD: 2% vs. 0.1%), as well as elevated rates of neurodevelopmental problems (13% vs. 3%) and autism (3% vs. 0.3%). There is a very similar picture with regard to educational problems, with increases in significant intellectual delay (11% vs. 1%), literacy/numeracy problems (34% vs. 10%), and statements of educational needs (23% vs. 3%) (Ford et al., 2007, p. 322).

The raised incidence of such problems is not simply derived from living in conditions of social disadvantage, because these problems are also between 2 and 10 times higher than in children raised within birth families facing significant social adversity. There are unique risks in being a looked-after child, over and above the well-known risks of social disadvantage. There is a long history of psychotherapy involvement in those populations of children who are identified as "severely deprived" (Boston & Szur, 1983). This work, and others such as those that have developed out of the work within the fostering and adoption workshop at the Tavistock Clinic, have made a contribution to a growing body of literature that has focused on theoretical and clinical frameworks for psychoanalytic approaches to looked-after children with complex histories (Bartram, 2003; Canham, 1999, 2003; Edwards, 2000; Hunter, 2002; M. E. Rustin, 2001).

These ideas have informed developments in wider CAMHS practices to meet the needs of looked-after children with a history of neglect and trauma. More recent work has focused specifically on children in transition (Kenrick, 2010; Wakelyn, 2008) and psychotherapy with children who have had multiple placements and who experience late adoption (Fagan, 2011). The greater understanding brought about by recent discoveries in neuroscience have offered another avenue for insight and the development of appropriate therapeutic interventions (Fagan, 2011; Music, 2011). This area of work has become extremely valuable in terms of the weight it gives to relationship-based interventions with looked-after children with histories of neglect and trauma. There is little doubt that neuroscientific claims about the post-natal development of the brain—in particular, the area of emotional regulation—is of particular importance for a greater understanding of the impact of neglect and trauma on the developing brain (Gerhardt, 2004; Glaser, 2000; Pally, 2000). It may offer a more secure grounding for the potential of ongoing, consistent, and relationship-based psychotherapeutic work to intervene at the level of neurodevelopment as well as at the level of emotional development.

Working with a child under 5 years is a required but often difficult-to-access part of a child psychotherapist's training. And yet, despite all of the research and literature to support earliest intervention, it is still quite unusual for a child to receive intensive psychotherapy before the child goes to school. One reason might be to do with the investment of time and money that intensive work demands. But it may also reflect the disbelief that the mind can already be subject to the kinds of insecurities and emotional pressure that is often observed during psychotherapy at this early point of a child's life. What is evident, however, from psychotherapeutic work with very young damaged children, is that once a young child is given the opportunity to recover and grow, things can often change for the better very quickly. The ramifications of early environmental failure have too great an impact on the ongoing relationships a child has with himself and others for us to turn a "blind eye" and await recovery through time itself. It is important to note that there are many models within child psychotherapy for working with very young children, some of which are impressively successful and support the development and protection of child–parent relationships, including the Parent Infant Project (PIP) at the Anna Freud Centre (Baradon, 2005). Other examples include work with families that utilize the Solihull Approach (Douglas & Brennan, 2004) and the Tavistock Under-Fives Service (Bradley & Emanuel, 2008).

Early intervention has become a buzz word in recent times in our field, and while there have been several very important developments such as "Sure Start", and other Early Years Intervention Services, the depth of the need at an individual and internal level can be overwhelming. There are many known examples of case histories by psychotherapists of individual treatments of children who have experienced early trauma, neglect, and abuse that show the often shocking and disturbing emotional impact of working with such children (Canham, 2003; Hoxter, 1983; M. E. Rustin, 2001). The descriptions of the countertransference responses aroused by children in these accounts may go some way to explain the struggle professionals in this field have to take on board the depth of the emotional problem that young children living with such predicaments present us with. A closer look at the clinical material of one single case, while it cannot provide generalizable and causal explanation, can draw our attention to the emotional impact of the child's internal world.

The grounded theory approach used in this research gave an opportunity to develop greater understanding about some of the themes and phenomena that lie at the heart of many child psychotherapy cases of very young looked-after children.

The case: emerging themes

The child in this case was removed from his birth parents at 18 months and was in foster care during most of the three-year treatment. In the latter stage of the treatment, and, I believe, in part due to the treatment, the foster carer who had initially taken him on a short-term basis became Joseph's special guardian and therefore permanent parent and home. Joseph had a diagnosis of an attachment disorder; he also had a diagnosis of global developmental delay and, at 3 years of age, reached the threshold for a statement of special educational needs. He was additionally thought to be at risk of developing ADHD. The network surrounding the case was vast, and there were, of course, many different points of view. There were high levels of concern for Joseph's emotional health, but additionally most professionals feared he would not be adopted or manageable in a temporary placement with the behavioural difficulties he was presenting at this early point in his life.

I identified two levels of inquiry in relation to my research material. The initial themes shaping the research frame were those that emerged in the clinical encounter and seemed to play an ongoing significant role in the therapy throughout the treatment. They were, in that sense, cumulative in that they emerged at several points in the material of the sessions over time and, as a result, became more apparent to the therapist as the therapy developed. Similar to Meltzer's (1967) description of the psychoanalytic process, I believe that the majority of these themes were there right at the beginning but perhaps only became more readily available to the mind once they had emerged again and again. Through the course of the psychoanalytic work these themes were elaborated, explored in their different guises, seen through different lenses, and related to differently and from different points of view. But as one might anticipate through the process of grounded theory analysis, with some consideration it became possible to condense these themes down to three key "higher level" concepts. These were "transitions", "boundaries", and "thresholds".

These three themes seemed to encapsulate several different important processes that appeared in the clinical encounter to be extremely significant from both a developmental and a therapeutic point of view, and they seemed, additionally, intrinsic to the context of therapeutic work with a looked-after child. The themes could therefore be understood and observed on many levels and also clearly related to Joseph's early experiences.

Transitions

In Session 4, for example, Joseph was brought to the room by his foster carer. She placed him down on the floor and reassured him she would see him at the end of the session. Joseph became distressed. As his foster carer left the room, he placed his head in his hands and cried. He then turned to the door and banged his head up against it. I went to the door and held Joseph's head in my hands. He calmed down and sat with his head in my hands and rocked back and forth. As his relationship with me and his foster carer developed, holding during transition seemed to be an important factor in Joseph's capacity to remain emotionally in one piece. While this rhythmical physical contact seemed to bring some relief and comfort to Joseph as his treatment progressed, he nevertheless remained destabilized by the process of moving from one place to another. In Session 24, for example, Joseph was accompanied along the corridor by his foster carer. As he proceeded along the corridor towards the door of the consulting room, he suddenly attempted to run as if in a state of panic, fell to the floor, looked up with terror and fear, and screamed.

From a theoretical point of view, I was struck by the relevance of Henri Rey's concept of the "space–time continuum", which, while focused on clinical work with adults, also describes the developmental and internal processes that seemed to underpin Joseph's disturbance. For Rey (1994), space and time are two dimensions of both external and internal reality, central to the development of a cohesive and orientated self in relation to others externally and to internal objects intrapsychically. This is a psychoanalytic developmental theory, which includes the idea that successful movement away and separation from the marsupial-like, maternal space in early infancy is a precursor to the capacity to tolerate the differentiation between, and the orientation within, self-space and non–self-space. The experience of seeking out in self-space the good and gratifying object is central to an individual's sense of security and the development of the self. Not being able to seek out the good object relationally in space and time increases the desire for such objects and can lead to anger and anxiety and to what

Rey describes as the "desire to deprive [the desired object] of the other space containing the desired objects" (1986, p. 22).

Following the terror that Joseph displayed in the corridor at the beginning of Session 24, on going into the room he calmed down and became quite still and watchful. He then started to kick the lid off the toy box, his gaze remaining fixed on me as he did so. Joseph tried several times to remove the lid with his foot, but eventually he decided to lean forward and remove it with his hands, doing this with a sigh of irritation. He then removed its contents in an angry and haphazard fashion. He moved to the couch and threw the blanket and pillow to the floor. Following this, Joseph squeezed himself in between the table and his therapist's chair and proceeded to separate some sheets of paper into separate piles. Following a short description—"that one there ... and that one there ..."—I introduced a greeting: "Hello, Joseph." "Hello, Ms A." Joseph repeated the greeting "Hello, Joseph" twice before collapsing onto the floor and stating, "Hello, Mum". Joseph then stood and squeezed himself into a small space in between the table and my chair. I remarked, "It's a tight squeeze". Joseph echoed this and then walked into the centre of the room and, holding his head between his hands, repeated "squeeze" again.

Through supervision and reflective analysis, I began to get a sense that there was a link between Joseph's fear that he was unable to locate the desired object in the transition from waiting room to consulting room, coupled with the separation from foster carer, and the way in which Joseph then turned his focus to the different spaces and objects in the room. Joseph systematically removed the objects that were linked to other objects from their spaces: the lid from the box, the toys from the inside of the box, and the blankets and pillows from the couch. This he did with anger and irritation. Following this, he squeezed himself in between the table and his therapist, removing space for any other potential object, and for a brief period he was able to think about dividing and separating the paper into two different spaces. When I used this rhythm to identify Joseph and me as two objects in space, like the two piles of paper, Joseph collapsed and seemed to be thrown back into the disintegrating impact of separation from "Mum". Again, recovery was sought through the squeeze into space, removing the gap between himself and me externally, but Joseph also went on to show the importance of the squeezing sensation to collect himself together internally when he placed each of his hands on either side of his head and stated, "squeeze".

One is reminded at this point of Temple Grandin's "cattle squeeze" and her understanding about the calming influence of deep touch pressure in children and adolescents with autism (1992). Theoretically, Winnicott's deep understanding of primitive anxieties is also hugely relevant here, particularly his conception of anxiety in relation to the earliest experience of infant care technique (1952). He describes such failures in what he calls the "environment–individual setup" as producing anxiety felt by the infant as states of

> Unintegration, becoming a feeling of disintegration; lack of relationship of psyche to soma, becoming a sense of depersonalization; also the feeling that the centre of gravity of consciousness transfers from the kernel to the shell, from the individual to the care, the technique. (Winnicott, 1952, p. 99)

I think this description of the movement of the centre of gravity from centre to the "shell" is particularly relevant in this case.

Needless to say, such ideas form and inform the backdrop of a therapist's thinking when working with children who clearly struggle with the levels and quality of anxiety that Joseph felt during his early years and his therapy. The anxiety Joseph was experiencing was both leading him to disintegrate at points of particular kinds of contact with the world and blocking him from developing the kind of inner security that would allow him to be in touch with the world in a believable and solid way. Losing a sense of orientation and losing a sense of self at points of transition and in relation to boundaries and thresholds seemed to be of paramount importance.

The combination of clinical examples such as those described above, the emergent themes, guidance from supervision, and theoretical concepts such as Rey's and Winnicott's, all helped to formulate a direction for the secondary level of enquiry and to begin to shape some research questions.

The sample sessions were theoretically and thematically selected, but the task of looking at each of the sessions in minute detail through the secondary analysis was primarily aimed at viewing the data with fresh eyes. This process sought to revise, review, and reconsider the initial thematic and theoretical formulations. In my experience, while this process is in some ways similar to the approach taken by psychoanalytic practitioners in relation to the material presented by their patients live in the session, undertaking the analysis post-treatment affords a unique opportunity to slow the process of analysis down and suspend judgement for longer than one would be able to do in the clinical situation. In general, the findings that have emerged from this process have confirmed the importance of the themes that were identified in the first level of enquiry as well as having helped to formulate a system for making sense of the data in relation to these initial themes. For the purposes of this chapter, I shall concentrate on two areas of development following from the secondary phase of analysis.

Expanding and deepening themes

The initial themes of *transitions, boundaries,* and *thresholds* that began as the focus of interest for the research were confirmed as a central organizing factor in the material through the second level of analysis. This analysis provided an opportunity to deepen my understanding of these themes, but it also highlighted the presence of two further themes that were as significant and as central as the themes already noted. Additionally, I became interested in the process of the therapy itself, and the analysis pointed towards an interesting way of clarifying and understanding this particular child's experience of therapy. I began to note the relationships between the observable phenomena, such as the identified themes, and the different processes and emotional responses that develop and unfold within the therapeutic relationship. I begin here by addressing the new themes that emerged from the detailed analysis of the sample of material.

One of the key aspects of the process of analysis was the re-engagement with the clinical encounter through work on the process notes recorded at the time. While primarily this involved a detailed consideration of the descriptions that I had recorded in writing, the very process of reading this material involved an emotional engagement that linked the research frame with the clinical frame. In my analysis of the sample, I was particularly struck that I had not identified *loss* as one of the central themes during the first level of enquiry. In my retrospective analysis, it seemed to sit at the heart of Joseph's state of mind. Loss therefore newly emerged as an important theme; it surprised me that this powerful emotional experience had not struck me so poignantly during the clinical observation itself. One could speculate about what might be the reasons, such as how much a clinician becomes focused on the management task of the therapy with a child like Joseph, as well as the impact of the overwhelming countertransferences. Following further analysis and comparison across the sample, I came to house the theme of loss within the wider description *"separation"* and added this to the three themes that had initially been identified.

Another theme that emerged at the point of re-engagement and analysis of the material were the phenomena that I felt I could begin to cluster within the concept of oedipal phenomena. Clearly there were overlaps between the other themes and this new emergent theme, but it also stood as a good measure for understanding a significant point of change within the material. For example, in early sessions, material that was representative of oedipal phenomena tended to be less associated with people and their coming and goings, and more about the movement in space and time of objects as well as highly emotive sensory experiences. For example, Joseph's banging and falling into and away from the boundary could be understood as a proto-oedipal sensory experience—a bodily reaction to the limitations experienced in the physical world. In a later phase of development, this limitation is experienced in relationships and expressed emotionally. Another example was Joseph's confusion over the size and order of the stacking cups, as discussed later. It was interesting to notice that at around the 50-session mark, these phenomena began to take the form of characters with characteristics. My hypothesis is that the introduction of these human aspects is one of the first signs of more stable internal object-relations and seems to suggest that Joseph was making a hugely important developmental transition. Alongside the increasingly object-related material was an increase in persecutory anxiety and identification processes.

There was an interesting occasion in supervision—interestingly, around the turning point that I am talking about—when my supervisor highlighted the theoretical difference between children one would better understand using theories developed by Frances Tustin and those who could be understood by reference to the ideas of Melanie Klein. The crux of such a contrast is the nature of development and the impact of early trauma on the capacity for object-relations. For example, for Tustin, premature catastrophic separation rendered certain children unable to identify with a primary object and therefore unable to make use of internal space for object-relatedness, seeking instead to relate to the surface of the object as if it were part of the self. By contrast, for Klein, the emotional capacity to withstand the rapid and intense oscillations between persecutory experiences of an object and a more loving experience is the primary factor in stabilizing inner-object relations in early childhood. It is probably fair to say that these early experiences are largely felt by the infant as physical experiences, and therefore the emotional capacity to sustain the fluctuations between good and bad encounters with the object relies hugely on the external experience of the physical world, including that offered by the parents. We thought that the child I was working with was a good example of how emotionally and developmentally one might move between the two theories, depending on the level of anxiety being experienced.

As I briefly mentioned earlier, the more I became familiar with the data it was evident that I could additionally cluster the codes and themes that were emerging from the material into different categories related to the clinical process. For example, where I had identified aspects of the material to be thematically described as related to *separation,* I noticed that at different times this material could also be described as related to *therapeutic processes.* Phenomena that had been identified in the material to be thematically related to *transitions,* such as falling, confusion, disorientation, and loss, could also at times be described as *primitive anxieties.* In this example, the first set of thematic codes—falling, confusion, disorientation, and loss—are described by Corbin and Strauss (2008) as "low level concepts" and are those concepts that are explicitly linked to the material; the latter, more general concepts of "transitions" and "primitive anxieties" are "higher level concepts" and lose their specificity in relation to the material. In total, five categories related to the clinical process emerged alongside the themes related to the clinical narrative: *therapeutic process, external process, developmental process, primitive anxieties, and defences.*

I now turn to an example from the second-level analysis and discussion to demonstrate the research exploration I have highlighted thus far. I shall take examples from the clinical material that emerged thematically in relation to *oedipal phenomena* and illustrate how these aspects interrelated clinically with *developmental processes.*

Oedipal phenomena and the developmental process

The first reference in the retrospective analysis to oedipal phenomena came in Session 1, when Joseph was exploring the objects in the box for the first time. At this point in the session, Joseph removed the stacking cups from the box. I responded with interest and described the process of waiting, choosing, and looking as Joseph looked inside the box, chose the cups, and then placed them onto the floor to look at them. It is noted in the first-level coding that this verbal communication offers something rhythmical to Joseph alongside my description of his actions. The rhythm contrasts with Joseph's jerky and hasty movements but then appeared to bring him into greater attunement with the task of exploration as he began to explore the cups sequentially. At the start of the session Joseph identified a numerical sequence and counted out 1, 2, 3. Despite the rhythmical quality of this, it nevertheless appeared to arouse Joseph's anxiety, as identified by his defensive jumping and jerky movements. Immediately following this, Joseph struggled to place the cups in size sequence and tried to fit two larger cups inside the smaller ones. He appeared to me to be confused. He was disorientated and appeared lost while he tried to physically insist that the threshold between the cups sizes can be denied.

After a while Joseph counted to 3 again, and I identified the 1, 2, 3 sequence again in relation to his three sessions. At this point Joseph made eye contact for the first time in the session and verbally agreed, "yeah", before putting his hand back into the box to search for further objects. This time he removed a bunch of pens held together with an elastic band. He handed the band to me. In the analysis it is noted that this is the object that holds the separated parts together. It appears to link with Joseph's eye contact and apparent orientation at the point when I make a link between the sequence and the rhythm of the sessions. Joseph proceeded to separate out the pens into smaller groups; two of the pens go onto the big table and three onto the smaller table. When one of the three pens on the smaller table rolled to the floor, Joseph was immediately alarmed and shouted, "Fall off". He then returned to the two that were left and threw them both in the same direction. There was a powerful sense that the loss of one meant the loss of them all. It may also have been Joseph's attempt at some kind of mastery over the situation, such as the sequence Freud described in relation to the cotton-reel game (1920g). In relation to there having been three, it would seem this might relate to a loss of the dimensionality of space, but it also appears to demonstrate that the third is separated from the couple.

Interestingly Joseph identified himself with the object that throws away, and he appeared to experience the fall as an attack rather than an accident against which he had to defend, through identification with the aggressor. Again when I verbally acknowledged what had happened, "They are all now falling off", Joseph made eye contact as he pointed to the pens on the floor, stating, "Fall over". This seemed to be a reference to a breakdown in continuity and appeared to powerfully identify Joseph's current predicament as a child who had lost his place.

There are several examples in the early sessions where collapsing and falling lie at the heart of Joseph's experience of oedipal anxieties, such as the stacking cups losing their sequence or, in the case of an example in Session 4, when Joseph lost all sense of dimensionality as he separated from his foster carer. In this example,

> Joseph repeatedly banged his head against a variety of hard surfaces in the room, primarily the door. He appeared terrified of what he feared lay inside the room and, in particular, of the proximity to me. In response to the rhythmical attunement of my vocalizations—for example, when I joined him counting to three, or when I sympathetically acknowledged his distress—he calmed down briefly before going to sit on the couch. From here, he looked over to me at the same time as sucking on his finger inside his mouth. Joseph appeared to be seeking internal security from the sucking, in the face of what he perceived as external dangers. He began to kick the toy box in a purposeful way.

In the retrospective analysis it is noted that the safety that I attempted to offer Joseph was experienced as an attack, which appeared to intensify his experience of claustrophobic anxiety. When Joseph collapsed again, I decided to take him back to the waiting room to reconnect him with his foster carer and then invited her to the therapy room.

> Joseph cried all the way down the corridor. As we arrived in the waiting room, he ran towards his foster carer (Carol), who received him with open arms. I asked Carol to join us. During this time Joseph had wandered off in the waiting room and had found a toy. Carol went and picked him up, and he said "Crying." Carol agreed, "Yes, you have been crying." As we walked up the corridor, Joseph said "Head", and he rubbed his head. In the room, Carol sat down with Joseph on the couch. I remarked on his need for Carol and that she and Ms A didn't want Joseph to feel too upset. Carol said she had been waiting for Joseph. I acknowledged that Joseph found it hard to believe that when Carol wasn't here with him, she was still waiting for him.

When Joseph was reconnected with Carol, he immediately recovered. All three of us returned to the room together, and the space appeared to open up for Joseph again. The dialogue offered to Joseph from by his foster carer and the therapist seemed to develop a triangular holding space, which regulated the emotional tension as well as offering holding and containment. During this time, however, Joseph explored the toy box and removed the scissors.

> Joseph then put the scissors in his mouth. Carol asked him to take the scissors out of his mouth, which he did. He then snapped them open and shut at the same time as saying, "Scissors", with his teeth exaggerating the "s" as he stated the word.

As noted in the first level of coding, Joseph is associating his mouth with the scissors, referring perhaps to an idea that it is the power of his own aggression (biting) that cuts and separates and therefore destroys. In terms of this material in the context of the oedipal theme, Joseph appeared to be demonstrating that at this developmental point, the experience of separation and therefore absence left him with a sense that the loss had been as a result of his own oral aggression, which might go some way to making sense of his anxiety when left with his therapist in the dyad. It also raised some important questions about how he had made sense of his early separation from his parents. It appears from this example that Joseph struggled to maintain a sense of place and lost a sense of spatial perspective in relation to the dyad when he and I were together, and his anxiety was raised by his concerns about his own aggression.

In Session 20, Joseph was still exploring this aspect of togetherness and separateness. In this session Joseph appeared to make a more explicit discovery of the potential separateness of the dyad as opposed to the object being broken in two. This material precipitated anxiety about falling and not having a place—previously discussed in terms of the material involving the crayon that did not fit with the others inside a cup. Joseph's anxiety about falling out and losing a place appeared then to draw Joseph to hold defensively on to seeking a sense of space through looking out of the window.

In Session 49, Joseph entered the room and, on noticing a ruler on the windowsill that did not belong to him or his box, immediately removed it and turned to me to show the offending item, while expressing a satisfied, "Ah-ha", as if the evidence somehow confirmed his phantasy that the intruders have indeed taken up residence in the space he claimed to be his. A degree of separation needed to have taken place in order for Joseph to allow for the phantasy of the intruders, symbolically represented by the ruler. One might interpret that this was a challenge to Joseph's "rule".

In Joseph's less structured and less ordered state of mind, there was still evidence of oedipal phenomena at the level of part objects.

The clearer identification of more whole-object oedipal phenomena marked a transition for Joseph into a more specifically object-related and symbolic expression of his sense of himself and his inner world.

Discussion and summary

It was only in the retrospective analysis that the oedipal phenomena in this material came into greater focus. Oedipal material at this developmental level is primarily experienced in terms of issues related to perception and dimensionality (Meltzer, 1975b) and part objects (Klein, 1946) as opposed to whole objects and parental roles.

Rhode (2011) has also referred to the "autistic" level of the Oedipus complex, which is experienced at the level of shapes.

With greater security in relation to his therapist, and a greater capacity to tolerate their separateness, came the inevitable concern about what happened and who was with whom when separated. Klein (1946) identified early oedipal anxieties within the first year. Rooted developmentally in the paranoid-schizoid position and when the infant is unable to perceive the whole object and its contrasting aspects, these early anxieties arouse ambivalence and confusion. Later, when the child is able to understand the varying natures of his objects without the fear of emotional collapse, the struggle to appreciate the variations in the relationships between objects and the different places to which they belong ensues and the oedipal situation emerges in the interplay between its different participants and whole objects.

Joseph's early development within his therapy can thus be seen to elaborate the difference between oedipal phenomena that are rooted in early part-object relations and therefore in relation to more primitive anxieties, such as the material involving the scissors, and those that emerge in relation to anxieties about whether or not one has a place in relation to another, such as the later material in which Joseph concerns himself with the evidence of intruders. One might suggest the former is experienced at a sensory and concrete level (Rhode, 2011) while the latter we might identify as taking shape in phantasy, when there is more of a mind to contain mental life.

The experience of therapy for Joseph aroused a great deal of anxiety about his own survival in relation to the relationships he was in the process of developing. In the first few sessions, there were moments when his anxiety was extremely overwhelming and additional support needed to be sought from his foster carer waiting in the waiting room. In the analysis of one of these moments in Session 4, the key feature of such a moment in terms of oedipal processes seems to be the triangular space that the dialogue and holding the arrival of Joseph's foster carer brings to the session. In his paper "Creating a 'Third Position' to Explore Oedipal Dynamics in the Task and Organization of a Therapeutic School", John Diamond (2012) discussed the need for "triangulation" in team work to support emotional growth in the extremely troubled and "multiply traumatised'" population of children who attend the Mulberry Bush School. He referred to the importance of the experience of "relationship-building" and observation of relationships as the stepping-stones towards a child's capacity to think about feelings, "to move beyond the 'blind eye' of self-interest and survival." Similarly, the use of the relationship between his therapist and foster carer in these early sessions appeared from the analysis to offer both holding and regulation to Joseph in response to his anxiety, but additionally offered him an experience of "relationship-building" between his therapist and foster carer, which he could begin to observe and take in from a "third position" (Britton, 1989). The greater stability afforded to Joseph in the external situation appeared to bring about a greater use of his internal space to think, explore, and play. The sample ends at the moment when Joseph began to use his therapeutic relationship to explore more openly his phantasies about the occupants he believed to take his place on separation from his therapeutic space. This is the level of oedipal anxiety, which assumes that there is an obstacle to one's occupying the internal space of the mother, but the obstacle is a lively and potent occupant, identified by Joseph as the owner of the "ruler" in Session 49.

This is a far cry from the frozen, empty space he stuck himself to in the face of fragmentary anxiety in Session 1, a place where nothing could grow and interact. The phenomena related to oedipal anxiety in the later sessions was rooted in the development of the relationship Joseph had to his therapist at the same time as the development of a greater internal cohesion that could allow him to locate himself in an external structure at the same time as explore the internal relationship between himself and his objects.

Conclusion

Recognizing the emotional ramifications of a child's experience of loss, separation, and abuse lies at the heart of the collection of papers entitled *Waiting to be Found: Papers on Children in Care*, edited by Andrew Briggs (2012). Briggs notes in the "Endpiece" that a policy identifying the need for continuity and stability in care and the provision of a "corporate parent", while understandable, nevertheless manages to "obscure from adult view, children's complex emotional lives". The case study presented here, together with the use of an in-depth research method, is an attempt to highlight some of the phenomena present in the clinical setting that point to the importance of noticing and responding to the emotional complexities in children who have had early histories of trauma and have been placed in care.

The themes of transitions, thresholds, boundaries, separation, and oedipal phenomena when taken together support the theoretical link between the development of a child's internal space and its occupants and a capacity to securely occupy and negotiate external space. Rey (1986) and Winnicott (1952) offer theoretical accounts that attend to the experience of inner security and its roots in an experience of spatial security provided by the maternal holding situation. While for Winnicott this is described as a "total-environment set-up", for Rey it is a "marsupial space"—a position from which an infant can remain within the maternal environment but begin to look outwards into the spaces beyond. In both theoretical accounts, this is a developmental and therefore transitional experience of space and the relationship to the caregiver. This transitional experience is essential for a capacity to experience separation and make a transition without internal space disintegrating.

Taking all of the in-depth outcomes into account, one might suggest that the emergent theoretical framework centres more singularly on how one comes to be at-home. My emerging hypothesis could be described in the following terms: *being at-home is a developmental achievement. It requires that a person has moved from a position of being held from the outside to having a greater sense of the capacity to hold oneself together from within.*

The material presented in this chapter highlights, I believe, a fundamental aspect of child psychotherapy practice in response to a child's developmental needs following early trauma. The development of a child's sense of place can be facilitated through the close attention of a therapeutic relationship.

CHAPTER THREE

The desert, the jungle, and the garden: some aspects of autistic functioning and language development

Carlos Tamm

This chapter is drawn from a retrospective qualitative study based on psychotherapy sessions with children presenting autistic features who use language in atypical ways. The purpose of this research was to explore what factors could hinder or enhance the development of communicative language and symbolic thinking. The study was based mainly on the detailed investigation of two cases. Two child patients (6 and 8 years old at the beginning of the study), in the range of autistic spectrum disorders (ASDs) and presenting idiosyncratic language use, were seen once weekly in 50-minute sessions of individual psychoanalytic psychotherapy for a period of two years. Although this was not the ideal frequency, it was difficult for their parents to commit to bringing the child to the clinic more than once weekly. Both families were also supported by parent work.

Methodological issues

The method of analysing two different cases was chosen because of similarities but, more importantly, marked differences between the two children's clinical presentations. Each was first studied as a single case using grounded theory methods. An attempt was also made to evaluate the clinical material using an adapted version of Bion's Grid (1977).

It is to be noted that my approach departed from a classical grounded theory procedure in two different respects. My previous experience with psychoanalytic clinical method had led me to acquire a theoretical mind-frame made familiar through habits of use, which informed my use of the grounded theory method (Glaser & Strauss, 1967). There was a second tool that had an auxiliary function in the first step of my evaluation of the clinical data: an adapted version of Bion's Grid. This tool is one of the most remarkable and creative endeavours to identify common aspects of the psychoanalytic method. It provides specific methods to evaluate its efficacy, the evolution of a treatment, and the development that happens (or not) during an analytic session according to the analyst's interpretations and the patient's response to them (Bion, 1963, 1965, 1962a, 1977, 1992).

An adaptation of the Grid (see Figure 3.1), including (–)β-elements (i.e., minus β-elements) to allow its application to work with autistic patients, was made to help to identify patterns of evolution or regression in the young patients observed, in terms of their emotional functioning and uses of language. The concept of (–)β-elements can provoke confusion, since β-elements represent the raw material of experience: therefore what I mean by (–)β-elements requires clarification. Following the Kantian concept of "thing-in-itself", Bion describes "β-elements" as "things-in-themselves"; β-elements are, therefore, "suitable for projective identification but not for thinking" (Sandler, 2005). The dominant use of projective identification is a characteristic of the first stages of development, when the infant does not have a psychic apparatus capable of containing distressing and disturbing sensations and feelings. The massive use of projective identification persists in psychotic patients. However, in spite of their primitive characteristics, β-elements are also defined as "the earliest matrix from which thoughts can be supposed to arise" (Sandler, 2005). We could say that the infant is experiencing the discomfort of something that needs to be evacuated somewhere. The discomfort that comes from the primordial helplessness of separateness gives rise to unbearable sensations and feelings that are projected into the mother, even when they are not yet forms of communication, as later they can be. What I am calling (–)β-elements then refers to the situation in which the infant, instead of projecting the β-elements that are exerting their pressure on the mental apparatus, does not even acknowledge their existence. The concept, thus, does not refer to the absence of this raw material—which would be logically impossible—but to the de-mobilization of the sensorial apparatus that would acknowledge its pressure on the psyche.

	Definitory Hypothesis 1	ψ 2	Notation 3	Attention 4	Inquiry 5	Action 6	n
A.a (−)ß-elements		A.a 2					
A.b ß-elements	A.b 1	A.b 2				A.b 6	
B α-elements	B1	B2	B3	B4	B5	B6	...Bn
C Dream Thoughts Dreams, Myths	C1	C2	C3	C4	C5	C6	...Cn
D Pre-conception	D1	D2	D3	D4	D5	D6	...Dn
E Conception	E1	E2	E3	E4	E5	E6	...En
F Concept	F1	F2	F3	F4	F5	F6	...Fn
G Scientific Deductive System		G2					
H Algebraic culculus							

Figure 3.1 This was based on Bion's original Grid (see Bion, 1984a [1962]). The only change I introduced was the division of A into A.a and A.b.

Bion's original Grid was elaborated having in mind projective identification as the earliest and most primitive kind of mental functioning, the massive use of it being something that Bion could repeatedly observe in his adult psychotic patients. The phenomenon later identified by authors who worked with autistic children, such as Meltzer and Bick, of "adhesive identification" (Bick, 1986; Meltzer, 1975a) or "adhesive equation", as Tustin (1984) preferred, added a new dimension to this perspective.

When using the Grid, each of the patient's expressions or behaviours is categorized, as well as the therapist's response. By identifying the category of the following manifestation of the patient, the therapist can know the effect of his or her interpretation, and the evolution, regression, or blockage that followed it, and at which mental level the patient seems to be at each point.

This adapted Grid was used as another source of information for triangulation in the data analysis. This was done before the coding and also helped in selecting the sessions to be coded and analysed. An example of its use is included below.

Example of use of the Grid

The use of the Grid involves categorizing each communication from the patient. The genetic (vertical) axis involves the evolution of the processes of thinking, while the horizontal axis relates to the use that is being made of the elements in the genetic axis.

In the clinical vignette shown in Box 3.1, what is observed is that there is basically *one* important evolutionary moment in the session, the one in which Sam's response can be categorized as B3. That means that the interpretation that triggered this response was the one that better reached the child in the session.

Theoretical sampling and coding

During the work with the children, when I was writing up my notes, occasional moments in sessions in which something particularly striking was happening involving language would already attract my attention. After the therapies were concluded, when reviewing all the notes for research purposes, I would pay particular attention to these specific moments and possible variations in the clinical presentation of the children before and after breaks, both planned and unplanned. These highlighted the way in which the children experienced separateness, an important feature concerning symbolic development, which underpins the use of language. The aim was to understand, through the interaction with the therapist, what emotional context, in terms of anxieties and defences, prevented the children from using language properly. This would be the basis for the later process of using theoretical sampling to select a few sessions of each therapy that would then be explored in detail. One important source of information about what was happening emotionally with the children at each moment was the observation of the transferential dynamics and the countertransferential response in the therapist. The final tier of evaluating the data involved using grounded theory and the Grid to analyse selected sessions. This provided a technique for analysing the data by grouping or categorizing what was

Box 3.1 Clinical vignette excerpt with a response categorized as B3

When he was answering his "calls", (from the imaginary mobile phone), he talked about "building", "I'm doing", "flat", "flattening", and many jumbles of words, a kind of cluster of words with no vowels, like "mmhngrn". I told him that it seemed that there was a lot of calls, voices, confusing noises coming from that mobile that made it difficult for him to focus on his play here with me. Maybe he feels the same way at school. Maybe those "calls" were coming from his own mind all the time.	**A.a2** (see Grid, Figure 3.1) Imperative voices. Copying adult speech: meaninglessness. Cluster of words with no vowels = instead of avoiding the separating consonants, he tries to copy the adult language, but without the vowels it becomes meaningless.
Sam stopped making calls, tidied up the table obsessively, and began to draw. He drew a rectangle with some lines in it, and some "round" lines on one corner. It was very similar to a drawing he made last session. He said it was a building. I asked about the round lines. He said they were the road.	Response to an interpretation = moment of an ordinary imaginative play. ***B3**

observed and described. Although the two children selected for the research presented language difficulties and had been previously diagnosed as being on the autistic spectrum, they had very different clinical presentations, as will be seen.

The whole process, including the discussion of the case, was carried out in respect of one child before starting with the other, and the systematic comparison of the cases was only made later. The reason for this decision was to try to avoid too much contamination in the analysis of one case by ideas emerging in the other. Two children with very different clinical presentations, behaviour, and personality were chosen for the study in an attempt to prevent unintended extrapolations from one case to the other.

From the analysis of the selected sessions some basic categories emerged. After further analysis, they were divided into three sub-groups, each corresponding to correlated phenomena.

Theoretical framework: autism

Autism is currently considered to be a syndrome with a multifactorial aetiology and there is still much to be investigated and discovered about it. Most researchers and clinicians agree that nature and nurture both play a role in its genesis, and that it has genetic, organic, psychological, and environmental factors implicated in it, to different degrees. There has been a significant amount of research in the field in the last three decades by neuropsychiatrists and developmental psychologists. Child analysts and psychotherapists have also accumulated significant clinical experience, observations, and conceptualizations.

The first known account of a psychoanalytic-based treatment of an autistic child is in Melanie Klein's 1930 paper "The Importance of Symbol-Formation in the Development of the Ego", written before Kanner's 1943 description of childhood autism. However, Frances Tustin was the first child psychotherapist to work extensively with children on the spectrum. She found that most of these children seemed to be terrified of the acknowledgement of separateness. She postulated that this terror provoked their "freezing" in a state of withdrawal from external and internal reality.

An important distinction needs to be made between the destructive narcissistic patients, described by Rosenfeld (1964, 1971, 2008) as being largely motivated by envy, and those we could call "autistic" narcissistic patients, who are terrified of the consequences of relating. As mentioned above, Bick, Tustin, and Meltzer described, in addition to projective identification, an even more primitive phenomenon that seems to predominate in some patients: "adhesive identification" or "adhesive equation". These patients' withdrawal from external and internal reality derives from another kind of primitive and terrifying anxiety, different from those present in patients whose main mode of functioning seems to be linked to projective identification and incorporation, a state of mind understood by Rosenfeld as connected to unbearable envy of the breast, the patient's confusion between self and object deriving from a ruthless incorporation of the object which denies the object's own reality. In these cases, there is already an object to be incorporated, denied, and there is somewhere to project what is undesirable, such as feelings of dependence. In the autistic patients, on the contrary, it is as if there were no object "out there" to be incorporated or into which to project.

Language development

Early non-verbal communicative experiences between mother (or carer) and her infant will pave the way for the later development of verbal language and thinking: this has been documented both by psychoanalysts—from Freud (1911b) to Bion in "A Theory of Thinking" (1962b), to Meltzer in *Explorations in Autism* (Meltzer, Bremner, Hoxter, Weddell, & Wittenberg, 1975d) and Bernard Golse in "Le Development du Langage" (1999)—and by developmental researchers (Stern, 1985; Trevarthen, Aitken, Papoudi, & Robarts, 1998). While children with autism experience separations as traumatic and protect themselves by blocking out awareness of other people's existence, communication and relationships spring from the acknowledgement of separateness, over whose vault language stretches out as a bridge.

As Colwyn Trevarthen suggested, "infant communication needs a partner" (Trevarthen, 1974). Quoting Wittgenstein's concept of language, we could say that the baby develops as a mind and an individual through his participation in a "language game" with the mother and the environment, which is initially non-verbal (Wittgenstein, 1953). Peter Hobson's research on child development leads him to a similar stance: "one needs experience of other people (with minds) in order to acquire concepts of mind in the first place" (Hobson, 2002, p. 242). Donald Meltzer, developing Bion's ideas about thinking, postulated that there are five essential factors for developing language (Meltzer, 1975c): the formation of "dream thoughts", the transformation of dream thoughts into language, the building of a vocabulary for describing the outside world, the finding of an object in the outside world, and the desire for communication. I would add to this the hope of being understood by this external object. The patients we are considering here did not seem to have anyone in their minds to talk to. We could say that over the abyss of separation experienced by the baby and his mother, both must try to build a bridge of gestures and expressions that will be the foundation of the later bridge of meaningful words.

Case study 1: Fred

Background

Fred's parents had moved only recently to the UK when Fred was born. Mother was feeling isolated and depressed. Father was out working most of the time. She felt he was "absent". Fred has a younger brother, Gabriel, who has had a normal development.

According to his parents, Fred had a delayed birth. When he was eventually born, they thought he was dead. He was put in an incubator and recovered. Mother observed that, since the time when he was a baby, Fred didn't make eye contact. According to her, Fred was not physically affectionate. At the age of 4, when Fred still could not speak properly, the parents realized that "something was definitely wrong about him". His speech was disjointed; sometimes he used just a jumble of words or noises, using an idiosyncratic language, including made-up words, and developing "nonsensical chat".

Fred was first diagnosed as presenting atypical autism, and later, when he was assessed through the ADOS[1] and ADI[2], it was considered that he met all the criteria for ASD: he showed limited eye-to-eye contact, poor language use, problems in the perception of the dimension of time, and very restricted capacity for understanding abstract concepts. The cognitive evaluation through the WISC-IV[3] showed that his performance was below average in all categories, although in most of them falling in the borderline range. His main handicap was his lack of verbal comprehension. Fred's social interaction was poor. He did not greet his peers or know their names, and he used to walk in circles or engage in repetitive play. It was also observed at school that he had involuntary tongue movements and was constantly licking his lips and the palms of his hands. Fred played *alongside* and not *with* other children.

Fred seemed to have had difficulties in learning from experience and in going from the particular to the general, which resulted in excessive concreteness in his use of language. For example, he used "peanuts" to indicate that something was salty. Or he could associate words with ideas in his own way, making it difficult for him to take part in shared language. For instance, it was reported that he could say "I'm five" to indicate that he was full, had had enough food—because he observed that the image of the number 5 had a curve, which could be similar to a belly. It was possible that the phonetic symmetry between the words "five" and "fine" played a role here. His insufficient grasp of abstract or conventional representations led him to resort to sensorial associations, visual or auditory.

First impressions

Fred was inhibited and did not clearly express any aggression. He was very disturbed by noises and sometimes used an idiosyncratic form of speech. His use of categories was confused: describing a drawing he had made, he said one shape was "round" and the other was "backwards". He seemed to have difficulties with the dimensions of time and space: he said his mum was playing with his brother when in fact his mother was alone in reception. He then said that his brother Gabriel was "upstairs, down. He's in year 9", while in fact Gabriel was just 3 years old. His communications were frequently enigmatic, as his parents had already reported. They would feel frustrated because it could take them a long time to understand what Fred meant.

Although Fred, over time, engaged in his psychotherapy in his own way, his attendance was patchy, because of mother's difficulties with child care. There would occasionally be long gaps between sessions. Since Fred was only coming once-weekly, any absence meant a two-week gap between sessions. What is interesting to note here are Fred's oscillations during his therapy in response to irregular attendance: after these gaps he was either more withdrawn or confused.

Outline of therapy

Fred could be sitting on the couch silent for a long time, without a word or any move to speak, draw, or play. It made it very difficult to be in the room with him without drifting away. In our first meeting, he brought a toy that was a kind of small green plastic pump with a straw, and he kept pressing the pump, blowing the air from it through the straw on his cheek. Only later in the therapy, when Fred seemed more able to express himself, could he play more imaginatively.

After one missed session, during a session to which he came 15 minutes late, Fred mentioned that there were things that "popped out" of his head. This seemed an acknowledgement of his difficulties and that he was feeling helpless and hopeless about them. In one of the following sessions, he said the Lego figures should be "protected from looking and thinking". Nonetheless, one of Fred's developments in the psychotherapeutic process was the increase in his feeling free enough to express his anger and aggressiveness.

The confusion in his mind about temporal dimensionality was in the session immediately following an Easter break, when he asked me if it would take "thousands of years" to get out from the window, after staring at a hole on the ceiling for a few minutes. It seemed as if he was always facing an empty and deadly object in his mind, which "sucked" his thoughts out of him, leaving his head "not working". I was always at risk of becoming this object. In the second year of his therapy, in the first session after the summer break—again prolonged because his mother had to cancel his two first sessions in September—Fred said that "when he was looking at the sun, he felt his eyes could melt, and so he stopped looking". It seemed that the sun, which needed to be strong enough to make light in dark spaces, like the "black humid things" that appeared sometimes in his communications, at the same time must not be so strong as to melt eyes. Could he also be afraid that his developing awareness of internal and external reality, the links that were being made between perceptions, feelings, and thoughts, could provoke a short-circuit in his head? Did he have a mind that could or wanted to contain all of this? Or would the dark hole want to destroy this light?[4]

In the session following this one, Fred seemed to be in a more developed position. He told me a well-ordered story in which there were three different places (these are described below). However, in the following sessions, Fred seemed to be progressively more anxious and persecuted. His mother was at work, sometimes away, and was not coming to see the parent worker any more. As we were approaching the Christmas break, of which I had forewarned him some weeks before, he grew more and more paranoid, fearing people in the corridor of the clinic and his own child-minder. He was afraid of losing parts of his body, scared of going to the toilet, and he kept touching his willy as if to confirm it was still there. He complained of tummy aches and said he was afraid of dying. Fred was also afraid of giants, of green slugs hidden in the toilet, of germs, and of parts of his body falling off, as we will see later. These expressions of terror provoked powerful countertransferential feelings in the therapist: was I really helping Fred? His helplessness and despair were painful to see, almost paralysing. What had the therapist done to Fred in bringing him out of his shell? Would he retreat again?

It later seemed to me that one key element in this narrative collection of nightmares was his mention that when *he looked up* (to the sun?) *his head could fall off*. The infant needs to look up to see his mother when being breastfed on her lap. The importance of this period of development has been emphasized by several different authors, including Melanie Klein, Winnicott, and Meltzer. What the baby finds there (in his mother's face and eyes), if he can bear to look, can be decisive in terms of his development, as is stressed by Winnicott (1967). This "looking up" is also an acknowledgement of the distance between the baby and the mother, when she is perceived as a person who is separate and different from the baby.

I quote here a vignette from one session from the beginning of the second year of therapy, following a missed session, in which he described three different landscapes:

> I have not heard what happened last week, when Fred could not attend. [...]
>
> He started saying something about "electric games", mentioned "IPod", "energy".
>
> I was reminded that sometimes he says that his "brain stops", his mind "doesn't work", he has no "energy". Maybe when he doesn't come here, like last week, he feels he needs some electricity to make his mind work, to feel alive. He wanted me to talk about something he was doing to confirm that he was alive. Maybe he also wanted to be sure that I was alive.
>
> He then said, in a heartfelt way, that he wouldn't "be ignored ever". He didn't like it when his mum ignored him. And now he talked to her when she did that, and then she listened to him.
>
> I said that he might have felt that our session last week was ignored, and then maybe he felt ignored and not listened to.
>
> He then started telling a story about three different places: "a jungle with bad, bad, bad animals", a "beautiful place full of trees", and "a desert where no one needs any help", spending more time on the last.
>
> I said sometimes he preferred to believe that he didn't need any help. When he felt he needed but couldn't have the attention he needed, he couldn't have his session, he felt as if he was in a jungle with bad, bad, bad animals. He wanted to arrive at this beautiful place full of trees where he could trust people.

When moving from his autistic refuge, his terror of bodily fragmentation and persecutory panic would be clearly expressed, as can be seen in the following excerpts from a session into the second year of his therapy.

> "I was moving my legs and then came this horrible sound."
>
> I said it seemed that he thought his moving his leg had provoked the noise, as if something terrible could happen. Maybe he thought he'd lose his leg, it was difficult to believe he could move his leg and not lose it. (…)
>
> After being silent for a few minutes, Fred said he had to hold his tummy so it wouldn't fall off.
>
> I said that maybe he was also afraid of losing parts of his mouth when he spoke, and this was why he was silent.
>
> He said he loses part of his eyes when he sees, part of his ears when he hears, part of his nostrils when he smells. He said when he looks high, his head can fall off.
>
> He added he needed to hold his hair so that the wind wouldn't take it away, and be clever so that his head doesn't fall off.

Later in his therapy, there was the emergence of a wish for a container to organize the fragments in his mind and for him to be recognized and listened to.

Discussion: basic oscillation

The analysis of Fred´s sessions revealed a basic oscillation in Fred's mental functioning among three different positions: these corresponded to three sites that were mentioned by him in more than one session. I simplified the names of these "places" to "Desert", "Jungle", and "Garden", each corresponding to a specific state of mind and way of using language. It is important to observe that these three states, although described separately here for the purpose of clarity, did not occur in a mutually exclusive way: elements of two or even three of them could be present, and fluctuations among them would occur in the same session.

Nevertheless, there was a clear predominance of one of them in each session. The "desert" was the dominant landscape of most sessions at the start of Fred's therapy, followed by an alternation between "desert" and "jungle". With the development of the therapy, the "garden" was more present, being still often replaced by "jungle" and by moments of "desert".

Desert—"A desert where no one needs any help"

The *mindscape* of "desert" involved experiences identified through line-by-line coding of the sessions: these were of *falling off* the couch, emptiness, auto-sensuousness, lack of self-orientation and spatial/temporal orientation, "on–off" functioning, absent or idiosyncratic communication, dispersion, difficulty in adding, and symbolic deficit. The communication difficulties involved very prolonged silences or moments of use of an idiosyncratic language. The lack of contact and of a mental context for using communicative language resulted in words being used only imitatively, the use of quasi-neologisms, and a lack of links between words that structure sentences—leading to words featuring as dispersed elements that could not be adequately joined. All of this indicated deficient symbolization.

In the first months of his therapy, Fred could be silent for long periods, and I felt I had to struggle to survive as a living person in the room: I could occasionally feel sleepy, or be tempted to withdraw to a day-dreaming state of mind. I then felt that I was being pushed into an autistic-like state myself, which made me acutely aware of the kind of internal landscape in which Fred lived.

Jungle—"A jungle with bad, bad, bad animals"

This mental landscape involved deep fears, a bodily terror of fragmentation, alarm, suspicion, and persecution. The language was less idiosyncratic, words were used according to their common usage, sentences could be structured, but an organized and meaningful narrative was lacking. The world was felt as scary and confusing, and it did not seem possible to make sense of it.

The jungle seemed to be a terrifying mindscape that was always there in the background of Fred's autistic features, and which he avoided by being in the "Desert". With the development of his therapy, sometimes these fears came up with painful intensity. Fred would be haunted by persecutory terrors, as could be seen in the session mentioned above.

The intensity of his terrors seemed to be linked to Fred's strong autistic defences, making him feel safer in the "desert".

Garden—"A beautiful place, full of trees."

This mindscape only appeared later in Fred's therapy. At these moments, he was more lively, showing a wish to be recognized and some hope of both understanding and being understood. His emotions and phantasies could be expressed in the sessions through play, drawings, and even verbalization without provoking too much persecutory anxiety. He would use more structured language, organized in meaningful narratives that could be followed without too much effort, and taking the form of sequences of interactions and play.

Mindscapes

These images delineated three different states of mind and ways of relating to internal and external objects—that is, three different levels of mental functioning. To arrive in the *beautiful place* he needed to cross *a jungle with very bad animals,* dealing with threatening internal and external objects. The "desert where no one needs any help", on the other hand, seemed to be a painfully accurate description of the isolation of his autistic encapsulation. However, his elaborate and imaginative description of those places, associated with his unconscious fears, and the sign of hope present in the "beautiful place" seemed to point in the direction of some progressive development in his symbolic capabilities.[5]

In terms of his use of language, we could say that Fred was moving from the earlier, predominant desert (his use of idiosyncratic language), through the fears and terrors of the jungle (a confusion of fragmented and disconnected, if scary, fragments of narrative[6]), to reach moments of meaningful communication of his feelings and phantasies through structured language (the *beautiful place full of trees*). This was not however a steady process of development, but was one in which there were evolutionary and regressive moments. In a later session in which he was silent and withdrawn, he said when I pointed this out that "when I didn't talk to him he stayed in his own world, he needed me to talk to him". He seemed to be expressing his need for me to help him to be born, to bring him to the world of relationships, as if he were not completely aware that he had already been born and was alive.

When we were approaching the end of his therapy, he started drawing some signs in horizontal rows, like hieroglyphs, and when I asked about them he said it was "a language of his own". This session showed a wish to regress to his familiar autistic functioning, probably caused by the approaching end of his therapy, but the regression was limited, since he was able to define what he was trying to do: to make "a language of his own". Although this could be seen as a threat to return to his isolation, since he felt he was to be left by me, on the other hand he was able to name it., Later in this session, he drew a big open-mouthed monster "down there", under the hieroglyphic lines. The monster was "eating them", but then "his brain could stop" and then "evil would kill him". This seemed to indicate a "jungle" moment in which the monster—the analyst?—was attacking his private world and making him enter a shared and terrifying world. However, in spite of the confusing material and the hieroglyphs, it is to be noted that his language was still structured and communicative. This kind of fluctuation was also clear in terms of his relationship with me. For instance, in one session he was agitated and told confusing stories full of explosions and strange creatures in a fragmented narrative.

> I connected this state of mind with the gap between the last time he came (he missed the previous session) and today, and reminded him of what he mentioned in a recent session about the "brain stopping" when he didn't come. He soon lowered his tone, was quiet and looking very fragile, and said he was sick. I said it seemed that I was reminding him of something that gets poisonous inside him when he feels I leave him. He said that he wasn't feeling sick any more. He then asked me: "How do you feel when I leave?"

It seemed that the oscillation between the "jungle" and the "garden" was now much more permeable and dynamic, despite the "garden" not being only a "beautiful place", but also a place of moments of deep sadness, vulnerability, feelings of loneliness and helplessness, which he was now able to experience in his contact with me. What is remarkable, though, is the difference in his use of language according to his predominant mood. The moments of highly enigmatic, sometimes idiosyncratic language of the beginning of the therapy were now less frequent, and there was a stark difference between the fragmented and confusing language that he could use when in a more paranoid and disorganized state, and the surprisingly thoughtful sentences he would use in moments like that at the end of the session above.

Case study 2: Sam

Background

Sam was referred for psychotherapy as an emotionally uncontained 8-year-old and presented as a child whose level of disturbance was quite pronounced. He was delayed in motor development and presented problems in writing and in the development of pragmatic language. He only started using sentences when he was more than 3½ years old. When he was 5, he had a language assessment which showed delays in expressive and receptive language. He was diagnosed as presenting pragmatic-semantic disorder, and although his assessment for autism was not completely conclusive, he had a provisional diagnosis of atypical autism.

It was reported that Sam was very delayed at school, and he was difficult to contain in the classroom and at home. He presented bizarre behaviour, such as licking, and his play was obsessive, lacking in creativity. He also displayed agitation and aggressiveness, which was worse at home. He would attack his younger brothers for no reason. He also had difficulties in accepting boundaries and showed little respect for his mother's authority, addressing her in a bossy way, yelling and swearing or even occasionally being violent towards her.

When Sam was around age 21 months, the family had been living in a foreign country, whose language they did not speak. Sam's mother who was then pregnant felt very isolated and depressed. They lived in a flat with no garden and there was no kindergarten around. When Sam was 2 years old, he already presented aggressive behaviour towards other children, biting and hitting them. He was very jealous when his next brother, Joseph, was born and became very "naughty" when his mother was with the baby. Until he was 3½ years old, he could only say a few words. When he wanted an apple, for instance, he would only say "apple" and would not use the correct links to structure his words into a sentence. He would say them out of the correct sequence, making it impossible for others to understand him. Back in London, in kindergarten, Sam presented difficulties in socializing with his peers, being either withdrawn or too aggressive towards them and the teachers. He still often made a strange use of words, according to his mother. She added that when he was anxious or angry, he tried to speak fast, and his speech and pronunciation became worse. The mother also confided that Sam had witnessed fierce arguments between his parents.

Outline of therapy

At the beginning of our work, Sam would often be very concentrated on the kind of obsessive play described. He ignored me or, alternatively, when not wanting to hear something I was saying, made animal sounds as if to scare me. He would stick plasticine on the table, forcefully flattening it into the surface in an obsessive way. He would use glue and Sellotape and try desperately to make sure that it would stick exactly where he put it. He would then straighten the plasticine and flatten it further, using a ruler. He fought fiercely against any perceived edges or gaps, once trying to fix a plank that had one end coming off the wall back onto it, using glue, Sellotape, and plasticine. On these occasions, he was silent and very focused on what he was doing, shunning any interference on my part. When speaking, he would often use jumbles of words with no separation between syllables or words and would sometimes utter unintelligible words made of consonants without vowels. It was as if he were also magically fixing in this way, symbolically mending things through sticking his words and syllables together in any order.

Later in his therapy, Sam was able to engage in less obsessive play. He would very often use variations of a theme: there would be a green field, made, for instance, of two sheets of paper painted green and linked to each other with glue and Sellotape. This would be placed at the end of the table, in the middle of which there would be a big lump of brown plasticine smashed and pressed against its surface, looking like a mud puddle. He would then place some animals at the uncovered opposite end of the table and bring them to the green field. Before arriving at the green field, each of the animals had to step deeply—almost to the point of being stuck—in the brown plasticine before leaving it with their dirty paws and finally reaching the green field.

On occasions he could eventually write a few words and speak or even listen to me—when something seemed to reach him, he would either protest loudly or look at me, surprised. His written or spoken words would still be difficult to grasp: there was no separation between the words in a written sentence, and although the letters would be clear, the spelling was usually very odd, with the suppression of some letters, particularly at the ends of words, as will be seen below, apparently avoiding the edges around words. His speech was congruent with that: his pronunciation was very unclear, but what made it more difficult to understand was the lack of separation between words, which could leave an impression of a jumble of mumbled sounds, when in fact there were some specific words but they were made difficult to distinguish owing to a lack of gaps between them. Approaching the end of the first year of his therapy, Sam could occasionally be in touch with his fragility and neediness, as can be seen in this vignette from a session that took place after a cancelled one:

> He then pulled a cloth from his shirt, sat on the couch with his feet on the little chair, and started sucking his right thumb and holding the cloth in his left hand against his left cheek.

In the same way that his aggressive behaviour on occasions could be off-putting, in his more machine-like moments he could occasionally make me feel tired and discouraged, making me daydream, sharing in his non-relational mode, which I was aware of. His usual avoidance of long powerful vowels, when he was behaving more obsessively, seemed to indicate that they were felt like holes through which the inside could fall through to the outside. I thought his flattening activity was related to this anxiety.

During the second year of his therapy, Sam could on occasions be thoughtful and talkative, occasionally asking for help with the spelling of a word—he could even show affection towards me. Nevertheless, there was a major setback for him when his rival brother, the youngest, started therapy at the Tavistock as well. Sam was enraged. He would kick the wall of the room several times while repeating that he wanted to kill his brother. It seemed that the wall represented a boundary that was experienced as the manifestation of the rival who inhabits the place and turns it bad. When he was attacking and dirtying the room too much in one session and I said it was better to stop now, because we both would have to clean up, he answered that I should clean it, since I was the one who had made the mess. This seemed to express very adequately his rage against me, my betrayal of him, and his feeling that I had been responsible for his brother's "arrival" at the clinic. After some sessions of this behaviour, he could again resume his evolution in the therapy. His aggressive regression after the next break did not last long, and he seemed thoughtful when I remarked that he now felt more able to put things together: letters, words, ideas, and people. When we were approaching the planned end of his therapy, the mess-mud threatened to take over again, with rage, aggressiveness, a mess of glue, plasticine, and paper spread all over the room, and things being hurled from his box. This state of mind persisted for a good few sessions.

A predominant theme in Sam's behaviour was the need for continuity of surfaces, the avoidance of lumps and holes, edges, gaps. He could spend long periods in his sessions flattening and straightening plasticine on the table. The search for continuity was also seen between consecutive sessions. He would check if some hole he had filled up with plasticine was still filled up, or if a piece of Sellotape he had stuck to the wall was still there. If I tried to intervene in his obsessional play with plasticine he would immediately react, squealing loudly as a piglet or roaring furiously as a lion. It seemed that if he was to be "pulled" from his mindless state of sticking and flattening, he would be in a jungle and needed to protest loudly. His persecutory anxieties seemed to be very close to the surface in spite of his defensive mechanisms and autistic traits. This "jungle" also had obvious anal connotations. Sam felt that his mess, when he was not controlling it by the sticking/flattening activity, could be too much: his mother could not control him, so who would be able to bear it? A cancellation, the dirt on the wall that could not be completely removed, made him feel panic.

Discussion: alternating states

Sam also oscillated between different states of mind, with his behaviour, his relationship with me, and his use of language varying according to which state of mind was predominant in each particular session, phase of therapy, or moment of a session. The first identified state of mind was evident mainly through his physical behaviour. In these moments he would be mostly silent, while obsessively sticking, flattening, and straightening not only the plasticine on the table, but everything that he found was loose in the room, or any hole that he felt *needed* to be filled or lump to be flattened in order to ensure a sense of continuity and to avoid gaps and edges, including between words in a sentence. I describe this mental pattern as the *Sticking Machine.*

The second state of mind corresponded to a limited space with a physical characteristic—the *Mud Puddle*—which was represented in his play mainly by brown or occasionally red plasticine that occupied the centre of the table, of the session, and of his mind. His communication here would usually be very aggressive, his anger and fear often felt as being beyond words.

The third of these patterns corresponded to a place—a *Green Field*—printed by him on paper and often including domestic animals and fences, like a farm. In these moments, there was a connection with a broader range of feelings. His spoken words and sentences would be clearly understandable. The written sentences would include increasing separation between words, in spite of the misspellings, with which he would occasionally ask for help.

The first two patterns were the predominant ones for most of Sam's therapy, and also patterns to which he would regress when there was anything that made him feel threatened. At the same time, the distinction between the *mud puddle* and the *sticking machine* was not always clear. The reason for this seemed to be that the *sticking machine* was a desperate effort to avoid the *mud puddle* that did not actually work. Sam seemed to be flooded by the mud, and even if he would on many occasions like to withdraw completely from it to a silent, detached, and mechanical place, he apparently could not succeed. The efforts, then, of the *sticking machine* were much increased and more strength was put into it in a very determined and anxious way, always threatened by failure. This made him enraged about anything felt as an interruption to his obsessive activity.

Sticking machine—"Mmhngrn!"

This mode of functioning involved the need to flatten surfaces, avoiding lumps, holes, edges, gaps, or any form of rupture that could indicate a discontinuity in space or time. There was desperate sticking activity, as well as straightening or filling any gap and a struggle to put things together suppressing their rebellious individual identity. The therapist needed to be there, but almost as an inanimate object, since he would otherwise be felt as a threatening presence. There was an anxious attempt to avoid the messy "mud", which seemed, however, to be already there. Language was rarely used, and, when it was, it was often like a jumble of words with no separation between syllables or words in a sentence. Occasionally the lack of vowels made speech unintelligible or meaningless. At other times, words were used with no discernible underlying context. In his speech and writing as in his play, he avoided edges and *lumps* or *holes* (the *highs* and *lows* given by vowels in ordinary speech). All of Sam's obsessive *machine* manoeuvres, nevertheless, also seemed to bear the character of forceful defences, which were rigid but not solid, like a fortress that needs constant vigilance. He needed to fill the holes or gaps in the wall through which the enemy—the acknowledgement of discontinuity and difference, and the persecutory fears engendered by them—could penetrate and take over. In a session after our first Christmas break,

> Sam spent some time sticking two sheets of paper together with the Sellotape.
>
> I said he wanted the gaps between his sessions, and between him and me to disappear.
>
> He then started to draw a building on another sheet of paper, using the first ones as a base for it. He felt the paper was too small and wrote: "papewastosmelsowerojustmakinitherecosthepapesnottaleranug".

> I wondered if he was expressing a feeling that there should be more sessions and less gaps between them, that he needed to fight hard to keep it together, or the building could fall apart.

He would play, using very few words or not uttering a single word, not responding to my interpretations or even acknowledging having heard them, while, for instance, wrapping his own arm or the furniture or me with Sellotape. In the above-mentioned second session after the first summer break, he was forcefully "flattening" the wall and filling its holes, concretely suppressing any gaps. He was also unable to listen to me, as if I should be flattened as well. I should not be something that disappears in the break, like a hole or a gap, or be allowed to stand out after it—as if my voice and comments were felt as sticking out from a flat surface.

Mud puddle—"Roarrr!"

This mindscape involved hate, terror, violence, a lack of boundaries or barriers for feelings impossible to contain or process, and a lack of differentiation between self and object. There was intrusiveness, mess, dirt, urgency, lack of time–space orientation, threats of having the space stolen by other creatures, and menacing voices. Its typical language included sounds of wild or cornered and dirty animals that he actually became, rather than merely playing at being one of them. When he used language here, it was more understandable and structured, even if on occasions it seemed more like copied language with menacing authoritarian and imperative voices, trying to control the chaos of his feelings of terror.

When he felt understood, he could at moments respond in a more communicative and organized fashion, as seen in the fragment below, in which not only did he speak properly, but also showed he was clear about the temporal dimension of the summer break.

> Sam was making noises copying the machine noises coming from works going on outside the building.
>
> I said he felt it would be safer to be like a machine, since he was feeling like I was treating him as a machine, not caring about him or his feelings and leaving him for such a long break, leaving him with no words, and he was afraid he could be very confused and furious.
>
> He stared at me silently for a few seconds. (…)
>
> When leaving, he said: "See you in September."

Green field—"The animals need to go to the green field!"

This mindscape, which in the beginning of his therapy could only be hinted at, involved an acknowledgement of Sam's own problems and fragilities—like his learning difficulties—a capacity to connect with his emotional need for important others who are separate individuals and who are not subject to his control. There was, therefore, instead of the de-humanized mechanical or animalesque behaviour, a capacity to connect with the therapist, even showing him affection, with a consequent fear of loss. There was pride in his developing powers of communication as well as a growing capacity to put things together, which implies a hint of oedipal organization. There was use of structured language here, in which the spaces between syllables and the adequate linking vowels were preserved. There were several misspellings, but he could ask for an adult's—the therapist's—help with them, showing that there was an effort to organize his mind.

In one session we had to change the room owing to the change in the session time that had taken place at the request of his mother, and Sam was more communicative. There was evidence of acknowledgement of his problems, and of his fear of losing the link with me, the therapy, and his evolution during the *gaps*: "This is the rechargeable hole" was the sentence previously confusedly written that he now struggled to read. This could mark a shift from an empty mouth experienced as a hole to one that can potentially receive something that can recharge him. In any case, it was as if he wanted to be sure that the input from the therapy could be rechargeable when he felt he was losing it.

> At the end of this session he drew a mobile that should be "waterproof, resist 200 meters under water", and so on.
>
> I then said he wanted a strong power of communication that could resist extreme conditions, that could work even when he was angry, worried, or sad. He did not want to lose his communication with me, which was developing.

In the second year of his therapy, and after the turbulent period connected to his brother's therapy, in the last session before our second Christmas break:

> Sam, after some initial reluctance in coming with me to the room, checked the toy box and proceeded to draw a Christmas tree, which he stuck on

one side of the box, and a symbol of his religion, which he stuck on the other side of it.

I wondered if the Christmas tree represented me and him, and it seemed that he wanted me to keep him in mind, and wanted to keep me in mind too.

He then wrote: "Merry Christmas" on the drawing of the tree, and "Happy ____ " on the other drawing, referring to the festival of his own tradition. The words were clearly written and separated from each other, and he asked for my help in spelling "Christmas" and the other festival.

Cross-case discussion

From the two cases studied, we can then make some observations about the nature of and fluctuation between different states of mind in both children and can relate the similarities and differences observed in their patterns with the general psychopathology of each child. This fluctuation between different states of mind occurred despite the initial impression of rigidity and impermeability and was manifested in their relationship with the therapist, in their mental functioning, and in their use of language.

One of the striking similarities between them was that both boys moved between three different mental states, uses of language, and modes of interaction in the sessions. It is important to make it clear that the distinction we are drawing here is schematic, in terms of the predominance of one mode of functioning over the other at a given moment. We are describing different capacities of the personality which coexisted simultaneously. Added to this is the fact that there was a move either from the more withdrawn state of autistic functioning to the persecutory or depressive anxieties that were being avoided; or, alternatively, from a persecuted state to moments of a more depressive working-through of these anxieties and then back to a more manifestly belligerent or terrified state of mind. Moreover, one of the children—Fred—described more than once three different landscapes that corresponded to these states of mind, as if defining a mental geography that included these features. Recalling these definitions:

» A "desert": "where no one needs any help".
» A "jungle": "with bad, bad, bad animals".
» A "garden": "A beautiful place, full of trees".

It was striking to note that, Sam also expressed this oscillation graphically through two different landscapes, the "green field" — and the "mud puddle" These two landscapes seemed to be closely related to two of Fred's landscapes:

» "garden, beautiful place, full of trees" = "green field"
» "jungle with bad, bad, bad animals" = "mud puddle"

Fred

During the first period of Fred's therapy, the "desert" was the most present mindscape, despite the fact that he could occasionally show a more sophisticated level of mental functioning. At the same time, as can be seen in his clinical material, the moments in which he was in a "jungle with bad animals" were absolutely terrifying, involving fears of fragmentation of his own body and its organs, and of persecution from external monsters. Compared with that, the desert seemed a safe place, "where no one needs any help". The desert also involved the notion that nothing can grow, as Fred himself could not grow, and wanted not to grow. The idea of growing itself implies something sticking out, becoming differentiated, an event that provoked huge anxiety, which Sam would fight fiercely with his flattening and sticking activities. This shows that in the desert as well as in the sticking machine mode, both children were searching desperately for an evenness of experience, a smooth continuity that could not be lost. The whole world needed to be an even surface. This is the experience of those autistic children who react against noises that stick out in terms of their auditory experience, or who seek to avoid physical contact. We can speculate whether the avoidance of protuberances and concavities has to do not only with the image of a catastrophic separation between nipple and mouth, but is also a denial of specifically masculine and feminine elements, the container and the contained.

Another aspect to be observed here concerns time. It is felt that sameness must pervade both space and time. Fred needed to believe that I lived at the clinic, and was always there. He also wanted to believe that he was always in the same room with "the same stuff". More than that, the difference between the topology of his mind and that of the building was blurred: where Gabriel was when Fred was here in the clinic was not clear. If, in his mind, Gabriel was in mum's mind, so he was in the building with mum. His confusion, or, more precisely, his indifference, about time could be seen in his lack of awareness of the length of breaks. As pointed out by Emmanuel Levinas, "The temporality of the interhuman opens up the meaning of otherness and the otherness of meaning" (quoted in Kearney, 2004). This "otherness" was precisely what needed to be avoided by Fred, due to the catastrophic feeling associated for him with separateness, and with his existence in time. As Tustin put it, autism works as a "protection against a terrible dissonance, mother and baby merge into each other, turning everything into consonance" (quoted in Korbivcher, 1995).

Fred's states of mind and behaviours suggested that his isolation and learning difficulties were in the service of keeping the terrors of the "jungle" at bay, while they were, at the same time, arresting his development. Only with the evolution of the therapy could these terrors emerge in all their dreadful intensity. The feelings evoked in the therapist when Fred was in these two states were of a remarkably different quality. While he was in the "desert" mode, the therapist felt often pushed to a state of isolation, incommunicability, passivity, discouragement, and alienation and was led to doubt the value of the therapy. This doubt about the therapy seemed to be associated with a doubt felt by the child about the real existence of the therapy and of the therapist. This appeared to correspond to the doubt Fred seemed to have about his own existence. The emptiness that accompanies the lack of introjection and differentiation present in autistic states leads to failure to define a sense of self. It is as if everything could be just an image or a momentary impression lacking substance. Fred could spend long periods in these sessions in a prolonged silence. When he spoke, it was always slowly and in a low tone, the meaning enigmatic, with words scattered apart from each other, lacking links and cohesion.

The gap between Fred and the therapist seemed to grow after breaks, and the mood in a session after a break could be very sparse, as if the child were a gas balloon that floated away further or higher and needed some time to land back in the consulting room and in the relationship with me. These seemed to be not only scattered allusions to distance and intervals of time—the break—but to the relationship as well—how long could it take to build it, and for how long could it resist gaps in time? But these elements were so dispersed that it was difficult to evaluate how much Fred could understand of interpretations that connected them, no matter how simple the words the therapist had used. This gaseous state of mind seemed to be related to avoiding putting things together. Such connections were felt to be potentially dangerous: it was better to lack energy than to risk a *short-circuit*, since there was no mental apparatus felt to be capable of containing and holding together these particles. Fred did not seem, from the start of his life, to have trusted that there was anyone who could help him to do this.

In the "jungle" mode, on the other hand, the therapist was put in a state of extreme awareness, alertness, and occasionally even alarm, triggered by the despair experienced by Fred. The "garden" moments, which became more frequent, were felt as a rewarding respite from this sometimes excruciating experience. When in the "jungle", Fred's communication was less idiosyncratic, and he would use sparse sentences that could be understood separately. Real dialogues would take place in these sessions. These revealed the extent of the terrors underlying his withdrawal and alienation, as could be seen in the session quoted above in which these terrors were poignantly expressed. It should be noted, though, that when moving from the peaceful "desert" into the "jungle", Fred's persecutory anxieties were of the very primitive kind found in autistic children, involving dread of losing parts of his body. Moreover, in his despair, he seemed to feel almost completely defenceless, invaded by terrors and without any presence in his mind that could help to organize these images into a meaningful narrative. The use of his senses and any incipient perception of a separation between him and the world brought a sense of imminent disaster. The difference in his mental dynamics when he came to feel he was more *related* to me, others, and himself became clear in a session in which his first communications had been connected with terrible fears of his body falling apart and of his potential disappearance. The following occurred after an interpretation that related these fears to his experience of separation from me during the break:

> Fred said he wished to be "a fish swimming in the dark forever".
>
> I said he wished not to have been born, not to see that he was separate from me, and from his mum, and not to have a relationship with me and now have to separate for the break.

He seemed occasionally terrified of his unpredictable therapist and he then drifted away, but he could return to contact. This previously rigid pattern seemed to be connected to his learning difficulties. He avoided hate and love so powerfully that he emptied his mind, turning it into a deadly deserted space that refused to accept thoughts. This was the very pattern from which he was slowly emerging. When we were approaching the end of his therapy, Fred could say in one session that the time until the review meeting was "way too long".

Sam

In Sam, similarly, the "green field" mindscape was more present in the later stages of his therapy. But, in his case, there was a remarkable difference in the pattern of alternation between the two other states described above. While the "sticking machine" was apparently the predominant mode, it did not show the peaceful deadliness of Fred's "desert". On the contrary, it presented features not only of obsessiveness but also of anxiety barely avoided. One could say that his autistic mechanisms of self-protection were not working as efficiently as Fred's, so his paranoid terrors were more accessible. When he uttered something, it would mostly be unintelligible sounds, jumbles of words with no clear divisions that could define syllables or words. He seemed to be operating with words in the same way that he operated with the objects he was constantly sticking together. I was informed by his mother that whenever Sam was anxious or angry, he would speak fast and his speech and pronunciation would become so much worse that only she could understand it, even partially. Perhaps in these moments Sam was merely manipulating the sounds in his mouth, rather than trying to speak to me. It is to be noted that such manipulation involves also attempting to do things with words at a concrete level—for instance, to regulate closeness and distance, to suppress gaps, and so on. Until the last months of his therapy, Sam's written sentences would not include spaces between words, or punctuation marks between different sentences. Moreover, his words would sometimes omit the last letter so they could more easily merge with the following one. It seemed that Sam did not feel he was really attached to any surface but was, nevertheless, desperately trying to bring such attachment about. The "mud puddle" seemed to be a constant presence, putting Sam in a state of alertness and threat that was barely controlled by the desperate determination of his flattening, straightening, and sticking activities. When in this mode, Sam would often reproduce the sounds of animals—sounding at times repellent, at other times extremely menacing with his eyes wide open in a furiously distorted facial expression—or shouting slogans that were apparently the copied speech of an authoritarian adult. This imperative voice seemed to be there, deceptively, to avoid mess or "mud", which was felt to be present and could potentially get out of control. This could be caused by himself when he intruded into me and the therapy room. This deep fear of disorder seemed to explain his great anxiety about dirt at the end of his sessions or at the beginning of a session when it followed one in which he felt he had left a mess in the room. Sam would, on these occasions, spend most of the session frantically trying to clean or remove something from the wall or the table, without uttering a single word while doing this and ignoring most of my comments about it.

The sense of *otherness* was then present only as a dangerous and threatening ghost that should be fiercely "shut up". "Shut up!" was Sam's answer to any interpretation that he felt to be an invitation to think and to make links between what was happening inside the playroom and his life outside it. He apparently needed to feel joined to the room and to me, with no space between us and no possibility of thinking and observing what was going on from a position outside it. This was connected to his furious reactions to breaks, indicating how anti-developmental tendencies take over when children like these are faced with the pain of separation.

Final considerations

I am suggesting that both patients showed a basic alternation between three different states of mind that were present in similar forms in each of them. These *mindscapes* closely correspond, in terms of the underlying anxiety, and apparent lack of or defence against it, to the paranoid-schizoid and the depressive positions described by Klein. There was, in addition, a third mode of functioning characterized by avoidance and terror, which I am naming *autistic functioning*. I do not postulate an "autistic position", in accordance with the view that Tustin expressed in her paper "The Perpetuation of an Error" (Tustin, 1994). What I describe is clearly a protective device, unlike Ogden's "autistic contiguous position" (Ogden, 1989), which seems much more akin to Tustin's earlier concept of "normal primary sensuousness" (Tustin, 1972). It seems to me that such strong features of withdrawal from external and internal reality only occur within states of arrested development. The idea of an autistic phase of normal development would imply accepting a non–object-related developmental phase. This is not to say that there are not what could be called autistic features present in neurotic or psychotic patients, or in normal development. Such momentary withdrawals from external and internal reality seem to permeate everyday mental life in parallel with other modes of relating to life, and they do not normally arrest development.

My study throws light on the nature of autistic defences. I also attempt to correlate particular uses of language, and thinking or non-thinking processes, with alternations between these three states. The evolution in the therapy seemed to increase and strengthen the "garden/field" moments of the two boys, and allow for more fluid fluctuation between the three states, diminishing the rigidity of their autistic defences. This was shown in the development of more communicative, object-related language, which slowly allowed thinking to develop.

Fred's "desert" and Sam's "sticking machine" each involved avoidance of awareness of separation and need, which would otherwise have provoked very primitive paranoid fears felt on a bodily level, or a state of depressive despair. Due to both children's autistic arrest, these primitive anxieties had not been fully experienced and worked through in the normal stages of their development, as if a large part of these children's minds had been frozen from a very early age. Only when the chaos and fragmentation of the "jungle with bad animals" and the "mud puddle" could be directly faced in their therapy could these anxieties be lessened, and a certain level of depressive integration and communication be achieved. This was represented by Fred's "garden" and Sam's "field".

Sam's mention that the animals needed to go to the green field, while at the same time sticking their paws in the mud after removing them from the box, seemed meaningful in terms of his own mechanisms now represented symbolically through the animals in his play. The box represented his refuge, his silent, straight, and closed world in which there were no gaps, a refuge that he had to work hard to keep like that, to avoid acknowledgement of the therapist as a person. To leave this world was to be in the "mud" and with the beasts. He had some hope of arriving at a better place, in the form of a "green field" and a realization that, in order to arrive there, he would need to face the "mud".

Sam's *stuckness* in the "sticking machine" was threatened by the emergence of disturbances from both outside and inside. Attempts at communication made by the therapist, when not avoided by *shutting the therapist up* or by his flattening/sticking/filling holes activity, could trigger outbursts of panic, rage, and animal roaring and his terror of "mess" and of "mud" getting out of control. He would then frequently try to resume his mechanical activity by annihilating the presence, meaning or importance of the therapist. Later in the therapy, these moments of anger felt towards the therapist were more frequent, alternating with moments of thoughtfulness—he would stare at me with eyes wide open following an interpretation that seemed to reach him.

Later still, there came frank demonstrations of affection. In other words, Sam seemed to be increasingly relating to his therapist as a real person.

Fred also moved, slowly and very tentatively, during his therapy from "desert" to "jungle"—moments of acute anxiety—and to "garden". Or, in other terms, from autistic defences and autistic functioning to primitive paranoid fears and, later on in the therapy, to moments of more depressive kinds of anxiety and mental integration.

Fred's parents' account of him in my first meeting with them, and the picture they gave of him one year later, were very different. In our first meeting, they said that Fred was unable to understand abstract concepts and could not make sense of words and sentences. His father also remarked that Fred did not know his classmates' names. One year later, they said he was more capable of taking part in shared games and play. Fred's mother added that he was telling less "crazy stories" and "nonsense", and that there was a major improvement in his use of language. This shows an interesting and important correlation: his new ability to take part in shared play, shared games, paralleled his increased ability to take part in a shared "language game", to use Wittgenstein's concept again. Moreover, he could occasionally present moments of sadness, which could be very moving. Sam, on the other hand, although usually at all costs avoiding thinking, could not remain completely unaware of his feelings of hatred. Yet in the evolution of his therapy, he showed a surprising improvement in his capacity to think, to communicate, and to relate to his therapist. He became clearly more capable of *putting together* things that could now be recognized to be separate. This was vividly seen in the session already mentioned when he brought together, in drawing, our two different religious traditions. This evolution was also noticeable in the session into the second year of his therapy in which he was very proud of his recent achievements and "new things".

In terms of their use of language, the oscillation in Fred's pattern could be described as going from silence or idiosyncratic language, with scattered words in search for a meaning—"desert"—to the more structured but painful idiom of the concrete persecutory terrors that involved, prominently, bodily fragmentation—"jungle". His use of integrated sentences seemed to indicate that, although expressing terrible and psychotic fears of disintegration, he was really *speaking* his mind and body, indicating that he was now more in touch with his real and separate existence and feelings. His previous use of language seemed to deny the existence of a reality outside himself or that he was outside anything. This denial affected his understanding of the dimensions of time and space and, apparently, even of his physical reality. This gave rise to my impression of the amazingly ethereal aspect of his presence and of his" "lighter-than-air" walk. This state of not being in touch with the natural weight of a human body might be related to the fact that his most terrible and primitive fears resided in his body. His use of words in this phase sometimes evoked the repetition of mere sounds, rather than conveying semantic meaning.

In Sam's case, the silent "sticking machine" would not usually allow space for more than the occasional compressed letters and syllables, which, denying any threatening gap or hole, would not make possible real communication.[7] Any sign of emergence of an acknowledgement of the other's—the therapist's—independent existence would be immediately responded to with animal sounds and imperatives, which were apparently the persecutory sounds that inhabited him. We can speculate that these children's intuitive realization that they had survived through the ordeal of facing their most dreaded terrors, allied to the new developments that they had achieved, was what stimulated them to remain engaged in their therapy.

To sum up these impressions:

» I believe that Bion's formulations on the links L(ove), H(ate), and K(nowledge) (Bion, 1962a, 1967) help us to understand what happens early in autism, where the denial of separation and of the reality of the external object as a differentiated person prevents the adequate development of symbolic thinking and language. The lack of development of links of love and hate with their objects causes problems in the awareness of internal and external reality and severe cognitive impairment. Moreover, in the moments when a patient does succeed in evolving from the shell-type defences of autism (Tustin, 1990a) into a relationship with an analyst, he then has to face the level of anxieties which he had not been at all able to deal with—namely, those of a persecutory and depressive kind.

» I consider that to the two important positions in mental functioning described by Melanie Klein—the paranoid-schizoid and the depressive (Klein, 1935, 1940, 1946)—we should add a third kind of mental functioning that exists in a dialectical relation with them and only becomes strong where there are developmental problems. This I call *autistic functioning*.

» In addition, I believe that specific patterns and levels of language development and language use correspond to different levels of emotional and cognitive development and object-relating, according to the different mechanisms present in each of these patterns of mental functioning.

» I also take into account Bion's very helpful description of the fluctuation between the positions, Ps ↔ D (Bion, 1970). Including the autistic functioning as a third factor, we could make a slightly different diagram:

↗↙ Ps ↖↘
Aut ← - - - - - - - - - - - - - → D

where Aut initially means a regression from the normal path of development to a kind of *pre-psychological birth* state, in the sense that the child refuses to acknowledge his individual self by refusing to acknowledge his mother as a differentiated and limited individual. There is significant overlapping of this solution to that of narcissistic patients, and this differentiation is not always simple. Nevertheless, in the narcissistic non-autistic individual, there is development of the notion of an object, whose existence is then denied by incorporation or by other means.

» I suggest that for these children the intensity of the terrors connected with psychic birth and bodily separation, associated with very primitive paranoid fears, contributed to keep them stuck in their mode of the autistic functioning.

From the clinical evidence described, there is one aspect that is not, at first sight, easily understandable. As mentioned, although being more in touch with his aggressiveness and persecutory fears, and to a certain extent less withdrawn than Fred, Sam showed at first no contact with depressive anxieties nor any kind of concern for the therapist. Fred, on the other hand, although being more encapsulated and avoidant of his persecutory anxieties, could show moments of affection, particularly with the development of his therapy, and even of striking insightfulness and thoughtfulness in the last stages of his treatment.

One way of interpreting this finding was that Sam's emotional functioning had the form of a to and fro between autistic functioning and strong paranoid features, with very little contact with depressive anxieties. Fred was clearly more encapsulated, with no structured paranoid defences, but with some underlying features of depression. It thus seemed that a small part of his personality which achieved some level of capacity for projection—and incipient introjection—could also put him in touch with hints of depressive anxieties. These elements were *there*, so to speak, waiting for the moment in which he, after facing more directly his paranoid fears and anger, would be able to develop them into some level of integration. Sam, on the other hand, was more in touch with a form of rough awareness of separation from his objects that involved massive intrusive identification. His personality was, however, less intensely dominated by adhesive mechanisms. Nevertheless, since his intrusive mechanisms were very rigidly established, there had been very little capacity for introjection, for concern for his objects, or for thinking, prior to his experience of psychotherapy. Moreover, since he did not suffer from Fred's inhibition of aggressiveness, he was by contrast at risk of developing antisocial tendencies.

It is important to note that, in these elaborations, I am taking into account Bion's important concept, following Freud, of the coexistence in every individual of psychotic and non-psychotic parts of the personality (Bion, 1967). Children on the autistic spectrum present to varying extents some level of psychotic and neurotic functioning in the same way that neurotic children—as well as adults—present not only psychotic but also *autistic nuclei* in their personalities, a phenomenon described by several authors—Sydney Klein (1980), Ogden (1989), Tustin (1986a, 1990a, 1990b), Winnicott (1974)—under slightly different names: autistic phenomena, autistic barriers, fear of breakdown, autistic enclaves, autistic pockets.

What therapy seemed to allow for these patients was, by freeing them from their terrors, a slow and progressive move from their rigidity and *stuckness* to a more dynamic to and fro between the parts of their personalities, which opened space for evolution, and for some level of recovery from an arrested development.

Conclusion

Dynamics of autistic states

The fluctuation in the children's emotional state and their use of language during their therapies demand some reflection. The sharp impoverishment of the mental and imaginative activity and of the emotional links with others which accompanies these states indicates, in Bion's terms, a deficit in α-function. In classically psychotic patients, this would mean an accumulation of β-elements, which are only manageable through evacuation. In these withdrawn patients, the normal processes of projection of β-elements through projective identification followed by re-introjection of these elements now digested by the mother's mental apparatus has not developed properly. The adhesive mechanisms employed by this part of the patient's personality do not allow the normal unfolding of the relationship between container and contained. The hypothesis is that these β-elements and the discomfort they could cause were not even acknowledged by these patients' perceptual apparatus: it is as if the β-elements were not there. This seems to be confirmed by the well-known increased tolerance or even indifference of autistic children to the experience of physical pain.

A sudden awareness of reality indicates that different capacities of the personality and different levels of development seem to coexist simultaneously even when the apparent picture is more evenly *flat*, as in Fred's case. We might then assume that some level of evacuation of β-elements, some level of exchange with the mother, and some introjection took place, leading to α-elements beginning to develop, even when this was minimal. This would then lead to the formation of scattered fragments of images, dispersed elements of a possible narrative, without α-function developed enough to integrate them into a meaningful whole.

The incipient formation of α-elements that residually underlies the overwhelming autistic condition can explain how some mute autistic children can suddenly start to speak sentences, or how Fred, from a formless mental state where words lacked context and content, could evolve to the structured and meaningful sentences quoted above. This would fall, in Bion's Grid, in the category of Dream-Thoughts.

It seems that, even where these processes were weakened so early on, their development can be at least partially resumed in the context of a therapeutic relationship with an analyst-container. Through the use the patient can make of the therapist's α-function, fragments can be transformed into meanings and crumbling and scattered bricks into tentative buildings. The analogy could be with film editing, when several dispersed scenes and sequences that, on their own would be lacking in meaning, are organized by an editor into a coherent whole. We could apply to our work what one of these professionals once said in a newspaper about his own, that *we repair other people's dreams*. When Fred's fragmented and dispersed language and mind were achieving cohesion in the context of an emotional link with the therapist, the anxiety about bodily fragmentation became experienced in all its terror and could be communicated to the therapist.

General formulation

1. Only a vocabulary of some sort can grant meaning to what is experienced through the senses. The pressure from this experience on the mental apparatus impels the development of a vocabulary to make sense of it.
2. Verbal language developed in due course can be the more sophisticated means of registering, remembering, and making sense of experience.
3. The possibility of these exchanges, which include projective identification as the more primitive form of communication, depends on the acknowledgement by the infant of his separateness from the mother's body and on the capacity to feel the experience of the sensory apparatus. Where this process is impaired, development of language and thinking is inhibited.
4. Psychoanalysis is in a privileged position to deal with this problem due to its nature as a particular language-game, which works on the boundaries and can link verbal language, bodily experience, and feelings.
5. Moments of withdrawal and of un-mentalized experience are present in every individual, corresponding to the limits of language. We could call these autistic nuclei, which will only interfere with a life of relatedness where they occupy a substantial proportion of the personality or exert a strong influence within it. In the case of autistic children, the autistic characteristics interfere with the development of the non-autistic part of the personality.
6. The move from an autistic refuge implies fully facing the catastrophic anxieties that were avoided until then. These are a primitive version of the persecutory anxieties described by Melanie Klein as typical of the paranoid-schizoid position. Depressive anxieties will then also have to be faced.
7. The *mindscapes* described by the children examined in this study, both in play and at a later stage in verbal communication, seemed to correspond to the characteristic anxieties and defences of the paranoid-schizoid and depressive positions, as well as of the lack of anxiety—accentuated in Fred—and the rigidity—noticeable in Sam—of an autistic refuge. Such mindscapes were for Fred called "desert", "jungle", and "garden", and for Sam "sticking machine", "mud puddle", and "green field".
8. During the psychotherapeutic work with these children, fluctuation was observed among the three mindscapes and the linguistic characteristics or dialects of each mindscape.

9. In a speculative way, we might compare these three mindscapes with the biblical myth of creation and the Christian depiction of Heaven, Hell, and Purgatory. In the Book of Genesis, God creates the heaven and the earth, the light, and all the creatures on the earth, and man formed from"the dust of the ground". Warning that man should not eat from the tree of the knowledge of good and evil, God makes woman from one of Adam's ribs. Tempted by the serpent, Eve and then, persuaded by her, Adam eat the fruit and are expelled from the Garden of Eden. Everything was peaceful when there was only Adam/Eden. The arrival of Eve as a separate being, despite the moments of delight, triggers catastrophe.

Although Christian doctrine implies that Purgatory is somewhere in-between Hell and Heaven, there might be another reading of the myth. It is when, out of the need for each other, Adam and Eve have intercourse that they are expelled from Eden. Their Fall presages the outcome of their relationship—the infant who will become mankind and human culture. Although they are banished from Paradise, they are no longer subject to the prohibition on being creative or thinking for themselves. We might call this Purgatory neither Heaven nor Hell. Their fall from Eden initiates a "brave new world"—the human world. Their progress is from Heaven through Hell to Purgatory, from the splendid self-sufficiency and isolation of narcissism, through the painful difficulties of relationships to the creative possibilities that relating also engenders. Once there is space between mother and infant for a third position, there is the capacity to observe and reflect: using my young patients' terminology, from "desert" through "jungle" to "garden"; in numerical terms, from one through two to three.

* * *

Tustin and Meltzer, when working with autism, came to realize that the previous formulations about the mental apparatus were not completely satisfactory for its understanding. As a result they opened a new field of exploration in psychoanalysis which provided tools not only to help these children and their families, but also to deeply enlighten our understanding of emotional development and human communication in general, and consequently refine our clinical approach. In this sense, autistic phenomena have in recent decades been a new vertex of thought which requires attention from psychoanalysts and psychotherapists.

Notes

1. The Autism Diagnostic Observation Schedule, first proposed by Lord, Rutter, Goode, et al. in 1989, is a semi-structured assessment of communication, social interaction, and play for individuals suspected of being in the autistic spectrum.

2. The Autism Diagnostic Interview, first proposed by Lord, Rutter, and LeCouteur in 1989 and revised in 1994, is a structured interview conducted with the parents of individuals who have been referred for the evaluation of possible autistic spectrum syndrome.

3. Fourth version of the Wechsler Intelligence Scale for Children, a cognitive-ability assessment of verbal comprehension, perceptual reasoning, working memory, and processing speed.

4. Here we are reminded of Tustin's mention of the traumatic disturbance in the infancy of autistic children of an early state of empathetic communion with the mother provided by the sensation of nipple-in-mouth in the suckling experience. What is left instead is an "unmourned sense of loss", the "black hole" described by her patient John (Tustin, 1966, 1986a, 1990b).

5. This was to be later confirmed, as will be shown in detail, by the reports from his mother and from the school.

6. This seems to relate to the anxieties that arise from moving from an autistic functioning, and an empty and half-alive space, the sense of a place where there is no certainty of having really being born, to the disturbed world of object-relations, with all the fears and anxieties of the paranoid-schizoid and depressive modes of functioning.

7. See, in relation to this, the paper "Sensory Aspects of Language Development in Relation to Primitive Anxieties" by Maria Rhode (2003).

CHAPTER FOUR

Curiouser and curiouser: researching the K link in psychoanalytic therapy

Emily Ryan

> In another moment, down went Alice ... never once considering how in the world she was to get out again.
>
> [Carroll, 1865, p. 1]

Like Alice's descent into Wonderland, for a clinician to attempt to research the unconscious through extra-clinical methods can feel like a headlong drop down a rabbit hole. You don't know what you'll find at the bottom, or even if there is a bottom. Unexpected discoveries send you off in altogether new directions. Frequently you find yourself blocked, and there are woeful moments when your limitations are starkly exposed. Yet the only way out seems to be to keep going, in the hope that you may find a key that can take you over a threshold and open up new perspectives on the questions that you have set out to explore.

In this chapter, I describe such a piece of research, based on a single case study of psychoanalytic therapy with a young ADHD boy in care, whom I call "Simon". I started with the idea of using theorized thematic analysis, a branch of grounded theory, as an approach to tracking the unconscious dynamics in the therapy to understand better Simon's internal situation and the shifts that took place in our work together. This involved close scrutiny of the clinical record and the evolution of a research methodology that could map the moment-to-moment dance between therapist and patient at a number of levels simultaneously.

Setting out, I did not think that my search for a conceptual key to guide the research would take me deep into Bion's theoretical thinking and ideas from complexity theory; that it would be an emotional journey, as well as an intellectual one; that I, like Alice, would have to think—sometimes painfully—as two persons, as the therapist immersed in the work and as the researcher at one-step remove.

Nor did I anticipate that this approach to the clinical record would yield such convincing evidence of Bion's claim, repeated by Britton and Fisher, that in psychic development the drive to Know stands on a par with Love and Hate as a primary and foundational force. By extension, the findings would add to the growing case for relational therapy for severely traumatized ADHD children like Simon, in place of more narrow medical treatment and behaviour management.

The patient

The research was motivated and shaped by a clinical experience with a particular patient, the first whom I saw in intensive treatment as a child psychotherapy trainee. It was my concern to understand him and the therapeutic relationship with him that led me to Bion, rather than a theoretical interest in Bion driving the research. Perhaps, with another patient, a different conceptual approach might have been indicated.

A brief description of Simon at the start of therapy may help to explain what I mean. I am choosing to say little about Simon's history before referral. Suffice it to say that his early abuse and presenting problems are shared by many children seen in CAMHS who are living in the care system. In this regard, he figures as a representative of a "family" of children with whom many child psychotherapists are familiar and whose levels of stress, aggression, and hyperactivity place huge demands on them, their carers, and the professionals who work with them.

When he was referred to me aged 11 years, Simon's behaviour had just dipped sharply with the move to secondary school. Both his school and foster placements were at risk. After two terms of weekly sessions, during which the situation deteriorated and there was a very violent incident at home, Simon began intensive therapy; he was then aged 12. At the same time he was diagnosed with ADHD and put on medication.

An extract from a session 15 months into intensive therapy, on the eve of an Easter break, illustrates some of the core features of Simon at this time. It also conveys his therapist's struggle with rigid, defensive thinking aroused by the sadistic, depriving identifications projected into her, and the inflammatory impact of her interpretations.

The session begins with Simon pushing boundaries by bringing food into the room and protesting his therapist's request that he leave it until the end of the session.

> He gets out the calendar we have been making and says with a flourish that he's going to mark off his first session—"now there are just nine left before Easter!" I comment that it sounds like he feels that's not much. Simon responds for a moment in a more ordinary voice, saying yeah, actually he can't believe it's only nine sessions until the holiday …
>
> He switches to his more hectoring voice to ask me what it was that we were playing the previous session. When I don't respond to this, he persists, louder—"Go on, tell me!" … Then he follows with another aggressive question—"And did you find out the May Bank Holiday dates?" I say that I haven't done this yet. "Why not? I bet you forgot, didn't you!"
>
> He has already repeatedly smashed his water cup against the table, spilling his water, and now picks a pencil out of his box and hurls it viciously against the far wall. I comment that he really wants to throw and smash things today, it looks like he is choosing things that will make a mess. I link this to him bringing in his nougat bar, knowing that I would object to this, and then going on to make a show of eating it, as if he was perhaps looking to get us into a fight. "Yeah", agrees Simon with emphasis. I suggest he wants to have a go at me today, and I wonder what he thinks this is about. Simon replies he just wants to play, that's all.

There follows an escalating attack on his therapist with paper planes and pellets.

> He orders me not to look at him, to turn my chair round and face the wall. I say I think he finds it very difficult when I look at him or speak to him when he's feeling like this. He comes across the room, saying if I don't move my chair, then he will! When he lays hands on the arm, I tell him to leave it be. He gives it a tug and says "Or what, what will you do, uh?" Then walks away.
>
> If I speak, he tells me to shut up, he's not listening. He talks about leaving early—he's got a party to go to at 6.30 and then at quarter to seven—he pauses, "What am I doing at quarter to seven …?" He stares at me, repeating his question over and over again, growing more strident. He starts twirling the cars around on the table, smashing them into each other, then hurling them as hard as he can across the room, making a tremendous and violent racket, every now and again shooting me a contemptuous look.

> "Don't cry!" he jeers, then breaks into a parody of crying, repeating this at different intervals. It feels horribly painful and hopeless.

The therapist is pelted with more, and harder, objects.

> I warn him that if he goes on throwing things at me, we will have to finish for today. He turns and throws them hard at the wall, then gets together two pencils. He drops them on the floor and orders me to "say goodbye to the pencils". When I don't respond, he repeats it louder each time, as he treads on the pencils and kicks them to the door, pushing them underneath. He opens the door to get them back and lined up again, before kicking them outside again. I talk about his feeling that he is getting closer and closer to getting himself "kicked out".

There is a brief return to vestiges of more friendly play, which collapses after a few seconds.

> He spots the wobbly table leg, kicking and tugging it, saying "it's broken, see!" He says any minute now I'm going to tell him it's time, and wants me to tell him exactly how many seconds he has left. When I respond that it's not long and I'll let him know when, he grabs my wrist, forcing it round to see my watch. I tell him to let me go. He jumps to his feet and goes to stand by the door. I tell him it is now time. He picks up some pens off the floor, saying "Freedom at last!" turns to throw them across the room, pulls open the door and turns off the light. I am left in darkness, with everything in the room spilt and overturned.

Simon came three times a week for two years and finally ended therapy aged 15. Therapy fell roughly into two phases: a repetitive/destructive phase of just over two years, and a phase of change/growth during the year and a half that followed. By the end of therapy, there had been significant improvements. There were no longer concerns about placement breakdown, and he had developed some friendships. He had been off ADHD medication for 10 months and off report at school for a term. He went on to get a good handful of GCSEs at C grade and above.

Identifying potential themes

The current research takes its general methodological principles from thematic analysis: "a method for identifying, analysing and reporting patterns (themes) within data" (Braun & Clarke, 2006, p. 79). Thematic analysis has much in common with grounded theory, but without the aim of developing theory out of data analysis. It postulates various stages in the research process, grounded in repeated examinations of the research data with a view to gradually refining a set of themes and the relations between them, with which to structure an analysis and final write-up of the clinical data.

> A theme captures something important about the data in relation to the research question, and represents some level of patterned response or meaning within the data set. (Braun & Clarke, 2006, p. 82)

The first stage of this process in the current study may be regarded as the review of detailed session material that resulted in the clinical paper on my patient, written for qualification purposes. The paper, based on transcripts of the 72 sessions written up for supervision during Simon's treatment, thus identified a research focus and what Braun and Clarke call a core group of "*candidate themes*" with which to revisit the data items in a more systematic way.

I summarized themes from the first phase of his therapy as follows:

» his appetite and destructiveness—constant messing and the consumption/spoiling of large amounts of materials;
» his attacks on the therapy and the sadomasochistic quality of his relationship with me;
» his intrusive, controlling behaviour;
» his concrete thinking and enactment in sessions;
» the inflammatory impact of interpretations;
» my own struggle with rigid, defensive thinking aroused by the sadistic, depriving identifications projected into me.

The second phase of therapy had different themes:

» lively, experimental playfulness began to develop;
» there was an increase in word play and imaginative interactive play;
» more reflective moments;
» a growing tolerance and reciprocity in the relationship.

As these themes began to take shape, I was drawn back to Bion's writing in two areas: first, his argument that thinking begins and takes shape in an emotional experience; and, second, his linking of symbolic capacity with emotional experiences of communication and containment. Would these ideas help make sense of Simon's presenting problems, given his early deprivation, and help me to research the change in his capacity to think/communicate with me during therapy?

Thinking as emotional process: the K link

Bion stressed the role of the parent in the child's development of symbolic function, communication, and thinking capacity. He expanded Klein's theory of projective processes in psychic development, to place projective identification at the heart of infantile communication. In giving her mind to her infant's earliest projections, the mother treats them as actions with meaning, which tell her about her child's internal state. The baby experiences its mother's understanding response as transformative. Its yell of hunger, which may first be aimed at physical expulsion of nameless all-encompassing torment, is, when understood and met by a soothing voice-and-breast, contained and made manageable. Bion emphasizes that it is not just milk that the infant then takes in, but an experience of an understanding mind, through whose operation something nameless finds an identity. If the mother gets it right, the baby's need is met—the hungry mouth finds the feeding breast—and then the baby has an experience of satisfaction. Bion described this as the baby's preconception of the breast meeting up with real breast and so acquiring shape and form. When a preconception meets with the necessary counterpart, a conception—or thought—is formed. Now the child is able to recognize what it seeks and, step by step, develops its own capacity to make sense of its experience and communicate it to others.

In Bion's view, the epistemophilic instinct is an emotional force in psychic development that stands on a par with Love and Hate and is not a derivative of them. Humans are born with an innate drive to find out, which is rooted in the drive to know and be known by another human mind. On this view, "the experience of knowing someone or something must express an emotional experience that can stand alongside the experience of loving someone or hating someone or something" (Fisher, 2011, p. 43). Truth, beginning in the area of such an emotional experience with another, is as important to psychic growth as nutrition is to physical development.[1]

> Being deprived of the truth of one's emotional experience is a kind of starvation since truth is essential for psychic health. [Fisher, 2011, p. 48, paraphrasing Bion 1962b/1984, p. 310]

Bion describes the process of getting to know and be known by another human mind as the K link. Thinking is thus "an emotional experience of trying to know oneself or someone else. … If xKy, the 'x is in the state of getting to know y and y is in a state of getting to be known by x'" (O'Shaughnessy, 1981/1988, p. 178). K develops "from emotional experiences with a nurturing object, functioning normally on the reality principle" (O'Shaughnessy, 1981/1988, p. 180)

It follows that infant thinking is contingent from the outset on the emotional quality of the parent–infant relationship. Where containment is "commensal", mother and infant "are dependent on each other for mutual benefit and without harm to either … the mother derives benefit and achieves mental growth from the experience: the infant likewise abstracts benefit and achieves growth" (Bion, 1962a, p. 91). The mother's K activity in this situation is internalized by the infant, leading to the growth of a K capacity in the baby. Bion sees such growth to occur within a climate where doubt can be tolerated and equates it with a developing capacity to learn from experience. It represents "the state of mind of the individual who can retain his knowledge and experience and yet be prepared to reconstrue past experiences in a manner that enables him to be receptive of a new idea" (Bion, 1962a, p. 93). A person in a K frame of mind, centred on a nurturing object, may be open to interactions with another, show curiosity, tolerate difference and uncertainty, and have freedom in associating ideas and experiences.

Impact of deprivation on cognitive and symbolic function: the concept of minus K

Where the container–contained relationship is what Bion termed "parasitic", mother and infant are involved in interactions characterized by misunderstanding, envious attack, and fragmentation. Bion considers many psychological disorders to spring from such an inversion of the K link, denoted minus K, when a person is under pressure to use his mind to attack/misunderstand links because these are felt to endanger the ego. Minus K can end in the collapse of K, when a person's mental activity becomes excessively concrete or fragmented (denoted "no K" by O'Shaughnessy, 1981).

In a parasitic container–contained relationship, instead of internalizing a capacity for tolerance of pain and self-reflection, the child internalizes the capacities of a "mindless" parent, who experiences the child's pain as an assault and acts to repel it, often through a counterattack on the child. The excessive mental pain of this experience adds emotional charge to the child's difficulty in thinking, giving it the quality of active resistance: the child clings to mindlessness because awareness is too painful.[2] Such a person is not curious to "know" himself or his object in the ordinary way, through "a human link—the endeavour to understand, comprehend the reality of, get insight into the nature of oneself or someone else" (O'Shaughnessy, 1981, p. 181). Instead, he substitutes the human link with something mechanical and indifferent; or, more extremely, he develops an increasingly violent and bizarre relationship with the world, which is imagined as peopled with animist objects hostile to the self.[3]

Bion observes that K is a process, not a fixed state of affairs, and attempts to capture or freeze K moments are doomed to failure: insight turns to dogma, "knowing" turns defensive, and K becomes minus K. K dynamics thus correspond closely with the oscillation between paranoid-schizoid and depressive states of mind, represented by Bion as Ps↔D.[4] Expanding this concept, Britton (1989) notes that such oscillation gives psychic development its structure, and it is when the subject becomes fixed in one or other position that thinking becomes pathological.

Minus K can then take the form of a "psychic retreat" to a pathological form of mental functioning, as a defence against unbearable psychic pain and anxiety (Britton, 1989; Steiner, 1993):

> [The patient regresses] to a ready-made, previously espoused coherent belief system ... to end uncertainty and the fears associated with fragmentation. [Britton, 1998, p. 72]

Simon, for instance, appeared to cling tenaciously to a "self-righteous state of chronic grievance" (Britton, 1998, p. 80) which—while severely restricting his contact with others—appeared to offer a psychic refuge from mental pain or a psychic container for holding things together.

Sampling the data items to refine themes

With these thoughts in mind, I turned to wondering whether the powerful concepts of K and minus K might provide the conceptual key with which to study Simon's progress in therapy and, in particular, the notable shift in his capacity to experiment with new ways of relating and to interact with me at an imaginative, symbolic level.

Two sample sessions were selected to get my thinking started. These sessions were chosen not at random, but because they were particularly representative of the sorts of behaviour and interactions I had identified, from among the 72 sessions, to contrast therapy at the beginning and end of treatment.[5] I reasoned that a study of the themes emerging in each of these sessions would then provide a useful template for approaching other sessions from the data items.[6]

Mapping process

I wanted the map of each session to track, for external inspection, the detail of interactions in the therapy room, and to be a means of following the conscious and unconscious processes at work between patient and therapist. Following Philips (2003), I divided each session record into a number of data extracts, or episodes of interaction between patient and therapist. Each episode comprised an act (or short sequence of acts/ communications) from the patient, evidencing his internal relationship to the therapist at that moment (transference projections) and sparking an internal reaction, a response (or sequence of these), from the therapist, which may or may not have been registered consciously and communicated back to the patient (countertransference identifications). The sequence had an outcome that could be read in what happened next between the two—that is, the content of the subsequent episode.

Analysis of data extracts

Using this method, data analysis began with a summary description of each episode or data extract, in terms of the dominant transference and countertransference activity (see Box 4.1).

Once the episodes had been clearly summarized, a secondary layer of themes could be examined in relation to the data. As the interest lay in examining the dynamic interplay of transference and countertransference states of mind, both patient and therapist aspects of each episode were classified. To start with, I used categories derived from Philps (2003).

However, I felt that I was not getting to the very primitive emotional dynamics of the interaction between Simon and me that seemed to characterize this particular therapy. I went on to experiment with a second matrix informed by child development research and the work of the Boston Study Group (Bruschweiler-Stern et al., 2002). I particularly liked their attention to the "local dynamics" of therapeutic interactions—a concept drawing on the unspoken, emotional, attunement-seeking activity described by infant observation research in mother–baby studies. Here the same categories are applied to both members of the dyad, so capturing the dance-like quality of the interaction. Their analysis also gave me a useful way of differentiating between types of activity between therapist and patient and linking this to processes of psychic change. I began to explore the interactions

Box 4.1 Summary description of each episode or data extract

Episode#	*Data extract*	*Summary*
3	There is a pause while he stands at the table and skids paper balls down it and into the bin. He adds a few planes, giving me a look and asking me if they are going in the bin.	P[atient] retreats to play, testing/checking T [herapist]'s readiness to follow him. Can T provide containment?
	I say that some are and some aren't. I add that I think it is very hard for him, not knowing how long he is going to be able to come here, and perhaps he thinks I'll be making these decisions without thinking about it with him, as if he'll have no say and could be just chucked out from one day to the next.	T registers the play but makes bid to return focus to uncertainty of therapy, and P's doubts about her commitment to holding a space for him.
4	His response is to round on me with a familiar question about who's the boss here, is it Mary or me or Jane? I say it's important to him to know who's in charge—he chips in to say Babette has told him Jane's in charge of one side of things, and Mary and I work on the other, so is that right?	P rejects T's redirection and signals issues of trustworthiness need to be addressed. Whose side is T on?
	I say I suppose it is about people doing different things and it all working together, but I think for him, he does feel someone has to be in charge.	T acknowledges importance to P of someone being in charge but misses link to here-and-now uncertainty.

between Simon and me in terms of mutual regulatory interaction, present moments, now moments, and moments of meeting. Subcategories of mutual regulatory interaction in the context of our relationship yielded a promising framework, allowing me differentiations with which to interrogate more closely what was going on between us at different moments:

negotiating, struggling, missing and repairing, mid-course correcting, scaffolding, and signalling. It drew my attention to the difficulties that Simon and I had in the first phase of therapy, in finding alignment with one another or establishing a shared space for being together, and to the severe limits of the comfort zone for interaction available to us at that time.

Yet trying to convert the nuanced variety of our positions, feelings, defences, and communications into a finite list of descriptors was not ultimately helpful to my study. I realized I needed an approach that allowed for flexibility and nuance and could capture the multiple levels/meanings—not always pointing in the same direction—of any one action and communication in the interplay.

This involved abandoning fixed descriptors as subcategories. Instead, I turned to thinking about a matrix that could be broad and abstract enough to encompass a range of multi-dimensional interactions, yet provide enough of a structure for the different strands of Simon's difficulties to be studied in relation to one another.

The basics of Bion's theory of thinking appeared to provide the appropriate conceptual principles for such a matrix, by placing thinking—his K and minus-K activity—in dynamic relation to Simon's emotional experience with his therapist. The aspects of my patient that had emerged as candidate themes were well organized by this approach, since they conceptually hypothesized a link between Simon's destructive repetitive behaviour, his difficulty in thinking and symbolic representation, his use of projection to communicate, and his need for his therapist to engage at a primitive emotional level to provide containment.

Each episode in the session was thus studied in relation to five categories:

1. A summary of the transference–countertransference interaction for patient and therapist. *Narrative memo*
2. Dominant self and other identifications in the process. *Identifications*
3. The primary emotional state active in patient and therapist during the interaction. *Feelings*
4. The responses/defences employed by patient and therapist during the interaction. *Defences/responses*
5. The K content of the interaction. *K content*

The tabular grid that resulted provided a framework for capturing and organizing data regarding the four salient features of this particular patient at the start of therapy—namely, his harsh inner-world persecutory feelings and identifications (1, 2, 3), paranoid-schizoid defences (4), and limited symbolic function (5). At an intrapsychic level, I had an opportunity to view the processes in each area unfolding side by side through a series of contemporaneous "snapshots" and thus a tool for finding repeated associative patterns, linking, for instance, shifts in Simon's emotional state or object representations to variations in his symbolic function from moment to moment. By including a corresponding focus on the therapist, it allowed me to consider the interpsychic dimension—that is, the therapist's part in reinforcing or challenging the patient's position, and how aspects of her own internal emotional, defensive, and K processes were active in shaping her patient's capacity for K at different moments. It was possible to pick out the different sorts of containment and projective identification active between therapist and patient and how these emerged in the modes of K link from moment to moment. The core of my research became a detailed reconstruction of each session based on this prior deconstruction of the interaction.[7]

Example of deconstruction/reconstruction process—session from Phase 1 of therapy

A sample from the final grid analysis shows its application to the ninth and tenth episode of clinical material from the Phase 1 session (see Appendix 4.1). Here, I illustrate how the elements identified in the grid were subsequently re-joined as building blocks to make a descriptive narrative of the episodes.

Episode 9/Phase 1 session

> The pen tops are thrown carelessly into the box, and Simon goes to the little table, near where I am sitting. He grabs hold of the toy basket and then turns to ask me if the wooden cars are in it. I say I think he is in a better place to see than I am. "No, but are they?" he wants to know, then turns back to rummage in the basket, complaining that they aren't there. After a few moments, he unearths the red one, then fishes out the blue and the green. I comment on him wanting me to know and find them for him. He pulls some fat felt-tips out of the basket and tells me he can send them flying across the room, demonstrating.

Reconstructed narrative

Simon moves closer to his therapist, telling her he needs her help to see things. He identifies with a helpless child without resources/

capacities. The rubbishing of the pens and rough grab at the toy basket carry an aggressive edge—as his assumed helplessness (he cannot see the toys) holds an accusation against a depriving mother. His therapist has become identified with a parent who, he hopes, holds something good for him, overlaid with the idea of a parent who refuses him.

His therapist is sensitive to his resentful, accusatory feelings, identifying with a beleaguered mother figure fending off a demanding, greedy child. She responds concretely with a refusal, missing the real need now symbolically equated with the vanished toys, as well as Simon's hope of finding a helpful parent in her; so, unconsciously, she falls into identification with the depriving mother projected into her. Simon experiences her reaction as a spurning of his needy self and redoubles his demand. His difficulty finding the toys he wants seems to express the difficulty he is having getting something good from the therapist—does she have something to give him or not? His complaint that the cars aren't there conveys the grievance of a child whose mother turns out to be disappointingly unavailable to look after his needs, to keep things safe over absences. His therapist draws attention to his neediness without being able to link it up with its counterpart—the disappointed hope of being accepted and understood. Simon's anger and despair at the breakdown in communication is evident in his retreat to body thinking and expulsion of messy destructive feelings in the treatment of the pens that follows.

In this episode, Simon shows his desire for K, which he experiences as lacking in himself and located in his therapist. His therapist's identification with the bad object prevents her picking up on the hope he is expressing and stifles K. Instead, she amplifies the splitting and aggression that accompany his projection, treating it as an attempt to expel responsibility rather than as an infantile attempt at communication via projective identification. Some fundamental misattunement is apparent between the two.

Episode 10/Phase 1 session

> I talk about so many things getting thrown around today. He sets the cars up on the little table and starts a game, which begins with the Sellotape roll crashing into them. When it goes off the table and flies across the room, he asks me to fetch it for him. When I don't obey, he abandons the roll and starts smashing the cars into each other, again and again, until one or other of them is pushed off the table. Occasionally he adds a few plastic or wooden bricks. It is repetitive and empty.

Reconstructed narrative

For a moment, the therapist is able to recognize the destructive turmoil engulfing the session and acknowledge it without immediately attributing it to Simon: something is happening in the room today, and observation is all she can offer at present. In response, Simon's activity acquires more play-like features—less an evacuation and more a concrete symbolisation of the situation between him and his therapist, a repetitive cycle of battering and collapsing contacts, as represented by the Sellotape ball and pens. Cutting across this scenario of connective torment between self and object, his request (or is it a demand?) for his therapist to retrieve the pieces/pens signals a renewed hope of finding a parent figure who can help him do something with the needy, aggressive feelings consuming him.

The therapist's deafness to the hopes conveyed by his demand show her still in the grip of an identification with a tormented/tormenting mother. Her refusal to meet Simon's demand pushes him back into his primary scenario, where relationship is figured as perpetual entrapment and conflict between a rivalrous, unreceptive self and other. He retreats to a physical bashing/expulsion of toy cars and other objects with only a vestigial resemblance to play.

K appears frail and fluctuating during this episode—the sort of K that might be common at Ps moments in the constant Ps ↔ D motion, which Bion used to describe the process of thinking. The therapist's fleeting K at the start lies in her negative capability to tolerate a situation of emotional turmoil that she cannot read. Simon's responsive K is again operating at the level of infantile projective identification. The strong Ps identifications on either side overwhelm both K moments: the therapist cannot pick up on Simon's K, seeing his play and the demand on her to pick up the pieces as a disavowal of his own capacity to think and his attempt to control her, rather than as an effort to communicate and explore an experience through her. Her misattunement demolishes Simon's nascent hope of finding K in his object, as shown by the collapse of his rudimentary game into concrete body thinking, with the mindless, repetitive quality of no K.

Example of deconstruction/reconstruction process—session from Phase 2 of therapy

So far I have only cited clinical material from Phase 1 of Simon's therapy. The following extracts come from a session in Phase 2 and illustrate some of the ways in which Simon's internal situation changed during the course of our work.

Therapist and patient were contending with two external events in the session: a change in timing, involving an early morning start, and the forthcoming reduction from three to two sessions a week, planned to follow the next holiday break. Themes of change, new contact, loss, and abandonment were prevalent, often working in counterpoint through the session.

Episode 9/Phase 2 session

> Simon says he's hungry, can't he go and get something to eat or fetch a drink. I say that he needs to wait until the end of the session. He comes over to the cushions beside my chair, grabbing a blanket and saying that he's going to sleep now—bye. He curls up on the chair across the room, as I comment on his wish to sleep through the last bit of the session. He talks about wishing he could go to the kitchen and put something in the microwave—the microwave would say "hello".

Reconstructed narrative

Simon signals his conflicting impulses, as he moves close to and then away from his therapist, as if wanting both more and less contact. The pull is to sleep, to exchange the live relationship with her for a more familiar, mechanical interaction, kept at a physical level (the feeding mother turned into a microwave). Yet his words suggest that the familiar may also be subtly changing—the world of inanimate objects is showing signs of life as he imagines the microwave saying "hello". His running commentary shows a wish to keep his therapist with him, hinting that this might not be a retreat from a hostile object but more like a rest in the safe care of a benign parental figure.

The therapist is in touch with the needy child Simon and, while holding the session boundary, is not pulled into identification with a depriving parent. She is receptive to his wish to rest. Her commentary is low-key, descriptive, signalling her availability while allowing space for Simon's thoughts and responses to unfold.

Awareness of loss and hunger are present but seem to be contained in the episode; they do not lead to a rupture; with his therapist's help, Simon is able to communicate the feelings in words without immediately evacuating them in action (he wants to go but is able to stay).

Likewise, the therapist can tolerate his need to take a break and follow his lead without defensive, foreclosing interpretation. The shift to more benign identifications and tolerance of limitations fosters the capacity for K in both, as evidenced in Simon's fluid, free-ranging associations and his therapist's attuned combination of low-key limit-setting and reflective observation. The emerging attunement between them recalls times in the pattern of early infantile K interactions: the moments where a mother allows and protects a space for her child to rest and digest between physical–emotional feeds.

Episode 10/Phase 2 session

> I wonder if this has something to do with his wish for a world of talking machines. Simon starts talking in a robotic, Dalek voice. I am not to confuse him for a human being, he says—robots aren't human and don't like being muddled up. I ask what robots do, what makes them different from humans? He replies that he cooks, cleans, drives … as I begin to say these all sound quite human, he adds that he can write a dictionary in a few minutes, and that robots don't have feelings, they aren't curious. He follows this with a robotic question and I point out that it sounds like this robot is curious after all. Simon says robots aren't alive, they are just a jumble of metal parts. He reels off a robot identity number, then adds "aka[8] Simon". I ask what they are, if they aren't alive. He hesitates and then says robots are dead. I talk about them being neither alive nor dead, perhaps? Simon says he is going to sleep until Monday. I think about him wanting to sleep his way over the weekend break, until his next session.

Reconstructed narrative

The therapist's opening comment is dreamy, meditative, playful, and Simon responds with a fresh flow of associations, keeping the contact going and expanding it. He plays with his own and his therapist's words, to draw out a thought. The play describes and explores the part of him that prefers a robotic identity—which wants to kill off curiosity and the capacity to feel emotion—to human contact. Yet the sequence seems to show him in identification with the robot's opposite: a lively, engaging child enjoying play with a receptive, responsive parent figure. The mention of sleep at the end of the episode may be, at one level, a response to the emotional effort of being in a live relationship, moving out of an old identity into unfamiliar territory. The robot's declared renunciation of life and meaning is slipping, and Simon's hesitation hints that he doesn't know what the alternative might be, if not death. Sleep, the giving up of consciousness, with its conflicts and uncertainties, beckons. At another level, the idea of sleep (lasting until his next session) could hold the fantasy of unbroken contact with his therapist, an infantile world where the child falls asleep, dreams, and wakes, out of a certainty in its mother's presence, a world where he does not have to experience the pain of separation, or of being on his own.

Simon's therapist supports this process with her own reverie, supplying words, questions, and associations to scaffold the emerging play. She slips into Simon's idiom of the robot, which flows from her opening association to a world of talking machines. The following dialogue acquires the quality of unfolding make-believe, creating an imaginative space for thought and feeling at one remove from reality. She observes how the Simon–robot is struggling with feelings of curiosity that it wants to disown; that it appears to exist uncertainly in a no-man's land, where things are neither alive nor dead. The therapist's ready responsiveness to the play evidences her unconscious attunement to the lively child directing it and her identification with a playful maternal figure. The same attunement is apparent in the ease with which she follows Simon's lead in switching out of the robot identity, to interpret his wish to lose the weekend break in sleep.

The dialogue in this episode is lively, with creativity and responsiveness in both patient and therapist. Persecutory anxiety has dropped into the background. They seem thoroughly engaged with one another, the mood is playful, tolerant, allowing ideas to flow and develop freely between them. K in this aspect is an experience bringing mutual enjoyment. A space has opened up for imagination and symbolic communication, reflected in Simon's new-found power to play with words. Likewise, acting (the make-believe quality of Simon–robot) has begun to take over from enactment. As in the previous episode, the interaction between patient and therapist has traces of the infantile quality of early mother–child explorations and is rounded by a pause to rest.

Episode 11/Phase 2 session

I call him "aka Simon" and Simon switches to being another robot, feigning ignorance of its predecessor—"Who said that? Who is aka Simon?" I suggest this robot has wiped its memory, as Simon does, too, sometimes, denying he's ever had a certain thought, or an experience we've shared gets obliterated. "No", says the new robot Simon, repeating this to each of my comments. I tease him about becoming a "No" robot, a one-word machine. We play with "no" and "know". I wonder if there's also a wish to be someone who doesn't—can't—make mistakes ...?

Reconstructed narrative

The play continues in the same vein as the previous episode, as the pair explore Simon's way of cutting off, disowning, his own experience and memories and attacking links. Play offers them a means of displacement so that the painful reality can be kept at a tolerable distance. The primary identifications of lively child and playful maternal figure hold good through the episode. The therapist picks up Simon's phrase "aka Simon", and Simon joins her in elaborating its meaning, through acting out the role of a robot that has many guises but no sense of self. A private language is evolving out of the interaction of free-flowing associations. The pair end up with the "no"/"know" play, bringing Simon's habitual denial, evasion of relatedness ("no") into humorous juxtaposition with the constraints on his freedom to think and explore ("know"). At another level, it may be that an underlying anxiety around allowing space for mistakes and misattunements—hinted at in previous episodes and active in both Simon and his therapist—is sparked into awareness.

Again, the episode is full of active K. The level of attunement and engagement remains high. Issues of control have been replaced by a receptive and creative interplay of ideas, where patient and therapist partner each other, insight and interpretation building off one another. Symbolic communication is enhanced, words acquire new layers of meaning, and some unconscious aspects of the therapy relationship are made available for reflection in a powerful and immediate way.

Secondary analysis

I am now going to discuss how I analysed the resulting narrative and briefly summarize the findings it produced in one of several areas explored in the research. I illustrate its potential as a research method for expanding understanding of my patient and of theoretical concepts like K.

I found it useful to study my material in three strands.[9]

First strand: isolating features of K and minus K

A first strand of study was to review the session narrative resulting from the deconstruction/reconstruction-by-episode process, noting emerging themes in each session. For example, in the first session sampled above, I picked up on the emerging features of K in relation to primitive paranoid-schizoid modes of functioning. I noted how, from a research position, it was possible to distinguish, across different episodes in the session, signs of K amidst opposing trends of minus K and no K. Yet, perhaps because paranoid-schizoid thinking has both a developmental and anti-developmental thrust at different stages and the therapist in this case was inexperienced and anxious, the signs of K in Simon were not always obvious to his therapist at the time.[10] In Episode 9, for example, Simon's search for K took an aggressive and controlling form, and his therapist mistook it for minus K. The concreteness of his demand suggested to her a wish to split off and deny his thinking self, forcing the therapist to take responsibility for it. She was unreceptive to the exploratory aspect of his projection and his wish for her help, which, in itself, was evidence of a new thought, barely formed, of a figure who might be available for him, help him to discover missing parts of himself. Simon was functioning at a level of projective identification and symbolic equation of an infantile kind in this episode, while his therapist was responding to him as a more mature ego in possession of a developed symbolic function. In other episodes, too, I found that concreteness, enactment, and literal thinking were frequent markers of a collapse of K in the therapist but often carried seeds of curiosity and unconscious linking in Simon.

By contrast, the themes to emerge from a review of the second session were very different. Paranoid-schizoid modes of relating had receded, and K was evidenced in the spontaneous evolution of ideas and language between Simon and therapist. Paraphrasing Ogden (1999, p. 230):

> certainty [has given way] … to tendency, knowledge … to a tentative, ever-sliding sense of things, fixity … to movement and transition.

The therapist had relaxed her rigid grip on analytic "technique", and her use of commentary was no longer controlling but had become descriptive, associative, grounded in emotional experience shared with her patient. She took up his words, playing with meaning in relation to the history between them, as in Episode 11, when she found in Simon's robot play a representation of his compulsion to disconnect and deny shared experience.

On Simon's side, the shift in K had other markers. The session maps his growing tolerance of separateness and frustration, which, in turn, allowed the later play sequences time to extend and evolve; there was a corresponding flowering in Simon's symbolization and symbolic communication. The continuity of play in Episodes 10 and 11 was in marked contrast to the staccato rhythm of the early sessions, when differences in meaning and understanding between Simon and therapist often halted an interaction. In the robot play, there was an acceptance and enjoyment in their different ways of taking up words, Simon tolerated the therapist's interpretative commentary, and it was elaborated into further play.

Seven or eight such emerging themes were identified in each session. My work to draw them out was key to isolating features of K-states-of-mind and their converse, which I gathered into a pair of modified quadrant graphs (Figures 4.1 and 4.2), corresponding to the two sessions.

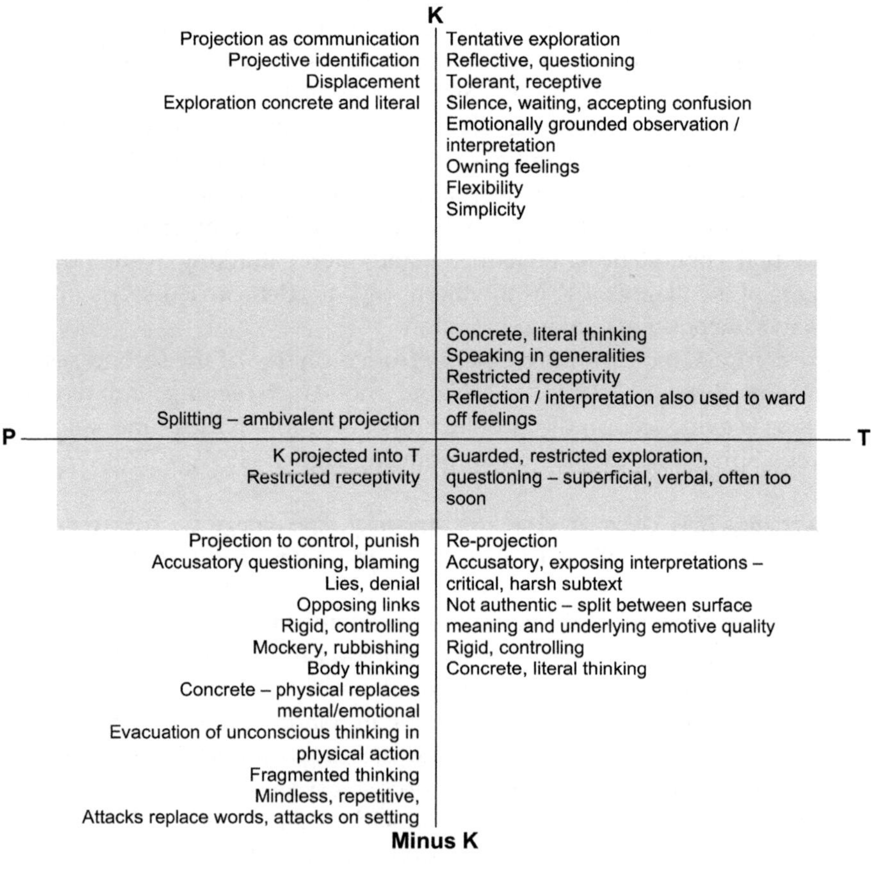

Figure 4.1 K states of mind and their converse for Session 1.

K

P	T
Curiosity Exploratory play / playfulness Imaginative free association Feelings/intentions owned Free flow and interplay of ideas, creative use of other, enriched communication / language Shift from control to partnering Digestive rests Attentive readiness / orientation to other Accepting of confusion/deficits Projective identification used to explore Active, discriminatory thinking Repetition to repair – sustain exploration Self reflection Increased awareness/acceptance of reality/limits/separateness Increased awareness/tolerance of warded-off parts Symbolisation / acting / "as if" replaces enactment Shift from two-dimensional to three-dimensional (from splitting to repression?)	Curiosity Exploratory playfulness Imaginative free association – reverie Feelings/intentions owned Free flow and interplay of ideas, creative use of other, enriched communication / language Shift from control to partnering Tolerance of digestive rests Attentive readiness / orientation to other Accepting of confusion / deficits Emotionally-grounded observation Descriptive, questioning commentary Adaptive pacing, prosody, use of displacement – responsive to P Flexibility Simplicity Tolerant, receptive – open – enhanced empathy Increased alignment / integration of conscious and unconscious identifications Non-persecutory boundary-keeping
Wary, cramped receptivity Vigilance limits receptivity Tentative equivocal readiness for change Suspicious exploration through projection	Wary, cramped receptivity Vigilance limits receptivity Interpretation to ward off uncertainty, evasive verbalisation restricts exploration Suspicion restricts exploration
Exploration turns literal, concrete to ward off uncertainty / aggression Use of symbolic equation to test for missing K	Rigidity interferes with exploration
Attack on change Denial and projection of disturbance Attack on thinking through physical enactment Envy Manic fragmentation Denial of separateness, via invasion, symbolic equation and projective identification Mockery, ridicule to punish, control Denial of meaning	Accusatory, exposing commentary / interpretation – critical, harsh subtext

Minus K

Figure 4.2 K states of mind and their converse for Session 2.

The graphs were organized around two axes, where the vertical line represents the continuum K to minus K and the horizontal differentiates patient from therapist. The shaded area midway between the K and minus-K poles indicates the area of slippage, which I label "restricted/defended K": this is the region of ambivalent, two-way-facing communications where K curiosity and the wish to know jostle for advantage with minus-K influences (particularly envy and anxiety).

The figures represented in graphic form my finding that K and minus K were not so much separated by a rigid barrier, as processes that could be seen to shade into one another; at times, communications wavered uncertainly between one and the other. Studying such a state of mind, it was not always easy to know who was doing what, where identifications originated, what was projection with an exploratory purpose, and what was projection as defence. Restricted/defended K emerged as an area of psychic confusion.

Second strand: triangulating my location of the patient's psychic position on a Ps→D continuum

In the second strand, I, together with three other qualified child psychotherapists, working blind, scored the two sessions under scrutiny, on the Personal Relatedness Profile (PRP) that has been used to distinguish Ps from D states of mind (Hobson, Patrick, & Valentine, 1998). The purpose here was to triangulate my location of the patient's psychic position on a Ps→D continuum. The results showed Simon in Session 1 to score high on the Ps scale, while in Session 2 he had shifted closer to a D position.[11] That is to say, there was broad consensus that data from Session 1 showed him to be in the grip of identifications with hostile, tormenting objects, in a controlling, sadomasochistic pattern of relationship, whereas in Session 2 the identifications involved more tolerant, sympathetic objects, capable of mutual concern and a receptive, cooperative mode of relating.

Third strand: identifying features of K and minus K in different psychic positions

The third strand involved bringing the two graphs into relation with the PRP rating for each session, in order to formulate a view of how basic modes of thinking/communication that carry K take a different shape depending on the patient's characteristic psychic state and mode of relating at the time. The prevailing mode of thinking/communication is seen to be markedly different between the two sessions, as shown in Box 4.2:

Box 4.2 Patient's prevailing mode of thinking/communication in Sessions 1 and 2

Simon's prevailing mode of thinking/communication	
Ps-dominated (Session 1)	*D-dominated (Session 2)*
» Enactment, projection, and projective identification primary means of expression/communication/exploration » Thoughts concrete/literal, two-dimensional » Fragmentary thinking, conflicted, disorganized, staccato; lack of connectivity in actions/interactions » Attention locked on primitive emotional content of interactions	» Play primary means of expression/communication/exploration » Move from two- to three-dimensional thinking—emergent capacity for self-reflection » Free association, creative flow of ideas » Imaginative verbal exchanges » Attention extended to symbolization, symbolic content of interactions

I found, in the Ps session, Simon's communication and thinking were largely through enactment, projection, and projective identification. Thoughts were concrete, literal, and two-dimensional. Thinking was fragmentary, conflicted, disorganized, and staccato. Simon's attention was found to be locked on the primitive emotional content of interactions. By contrast, in the D session, play was his primary means of expressions and exploration. There was a move from two- to three-dimensional thinking and moments of self-reflection. The thinking was discursive and free-wheeling. We communicated through imaginative, verbal exchanges, and his attention had extended to the symbolic content of our interactions.

As well as providing perspective on Simon's K activity, the research threw up interesting observations regarding the therapist's role of container. In both sessions, lack of containment was closely correlated with the therapist's emotional unavailability, defence, or avoidance. But the form of her *containment* was seen to vary with the change in the psychic situation between sessions (Box 4.3).

Box 4.3 Features of the therapist's containment in Sessions 1 and 2

Therapist's containment	
Ps-dominated (Session, 1)	*D-dominated (Session, 2)*
» Silent, receptive, patient » Thinking conflicted, uncertain, tentative » Inside space for feeling to unfold » Attention to emotional content of interactions » Thinking emotionally grounded	» Joining patient in free association—flow of ideas » Integrative, declarative, interpretative commentary » Expansive symbolization and playful exchange » Thinking emotionally grounded

Where Simon is operating from a Ps position, my containment tends to be associated with silence and "patience"—the word used by Bion to describe the Ps pole of psychic growth (cited by Britton, 1998). My thinking is uncertain, and I do not have answers. I allow space in myself for feelings to unfold. By contrast, in the second session, where Simon shows more depressive features, my containment is associated with playfulness, free association, expansive interaction, and commentary. Such patterns show primitive K and/or Ps-dominated K to call up a different brand of containment from D-dominated K, and that where there is a mismatch, containment fails. So, for instance, integrative, interpretative commentary from the therapist was inflammatory in Session 1 and containing in Session 2.

The analysis went further to show that a quest for emotional truth was an irreducible factor at work in many of Simon's interactions with me, though often at odds with, or overwhelmed by, Love and Hate. In Session 1, Simon behaved like a child who has been so starved of emotional truth that his capacity to experience more than a limited, largely negative range of emotions appeared stunted,[12] along with his capacity for more abstract, complex communications. Yet his sensitivity and drive to expose emotionally false notes in his therapist, although repeatedly interfered with by cross-currents of suspicion and envy, offers insight into the instinctual questing after truth at the emotional level of preverbal thought, which, Bion argues is the K-state-of-mind in its most primitive form.

A sample of the final grid analysis is presented in Appendix 4.1.

Implications for practice

Alice's curiosity turns out to be her strength, seeing her through all sorts of strange and alarming reversals down the rabbit hole. Through this study, I, too, came to appreciate the extraordinary power of curiosity, the K drive, in the different psychic situations represented by Klein's paranoid-schizoid and depressive positions. K emerges as a profound emotional experience for both patient and therapist. The hunger for truth, the desire to know and be known by another human mind, and the contrary envy and fear this desire arouses are shown to be fundamental factors in the interaction.

Simon stirred up strong feelings of exasperation mixed with concern in the adults responsible for him. Such feelings are very common among carers and professionals who live and work with deprived children who are hyperactive, attention-seeking, challenging, controlling, and often cruel and destructive towards others. As I found in Simon's therapy, the pressure to control such children and limit their demanding, destructive behaviour can drive out curiosity about why they re-create damaging relationships around themselves and appear unable to self-regulate or learn from experience. Sometimes it can seem as if all the available resources are going towards putting in place external limits, and there is no longer any real hope among carers and professionals of the child's internal situation improving.

NICE (National Institute for Health and Care Excellence) guidelines and current clinical practice for older school-age children with ADHD and conduct disorders focus on strategies for managing the condition. They recommend first-line parent education/group work, and cognitive behavioural therapy (CBT)/social skills work with the child. In the case of severe ADHD, medication is regarded as the superior treatment. While NICE guidelines are clear that medication should not be offered in isolation from psychological, behavioural interventions and educational advice, in practice such interventions are often minimal and linked to medication reviews. Large numbers of children with an ADHD diagnosis are medicated through to adulthood.

The current research investigates a different treatment option, not excluding medication but relating change to processes occurring in parallel with medication, within an intensive psychological, relationship-based therapy. Despite the severity of his presenting symptoms, Simon was managing without medication 10 months before the end of treatment. Change was apparent in his more open, receptive relationship with his therapist; a new curiosity and playfulness with language and ideas; less extreme emotional outbursts; a reduction in hyperactivity; more extended periods of play and attention; and greater awareness of himself and others. These changes extended beyond the consulting room to Simon's home and school life, where improvements were noted by both carers and teachers. He held on to his foster placement and completed school with several GCSEs, as well as developing some friendships and a secure relationship with the new baby in the family. Such outcomes raise speculation about what helps a deprived child to find a different position for himself, even in cases of serious deprivation and after a lapse of several years.

It is seen to be a struggle for patient and therapist to free themselves from the shadow of Simon's early years with his birth family. Indeed, the evidence suggests that psychic movement happens in the context of a slowly evolving, emotionally live relationship with a regular therapist, who is helped through supervision to

» stick with the child even when the only relationship possible seems a damaged and damaging one;
» stay curious;
» put up with doubts, confusion, and repeated disappointment;
» hold safe boundaries around the child while remaining flexible and attentive to the unexpected as well as the expected;
» acknowledge destructive feelings and repair mistakes and misunderstanding;
» tune in to the child's level of emotional development and ways of communicating;
» make space for feelings and thoughts to develop.

On this analysis, the disturbance, sense of failure, and damage that carers and professionals can feel around children like Simon are seen to be linked to the child's sense of self and others. Being receptive to such feelings, without losing the capacity to reflect on them or hold safe boundaries, is found to be an indispensable aspect of a therapeutic relationship with the potential to help deprived children grow and change. The model of psychic development occurring within a relationship, which develops over time through a process of attentiveness, emotional exchange, attunement-seeking interactions, and reflection, is hypothesized to hold good in a clinical context and have therapeutic value for addressing emotional and cognitive damage caused by early deprivation.

In contrast to the treatments referred to in the NICE guidelines, these findings suggest that *therapy* with deprived children (as distinct from the day-to-day management of their behaviour) is concerned less with having a package of social and behavioural strategies to hand, and more with being emotionally alive to, and curious about, the interactions that form in therapy. This links to the view that the deficit being addressed concerns an area of mental functioning (the capacity to mentalize, to process experience) rather than a skills base (area of know-how). I bring forward a systematic, empirically based account to support the hypothesis that, with children like Simon, starting from a position of certainty about interpretations, solutions, and strategies interferes with the therapist's emotional availability, attention to the unexpected, and thoughtfulness about what is happening in the here and now. I found, through detailed analysis, that such a stance was often associated with disengagement, stagnation, or a battle for control between me and Simon.

Finally, how patient and therapist experience and manage the conflict between K and Love and Hate were found to be core determinants in Simon's gradual emergence from psychic retreat and towards development of his mind. The research thus begins to formalize a systematic evidence base for Bion's claim, repeated by O'Shaughnessy, Britton, and Fisher, that K stands on a par with Love and Hate as a primary and foundational force in psychic development. Furthermore, it points to the central relevance of therapy, which addresses the nature of internal and external object relationships for severely traumatized children like Simon, who, under current guidelines, are often offered only medical forms of treatment and behaviour management. Limiting treatment options in this way may be argued on resource grounds, but, as the evidence accumulates, it is increasingly hard to deny that what works for this group of children, and what they need, is long-term, relationship-based therapy.

Notes

1. My patient Simon's striking persistence in asserting the truth of his early abuse in the face of parental denial and rejection, his insatiable, intrusive curiosity, his attunement to the feelings behind my words, are all perhaps expressions of this drive to know in someone who has been denied emotional truth and fed lies at a very young age.

2. Simon's dedication to repetitive games of chance and his retreat in sessions for long periods at a time to a world of mindless, mechanical objects had this quality.

3. See the case of Salomonsson's ADHD patient Anthony (Salomonsson, 2004).

4. Ps here denotes the stage of un-integration, where the mind may be occupied by confusing, disconnected, sometimes conflicting thoughts and feelings. D refers to the stage of integration where thoughts come together in the mind of the subject: confusion acquires shape, turned by containment into meaning.

5. My selection was approved by the case supervisor, a senior child psychotherapist with detailed knowledge of the patient.

6. Retrospectively borrowing from Mandelbrot set theory, such selection might be considered a "fractal" approach to the data, on the theory that zooming in on any point of a complex, irregular phenomenon will reveal the same (though never exactly repeated) emergent pattern and contributes vital understanding to more macro-analysis of the phenomenon as a whole.

7. The underpinning provided by the tabular grid made my reading of events available for external scrutiny and consensual validation, as recommended by Spence (1993). It provided a clear demarcation between thoughts in the session and my later reflections, such that a helpful line was drawn between the clinical material and the possible theorizing around it, allowing space for alternative constructions to emerge, in place of a single narrative. As a result, I was in a better position to engage with challenges to my necessarily subjective account of events. The first detailed grid analysis of the two sessions was closely read and examined by two senior psychotherapy colleagues acting as research supervisors and a third independent training analyst. Their contributions, integrated into the final grid analysis, qualify the inherent subjectivity of my account, as noted by M. J. Rustin (2001).

8. Aka is a common abbreviation for "also known as".

9. The strands were not sequential, and the order given them here is not intended to be understood as chronological.

10. Klein points out that paranoid-schizoid thinking is, first and foremost, a developmental response of the infant to the torrent of early inchoate experiences that threaten to overwhelm it. It splits and projects in an attempt to organize and distinguish good from bad, to protect the self from collapse into chaos. Splitting and projection are, in this regard, the earliest forms of thinking. They lay the foundations for a later shift in the opposite direction, towards integration, when the ego has grown strong enough to tolerate its powerful, often competing emotions without being torn to pieces. The shift towards integration is important for the self to be able to form relationships with, and within, the real world. Continuing to split and project beyond a certain point becomes minus K, an evasion and distortion of reality, perhaps because early experience of relatedness has been traumatic and the child now feels compelled to keep reality at bay. Paranoid-schizoid thinking thus always carries a potential for K and minus K.

11. There was an exception to this: one therapist scored Session 1 high on depressive features, on a par with the same therapist's score for Session 2. In subsequent conversation, it emerged that it was this therapist's sensitivity to the *object-seeking* quality of Simon's activity in Session 1 that underpinned the therapist's high "D" scoring of the session. I wonder if this therapist was picking up and amplifying the depressive, object-seeking aspects of Simon's communication, which could often

be drowned out within the strong Ps identifications active between him and his therapist, as I discuss below.

12. Fisher writes: "It is the K-state-of-mind that makes possible the experience of the full range of human emotions … paradoxically certain emotions—such as anxiety, envy and hatred—attack and makes impossible the experiencing of other emotions. Actually, rather than envy, perhaps we should put fear at the head of the list of the minus K factors, the fear that emotional experience is not survivable" (Fisher, 2011, p. 60).

Appendix 4.1 Sample of final grid analysis

No	*Session 1*	*Narrative memo*	*Identifications*		*Feelings*	*Defences/ responses*	*K content*
			Patient	*Therapist*			
9	The pen tops are thrown carelessly into the box, and S goes to the little table, near where I am sitting. He grabs hold of the toy basket and then turns to ask me if the wooden cars are in it.	P looks to T for something more	helpless, needy, deprived child	withholding mother	aggrieved, deprived	assumed helplessness; pushing for more	K projected into T; P splits K, disowning K in himself, looks for K in T
	I say I think he is in a better place to see than I am. "No, but are they?" he wants to know, then turns back to rummage in the basket, complaining that they aren't there. After a few moments, he unearths the red one, then fishes out the blue and the green. I comment on him wanting me to know and find them for him.	T sidesteps challenge, reminds P he has resources of his own	demanding, greedy child	beleaguered mother, withholding mother	under pressure, pushed out of role	challenges P's helplessness	K lost—literal thinking

	He pulls some fat felt-tips out of the basket and tells me he can send them flying across the room, demonstrating.	P shows resentment, frustration with T's refusal to respond to his demands. Unsafe when left on his own.	rubbish, rubbished child	rubbish, unresponsive mother	angry, abandoned, deprived, unsafe	evacuates feelings in messy play; attack on rubbish resources	body thinking; no K
10	I talk about so many things getting thrown around today. He sets the cars up on the little table and starts a game, which begins with the Sellotape roll crashing into them. When it goes off the table and flies across the room, he asks me to fetch it for him.	P responds to T's acknowledgement with shift to "game"	destructive, needy child	rubbish, unresponsive mother, alongside more receptive mother figure	abandoned, deprived, unsafe; partly understood	destructive play; assumed helplessness; pushing for more	T's observation—negative capability—momentary K. P's body thinking/no K turns to projective K and simultaneous experience of loss.
	When I don't obey,	T becomes passive —withholds help	over-demanding child	tormented, tormenting mum	withholding	back off from contact	early K disappears, fractures
	he abandons the roll and starts smashing the cars into each other, again and again, until one or other of them is pushed off the table. Occasionally he adds a few plastic or wooden bricks. It is repetitive and empty.	P retreats to increasingly destructive play	mindless, fragmented child	mindless, unreceptive mother	angry, abandoned, deprived, unsafe	cutting off in destructive empty play; evacuating feelings	body thinking; no K (K evacuated); H.

CHAPTER FIVE

A comparison of process notes and audio recordings in psychoanalytic psychotherapy

Miriam Creaser

Psychotherapists typically use process notes—written descriptions of a session produced shortly afterwards from memory—to record their work. These process notes aim to capture, in as much detail as possible, both the external action of the session (what the patient and therapist said and did) and the internal action from the therapist's perspective (what the therapist thought and felt). Through this, process notes should provide insight into what happened in a session and into the therapist's internal thought processes and emotional reactions during the session.

Writing detailed notes from memory is a skill first developed by child psychotherapists during their pre-clinical training in infant observation and in work discussion. This skill is later transferred to the recording of clinical sessions in process notes. Such notes hold a significant role in child and adolescent psychoanalytic psychotherapy. They are central in training, in supervision, and in developing understanding through self-supervision and some forms of psychotherapy research. Yet, how often do we stop to consider the process notes we write or read: asking what has been remembered and what changed or was forgotten and why? Using grounded theory, my doctoral thesis examined such questions through a comparison of process notes with audio recordings of the same sessions.

The study started with the basic assumption that significant differences between what was said and thought by the patient and therapist in a therapy session and what the therapist managed to record afterwards were inevitable; it seemed impossible that anyone would be able to remember an entire 50-minute session with all its twists and turns, and one in which they had been a participant, and then record it accurately afterwards. This assumption is borne out by five earlier studies that compare process notes with recordings of therapy sessions (Bailey, 2000; Bonnin, 2011; Covner, 1944a, 1944b; Knapp, Mushatt, & Nemetz, 1966; Wolfson & Sampson, 1976). These studies all sought to quantify the differences between these two forms of recording psychotherapy sessions and had broadly consistent findings of substantial differences between the two. The earliest study found that 75–95% of the material in session notes was accurate, but that more than 70% of the session content was missing in the notes (Covner, 1944a). The most recent study also found that a significant amount of information was omitted from the therapists' notes: 57.2% of clinical facts—units of verbally communicated information—was missing; there was an average of three facts in the notes that were not in the recordings; and there was an average of nine distortions per session (Bonnin, 2011). Bonnin's interpretation of clinical fact as a unit of verbally communicated information is part of a wider debate on what the nature of a clinical fact actually is, as captured in the 1994 Special Issue of the *International Journal of Psychoanalysis* on clinical facts, which presented a range of papers exploring the nature of a clinical fact. In my study, the child psychotherapists' understanding of clinical facts is likely to have been different from Bonnin's. Instead, their approach appears to have been informed by an understanding that a clinical fact stems from the "immediate emotional reality of the session" created between patient and analyst (O'Shaughnessy, 1994, p. 945), or, as Paul and Anna Ornstein express it, "In psychoanalysis, clinical facts are 'created' by both participants ... it is this on-going negotiation between patient and analyst (with all that its turbulence entails), that shapes the clinical facts and captures their meaning(s)" (Ornstein & Ornstein, 1994, p. 978). Such an understanding of clinical facts as located in and created by the transference relationship between patient and therapist would partly inform the process that therapists go through when they select what to write in process notes.

Unlike the earlier studies, I did not want to quantify differences between the two forms of recording; rather, I sought to explore the meaning of any differences and what might have led to them and to investigate what they could illuminate about the process of psychotherapy. Given that the therapist's experience of the session would inevitably not be an exact replica of the session, the central question became: why are particular things remembered while others are not? Freud's understanding of forgetting as a form of "parapraxis", or an unconscious slip that informs the subject's unconscious meaning or experience (1901b), was central, and I posited that analysis of the differences could develop understanding of the processes at work in psychotherapy.

My study also has a bearing on the debate about the validity of process notes as an evidence base for psychotherapy. The reliance of psychotherapy and psychoanalysis on such reports has led to several significant criticisms, with writers pointing to the fallible nature of human memory and to the inevitability of selection when writing process notes (Spence, 2007; Wallerstein & Sampson, 1971). Indeed, a brief review of the literature on memory function indicated that "memories are records of how we have experienced events, not replicas of the events themselves" (Schacter, 1996, p. 6). Spence, in particular, makes reference to Loftus's experiments proving the unreliability of eye-witness accounts, which demonstrated that eye-witness reports could be permanently altered by something seen or heard after the incident (Loftus, 1979). Drawing a parallel between Loftus's findings and process notes, Spence argues that the analyst's or therapist's memory is likely to be altered after the session as it becomes shaped in accordance with the analyst's dominant theories (Spence, 2002). He maintains that the analyst's memory is influenced subtly in order to fit the received theory, as the parts of the session that fit with theory become remembered and reinforced, while other aspects of the session, which might challenge certain aspects of theory, become forgotten (Spence, 1982, 1998, 2002, 2007). Thus, through this mechanism, the therapists' sense of what they should be doing might serve to inhibit their ability to remember what they actually did (Spence, 2000). Perhaps in keeping with this, there is also the charge that mistakes, technical errors in particular, will be forgotten when writing up the notes (Spence, 1998, 2002, 2007).

Spence also draws our attention to the narrative pressure underlying both process notes and those more substantial case reports in which the analyst is conceived as a "performer" rather than an "historian", telling a story of analytic endeavour and struggle that leads, ultimately, to success (Spence, 2002). This is felt to operate on a detailed level in which "broken accounts that seem hard to follow during the hour might easily be changed, in memory, to complete sentences" (Spence,

2007, p. 609), as well as on a meta-level in which the overall session, or indeed the whole treatment, is given in memory a more coherent and persuasive argument. The irony for Spence is that the pull towards a more persuasive argument ensures that case studies become less persuasive arguments for psychoanalysis, by actually restricting access to the raw data of the sessions (Spence, 1982). In turn, this lack of access to raw data and the narrative pressure are seen to limit the development of psychoanalysis as a theory by restricting access to new discoveries, which remain unnoticed (Spence, 1982; Wallerstein & Sampson, 1971).

My study, by comparing the "raw data" of the session recordings with the process notes, introduces a significant new dimension that is not explored in earlier literature, in which it is possible to really examine what has happened in the process of writing up the session and to explore the possible reasons why this took place.

In this chapter, following a brief discussion of my methodology, I focus on one of my findings: that there are changes in how patients are represented in the process notes from how they appear in the recording. In particular, I explore the presence of an idealized parental transference relationship manifest in the sessions studied and suggest that this relationship between therapist and patient influences what is changed or forgotten in the process note and that by comparing the two forms of recording (process notes and audio recordings), the therapist or researcher can gain a deeper understanding than would otherwise have been available of the transference processes at work in the psychotherapy session.

Methodology: developing a comparative method

The audio recordings and process notes studied were produced as part of the Improving Mood with Psychoanalytic and Cognitive-Behavioural Therapy study (the IMPACT study), a national randomized controlled trial into treatment of adolescent depression, which compared the outcomes of cognitive-behavioural therapy, short term psychoanalytic psychotherapy and specialist clinical care. The study was led by Professor Ian Goodyer of Cambridge University and funded by the National Institute of Health Research Health Technology Assessment programme (Goodyer et al., 2011). The IMPACT study offered randomly allocated adolescents with a diagnosis of moderate to severe unipolar major depressive disorder 28 weekly sessions of psychoanalytic psychotherapy [short-term psychoanalytic psychotherapy (STPP)]. As part of the study the psychotherapy sessions were recorded by a Dictaphone in the room. The therapists also produced process notes of each session, written after the session and without the use of the recording as an aid to memory. These process notes formed the basis of the supervision of the work done with these patients and are not part of a full case write-up. Therefore, the data analysed for this doctoral thesis were not gathered specifically for it, and the therapists at the time of writing their notes were not writing with a study comparing the notes and the recordings in mind. Additional data for the study came from interviews with two of the therapists. These interviews aimed to gather data on the therapists' understanding of their patients, their experience in writing the notes, and of being in a research study.

The data for the study comprise nine recordings of psychoanalytic psychotherapy sessions and the accompanying process notes. The therapies were conducted by a male therapist in his final year of training (called Therapist 2) and two female therapists (Therapist 1 and 3), all working in the NHS. I studied a total of nine sessions, three from each therapist. The three sessions used from each therapist were all from the same case and, as far as possible, were spread across the duration of the treatment. All the cases were completed prior to this study starting. I did not read the sessions before choosing them. All the patients whose sessions were studied were female (not intentionally) but were of different ages: 14, 15 and 17.

It was essential that my research methodology allowed me to have access to the two different forms of recording of psychotherapy sessions together and thus be able to compare the differences between them. Furthermore, the methodology needed to enable me to develop theory rooted in the data I gathered, rather than to test existing theory. Grounded theory was indicated because it enables theory generation from a qualitative analysis based on a small sample size. I had to identify missing material that I felt was significant enough to form the raw data for my grounded theory. Such material fell into three groups: "material not found in the process note"; "material not found in the recording", and "material which appears in both, but with significant differences".

The data from these three categories were then analysed, with material from the third category ("material that appears in both, but with significant differences") contained in a chart, so that the two forms could be examined in tandem. A straightforward application of line-by-line coding, again, appeared to lead the study away from the comparison between the two forms of recording and into an analysis of the sessions themselves as represented by each. Instead, it became necessary to develop a form of "incident-by-incident" coding—described by Charmaz as a "close cousin" of line-by-line coding—in which incidents rather than lines become the unit analysed (2006, p. 53).[1] In this development of analytic technique, each unit of information that was missing, inserted, or different became an "incident" for coding. In order to include codes in my analysis, they needed to be applicable to the data from all three therapists.

My study was undertaken within an interpretive framework. As such, it is important to acknowledge that the data analysis undertaken represents my interpretation of the data. I did not interact directly with the therapists during the period in which the data were generated, and they had no knowledge of the study at the time they wrote their notes. As the researcher in this study, I have influenced the findings in two main ways. First, in the identification of the data—that is, in identifying the differences between the two forms of recording to be studied. In order to compile these classifications, I had to judge what I felt was a significant difference in the following classifications: the emotional tone or the meaning, or the location of the material within the order of the session, or a combination of any of these.

Secondly, my own interpretive stance and conceptual framework influenced the analysis of the data. Psychoanalytic researchers using grounded theory, as Rustin explains, "have usually chosen to work within a psychoanalytic frame of reference from the start, while remaining open to new conjectures or 'grounded theories' that are informed by it" (M. J. Rustin, 2009, p. 46). Indeed, Burstall argues that "every researcher, equipped with the basic premises of grounded theory methodology, goes on to develop their own variation of grounded theory technique, adapted to the context and purposes of the study and the individual's mind-set" (2004, p. 81, cited in Wakelyn, 2011). It could be argued that approaching the data with a psychoanalytic framework would limit theory development. Even so, given that my research specifically set out to explore the processes at work in psychoanalytic psychotherapy, it was felt to be essential to maintain awareness of such concepts while analysing the data. Theoretical ideas of particular importance that informed the interpretation of the data in this study include: an appreciation of the importance of the relationship between the therapist and patient and of what type of relationship that should be; the understanding that key aspects of the patient's internal situation can become re-enacted within the relationship between therapist and patient; a central understanding of the presence and function of an unconscious part of the mind; and an understanding of psychoanalytic ideas about how difficult or painful ideas are managed. These ideas form part of my own psychoanalytic, transference-informed approach to clinical practice as a child and adolescent psychoanalytic psychotherapist and therefore informed my data analysis.

Findings: changes in the representation of the patient

Although I had assumed there would be differences between the process notes and the recordings, I nevertheless found the nature of the differences striking: I noted significant changes in the ordering of material within the sessions, sections of the session entirely omitted from the notes, interactions of several thousand words summarized in a hundred, misattributions of things said, as well as more subtle changes of language that nonetheless created a different impression. My study generated as many as eight core categories of findings, but in this chapter I focus on just one particular category: changes in the representation of patients in the process notes.[2] I explore how the relationship between the patient and therapist may influence what is and is not captured in the process notes and what that could indicate about unconscious aspects of the transference. For all three therapists, my study found that in all the process notes of sessions studied there was an enduring representation of the patients in which certain aspects of their presentation were privileged over others. Box 5.1, an extract from Therapist 2's session with his 14-year-old patient, is a good example: the comparison identifies a pattern of minimizing the levels of violence in the patient's behaviour and in her environment:

Box 5.1 Extract from Therapist 2's Session 9

Recording	*Process notes*
Patient: And my little cousin, he's 13, he wouldn't do nothing because of his dad. I got there, he strangled me, and I went bright red, and I don't know why I just lost my temper. And then I see him trying to strangle Lucy, and I just like I had to double look to make sure I was right, and I lost it. He just went total mad, because his dad weren't there, he thought he could take advantage of his mum.	She was talking about being at an Uncle's and her cousin had strangled her and there had been a big fight between her and her cousin where she had lost her temper.

And then he's obviously got two older brothers, and it took both of them to take me off of him, I was that angry. And normally all they'll have to do is stand up and he'll stop, and he never stopped like when I stood up. So as they went to stand up he went to stop but then carried on because he saw that I was going to stand. So I lost it. And all they were going to do was punch him so that he knew to let go, because she's a girl, you can't really do that to people that you don't know. Obviously I know he's younger, but he fancies her as well, which made it harder, and then I just lost it and I just started like beating him up, not bad, not like he had bruises or anything, but I just went mad at him and started pushing him off of her, slapping him. He booted me in my stomach. I just went mental.	

The changes in the language in the process note above indicate the pattern of minimizing violence and sexuality; for example, "I just went mental" in the recording becomes "she lost her temper". The patient's language is quite rich as she describes this violent altercation, with words that convey the physicality of the fight: "beating", "pushing", "slapping". Such words imply some element of savouring the violence. This possible enjoyment, or indeed excitement, in the physicality of the violence is lost in translation to the process notes. The therapist seems determined to keep his patient out of the perpetrator role, moving her from the one who is launching the attack in order to protect her friend to keeping her as the victim who is strangled. While it may have been difficult to follow the level of detail as the patient talked fast, it is consistent with the wider tendency to downplay the level of the patient's violence. In other examples from all three sessions, the same patient's repeated declarations that she is aggressive—that she will "explode", "hurt" people, and leave a "mark"—are strikingly absent from the notes, and at other times the necessary summarizing in the process notes serves to write out the sense of threatening swagger with which the patient speaks.

As well as her own violence, the violence of things happening to the patient is also reduced; in one session she describes being bitten by a dog, saying: "It took that whole bit, where is it? Yes, you see that lump, it took the whole bit of my hand off and it was hanging. It looked disgusting. It was horrible at the time, it hurt." In the notes this rather graphic image of the dog bite is summarized and sanitized with the gore removed: "She then went on to tell me about how she had been bitten and the owners had felt so guilty that they had 'got rid' of the dog."

The comparison between process note and recording for this patient and her male therapist identifies a parallel process in which the reduction of violence in the notes corresponds to an emphasis on the patient's vulnerability and her capacity to evoke the wish to look after her. The therapist was aware of her vulnerability from the very start of their work together, writing in his first process note: "I immediately felt she needing [sic] caring for … she stretched and yawned, looking much younger than she is." This continued through to what was to become their last session together, where he noted:

> She … looked as if she was taking better care of herself than usual, but [her jeans] made her look even skinnier than her usual jeans do while showing off more of her body than I felt most fathers would want their daughters to be showing off. I wanted to give her some proper clothes.

Changes in representation of the patient influenced by the transference

I suggest that the tendency to notice the patient's vulnerability at the expense of recognizing her violence appears to be determined by the transference dynamic. In the extract above the therapist's mind goes to how fathers would want their daughters to be dressed; indeed, he himself seems to be regarding her with a paternal eye—taking pleasure in the fact that she looks better, but wanting to protect her by making her cover her body more. The therapist seems, in this, to become an ideal father who is able to both appreciate and protect his daughter. This transference position was prevalent in all three sessions studied: a vulnerable daughter relating to an ideal, protective father. The therapist was, to some extent, aware of this position, as he said in his interview:

> I was aware of lots of feelings of really wanting to take care of her and it felt more paternal … I would have been quite happy in one way to sort of take her home and look after her properly.

What he was less aware of was that the powerful pull of this transference position restricted his capacity to notice. For it seems that the very fact of being in the idealized father position serves to impinge on the therapist's ability to take enough note of the other more aggressive aspects of the patient, as demonstrated by their absence from the process notes.

There are clear links between the transference relationship and what remains unnoticed in Therapist 3's sessions with her 15-year-old patient, this time with the pull towards an ideal maternal transference. The patient's mother has a significant presence in the sessions, with the patient often talking about her and, importantly, the therapist often introducing her in to the conversation. The patient represents herself as consistently ignored by a mother who is only interested in her brother, who is much more the favourite. In contrast, the therapist was interested in her and wanted to help her patient. The recordings demonstrate that the therapist often took up a more solution-focused approach. For example, in Box 5.2, the therapist makes a suggestion aimed at supporting and helping her patient at a parents' evening.

This comment is not in the process notes: could this be because it was harder for the therapist to remember this helpful moment? Or is it because—in line with Spence's criticism—as a moment of non-analytic technique, it is omitted?

For Therapist 3 and her patient, the most significant points of change between the process notes and recordings are often found in the representation of laughter. On listening to the sessions, I was struck by the high levels of joint laughter, often at times where potentially painful topics are being discussed. The overall impression is of a friendly, indeed even cosy, interchange enjoyed by both parties, yet this quality of the interaction, their joint laughter, is repeatedly recorded as just the patient's (as marked in bold in Box 5.3):

Box 5.2 Extract from Therapist 3's Session 10

Recording, not in process notes

Patient: I've got parents' evening with her soon, so she's [the teacher] going to be bring that up again with my mum, that's going to piss my mum off, just when things were getting better it's going to get worse again.

Therapist: But could you not talk beforehand with your mum?

Box 5.3 Extract from Therapist 3's Session 14

Recording	*Process notes*
Patient: Oh no, no, no, no, no! ***(Therapist laughs.)*** Oh I've just remembered something they've got a nasty cat, nasty, oh it's horrible, they've got a horrible cat, seriously I don't want to go there now. ***(Therapist laughs.)*** No, it's fine, I'll kick it. ***(Patient laughs.)*** It's like "come near me'! My cousins, they're both twins, one of them's got a massive scratch going down there from the cat, they're like three and they don't keep away from the cat. Ellen will just let them run around the cat, whoa the cat, feisty, it keeps on clawing and biting everybody and if you're just standing there it'll come and attack your legs. It's horrible! I was just sitting on the sofa with my legs up, the cat was under the sofa and I didn't know it. I put my legs down and ended up with claw marks all over my legs, it bloody hurt. I'll just stay up in my room all day. ***(Therapist laughs.)*** I won't be there most of the time. ***(Patient laughs.)*** *Therapist:* That won't be much difference then. ***(Therapist laughs.)***	Grannys, My aunts face and cousins massive scratches from cat [sic]. She doesn't want to go there anymore. **She laughs**. She stays in her room all day. Won't be there most of the time. Not much difference then. But then **she laughs** and says she will go out and meet Ben.

As with Therapist 2, the process notes appear to diminish the extremity of the patient's painful emotional experiences. In the extract presented in Box 5.4 the patient tells a very lively story about how her friends threw her shoes out of the window into the snow:

Box 5.4 Extract from Therapist 3's Session 10

Recording; not in process notes
Patient: My friends threw my shoes out the window. *(Patient laughs.)*
Therapist: You what?
Patient: My friends threw my shoes out the window. *(Therapist laughs.)* It proper annoyed me, I mean like Kate, Mike, and Carys, they're starting to get on my nerves, I never thought I would say this, but they're really starting to annoy me.

Therapist: You said last week that Mike and Carys are quite annoying.

Patient: I mean, yeah, don't ... It's not Kate, it's Carys and Mike, they're so annoying, like Carys was just like holding my shoe out the window, and Mike went up to her and went like that and my shoe went flying out the window and then Carys throws the other one out. I was like: "Cheers guys, do you want to go get my shoes?, "No, no", "Go and get my shoes", "No, I can't go out there", she just goes "Why not?, "Cos one, I don't have any shoes and two, look who's outside, I'm not going anywhere near them thank you very much!" And, yeah, she wouldn't get my shoes.

As the patient relays this story in a laughing, lively manner, as if telling an entertaining tale, she does not acknowledge how unpleasant it could have been to have had her friends gang up against her and force her into the snow in her socks; instead, the laughter conveys anxiety and avoidance of distress. It may be that the patient's determinedly jovial retelling is so powerful that it draws the therapist into it; the therapist also laughs, and her comment moves the focus away from the incident. This process of moving away from a painful incident is furthered in the process notes, as the interaction does not feature in the notes at all. In fact, the entire process note from this session concentrates solely on the patient's improved interactions with her mother.

I suggest that the warm joint laughter and the focus on a supportive approach indicate a pull towards an idealized maternal transference. As with Therapist 2, the idealized parental transference seems to link to "blind spots" for the therapist, in which, for example, the patient's painful experiences are omitted from the notes.

Analysis of the recordings and process notes from Therapist 1 and her 17-year-old patient also indicates a pull into an idealized relationship. The transference relationship with the strongest pull in Therapist 1's sessions seems to be between the patient and an idealized elder sister. Thus, the therapist is positioned more as an idealized elder sister who will chat in a friendly way with the patient. In her interview, the therapist seemed to be aware of this to an extent:

> "Her transference, I think to me, was a friend, that was the first, she was relating to me like an older, wiser friend and she was having very overblown hopes which she directly voice[d] of this turning her life around and at the end of the therapy living happily ever after."

The therapist is aware of how hard this dynamic made it for her to "elicit the negative transference" and reported very much enjoying working with the patient, saying "I did feel quite energized and I did look forward to [the sessions], she was really a pleasure to be working with, because you could really see from each week, I could see a development." While the therapist was clearly aware of wanting to seek out negative transference, as well as negative countertransference, it may be that this pleasure in a patient who developed and the pull into the idealized transference role made it harder to notice the uncomfortable aspects of this position. Even though the therapist mentioned this in her interview, the transference still appears to relate to elements of the sessions that become forgotten in the process notes, as shown, for example, in Box 5.5.

Although the patient does agree with the therapist in the process notes, the word "exactly" does not appear in the process notes, and there is no sense of the frequency (on average, every minute and a half). In the light of the idealized elder sister transference, it may be that the repeated "exactly" becomes uncomfortable, as if the patient is trying to adhesively identify with the therapist, by agreeing too quickly with the admired older figure (Meltzer, 1975a). The patient's use of "exactly" may also convey her search for an "exact match" with her therapist, in which she would not be disappointed by her therapist.

From the start of this therapy it seemed to be hard to end the sessions on time: as if the reality of the limit of 50 minutes was difficult for this patient. (This is shown, for example, in Box 5.6.)

This struggle with the therapeutic boundaries may represent a pull towards the more relaxed, informal sibling mode—a conversation that is not bounded by a professional time frame and one that avoids any potential hatred in response to limit-setting. In keeping with this, there is also a pull towards being conversationally chatty with this patient,

Box 5.5 Extract from Therapist 1's Session 11

Recording	*Process notes*
The patient says "exactly" 35 times throughout the session in response to the therapist's comments.	There are four times the patient says something like: "yes she thought that was right" or just "yes" in the process notes.

Box 5.6 Extract from Therapist I's Session 4

Recording	*Process notes*
Therapist: We're going to have to stop talking. We've done it again, haven't we? *Patient:* It's always the same. (*Overtalking.*) *Therapist:* We've decided to always go two minutes over. *Patient:* Yes, it's becoming our routine now. *Therapist:* So I'm going to see you not next week but the week after. *Patient:* The week after, yes. *Therapist:* Okay.	We had to stop there—having gone a minute or so over time as seems to have become a pattern.

an aspect that is not captured in the process notes. In one example where the therapist and patient are discussing the patient's father's sweet tooth, the therapist in the recording asks questions: "Really?", "So he'll eat a lot?", "That's very extreme isn't it?" And expresses her surprise, saying "wow" twice. Yet in the notes the only thing she is recorded as saying is that the patient "was remembering really sad and disturbing things from her childhood"—perhaps a more traditional "therapist" comment that is not actually in the recording.

Other examples of a more conversational tone seem for this dyad linked, in part, to times when the therapist may have anticipated potential criticism from the patient. In the extract shown in Box 5.7, the idealized elder-sister transference is challenged by potential complaints about cancelled sessions.

It is interesting that at the point when the therapist feels most under attack by what the patient is saying—and, I would argue, by the unspoken attack with regard to the missed session and complaints about the cancelled sessions—she starts asking lots of questions herself and involves herself in quite a chatty way with the patient's world. It could be that the questions are the therapist's attempts to protect herself against the feeling of bombardment or her way of seeking to make

Box 5.7 Extract from Therapist I's Session 11

Recording	*Process notes*
Patient: I'm really sorry I couldn't come last week. I was just so busy with work because they gave us extra work to do because we didn't have college.	She went into a lot of detail about her different projects and I was finding it hard to think, it felt like being bombarded with a barrage of words.
Therapist: Is this over the half term? So you had more work than usual?	
Patient: Exactly, yes, because as well as that we had to catch up on other things that we were doing. So it was just so much I didn't get time for anything. I certainly didn't hear from any of my friends last week.	
Therapist: Really? And you were going to do quite a bit of that, weren't you?	
Patient: Yes, I was. There was just no time for it.	
Therapist: Didn't have a proper holiday.	
Patient: Exactly. It was just a lot of work, and I think it went really quickly as well because, usually, we need like a week to get into the whole like holidays and then have a holiday but I think there is one coming up soon, Easter holiday.	
Therapist: The Easter holiday is coming up in April. That's right, yes.	
Patient: Ah, it's still quite far.	
Therapist: So there's still a whole month to go.	
Patient: Yes.	
Therapist: That's quite bad though, isn't it, that they give you so much work over the holiday?	
Patient: I know. They do give us a lot.	

Therapist: I mean, just to say from the point of view of the therapy, because it was a session cancelled by you but offered by me, we do need to count it. But that session ... Like next week, I don't know if you remember that next week is a week when I'm not here. So that won't, that's not counted in the numbers.	
Patient: Okay.	
Therapist: So you've spent the whole week just doing work, obviously?	

the bombardment manageable; alternatively it could be that in the questions the therapist has unconsciously become drawn into the patient's own transference-wish to be sisters chatting together about the difficulties. In the recording the therapist also seems to join in with the patient's view—criticizing the college for giving them so much work. This is not captured in the process notes, as if perhaps the therapist did not realize that she had entered this position.

Generating theory: developing the idea of the core transference dynamic

For all three therapist–patient couples studied, the comparison between the process notes and recordings indicates that there were dominant transference positions in all sessions. I have termed the dominant position the core transference dynamic. Such core transference dynamics seem to function as a lens through which the patient is seen, meaning that some aspects of the patient come to be focused on, while others, which do not fit within this picture, become harder for the therapist to capture in the process notes. For all the therapist–patient couples in this study, a core transference dynamic featuring an idealized relationship was observed. Needless to say, given the patients' experience, this was not necessarily a transference in which past relationships were straightforwardly being brought to life within the therapeutic relationship but, rather, a more Kleinian understanding in which current unconscious phantasy is also encompassed by the transference (Klein, 1952) and where the transference becomes "part of the continuous stream of unconscious phantasy accompanying all libidinal and destructive impulses, with the therapist now as their object" (Rosenbluth, 1970, p. 74).

The study suggests that overtly "positive" relationships seem to restrict the space for noticing "negative" emotions. The core dynamic identified for Therapist 2 was the idealized father/daughter relationship, which was seen to link to the therapist's keen appreciation of the patient's vulnerability. Yet this very appreciation of vulnerability was seen to impinge on the therapist's capacity to see the patient's non-vulnerable violent and sexual aspects. For Therapist 3, we noted an idealized mother–daughter relationship, evidenced by the strong didactic impulses in sessions and the warm mutual laughter. As with Therapist 2, this idealized parental transference was inexorably linked to a difficulty in noticing the patient's pain hidden behind the laughing, lively atmosphere. Finally, for Therapist 1, the core dynamic of idealized elder sister–younger sister relationship was seen to limit the capacity to observe certain aspects of the patient's presentation. This was seen most clearly in the absence of the patient's repeated "exactly", understood here as an attempt by the patient to adhesively identify with the therapist. This wish to be "stuck to" the therapist was then seen to link to the difficulty the therapist had in ending the sessions on time, as if breaking the illusion of closeness was too painful.

Why, then, should this core transference dynamic be so visible in the points of comparison between process notes and audio recordings of a session? I suggest two potential reasons: the first through enactments that the transference position creates and the second in the form of countertransference responses they may provoke. As we have seen, the core transference dynamic presents a powerful pull to the therapist to respond by, say, encouraging the patient to speak to her mother before parents' evening, thereby enacting the patient's phantasies (Akhtar, 2009). It now appears that such moments of enactment can be difficult for therapists to notice and record in the process notes. While the therapist strives to maintain an observational stance towards the patient's communications, the patient's projections often seek to create an impact on the therapist that can threaten this very stance. I argue that the attack on the observational stance is made manifest in the changes between recording and process notes.

Second, if we consider the therapist's possible countertransference response to the core transference dynamic, another understanding becomes possible. Heimann's conception of countertransference as "an instrument of research into the patient's unconscious" (1950, p. 81) describes countertransference feelings experienced by the analyst as the "the patient's *creation*" (p. 83). There is, however, debate about how much of the countertransference the analyst or therapist can really be aware of. In "The Dawn of Oblivion", the third part of *A Memoir of the Future,* Bion has the character P.A. say:

> Do not forget that the "counter-transference" is by definition unconscious; it follows that I do not know the nature, in reality, of my counter-transference. I know theoretically, but that is only knowing *about* counter-transference—that is not knowing the "thing itself". [1991, p. 515]

Segal follows this, arguing that if much of the countertransference is unconscious, much of the analyst's conscious feelings about the patient will be derived from unconscious ones (1997). What if one way that the unconscious transference expresses itself were through just what is remembered or forgotten as the therapist writes the process notes?

The transference is, of course, a subtle multi-layered phenomenon, and while the idea of the "core transference dynamic" was most evident in this study, there were also examples of multiple transferences. This was seen most clearly with Therapist 3, where the constraints created by the idealized mother position—the difficulty in noticing the pain—essentially caused a form of re-enactment of a different transference, that of the actual—or described as actual—relationship between the patient and her mother. The patient represented her mother as someone who had habitually ignored her needs; the therapist aims to be—and to a large extent is—the opposite: interested in and focused on her patient. Yet, as the therapist's acting-in with the idealized mother transference restricts her capacity to notice the more hidden pain, on one level she does become a mother who ignores (aspects of) her daughter, as we saw when the therapist laughed as she was told about the patient's friends ganging up on her and throwing her shoes into the snow.

Although the transference would be rooted in the patient's psyche, my study also indicates a further explanation for the strength of the core transference dynamic evidenced in the sessions: the therapists' feelings about their patients' parents. This is in keeping with Money-Kyrle's statement that "the analyst's unconscious can hardly fail to respond in some degree by regarding the patient as his child" (1956, p. 360). The interviews with Therapists 1 and 2 indicates that both were aware of their patients' parents' limitations; in the light of this, the "parental" response to the patient seems likely to foster an unconscious wish to mitigate the actual deprivation, in turn predisposing the therapists to act-in to the idealized relationship offered by their patients. Indeed, the therapist's role in relation to the patient's external relational deprivation has led to debate about whether psychoanalytic work resides primarily in interpreting the transference or in the possibility for the patient offered by the therapist as a real, developmental object (A. Freud, 1978; Greenson, 1967; Hurry, 1998; Joseph, 1985; Strachey, 1934).

Conclusion

This study shows that the grounded theory comparison of process notes and audio recordings provides greater insight into the processes present during the session than either form of recording on its own; in particular, the comparison allows a far deeper understanding of the transference dynamic's impact on therapists and their capacity to perceive and record. Indeed, the comparison of process notes and recordings captures aspects of the patient–therapist relationship that the therapists were not conscious of as they wrote the notes, and so invites the reader inside an aspect of the session that would normally remain hidden. I had originally hoped to have access to supervision records for these same sessions to see what, if any, of the material lost in translation to the process note and the dynamics behind it became apparent during the supervision, but this further dimension might need to be explored in another study.

This method of comparing process notes with audio recordings (developed in this study and termed the comparison method) suggests a new approach for learning about the patient and about clinical work. Such comparisons between process notes and audio recordings offer a deeper level of understanding of a session and a much more rounded appreciation of what actually occurred on a conscious and unconscious level in the session than looking at either process notes or session recordings do on their own. The comparison method's ability to bring to light how the transference is functioning as it influences what is—and, crucially, is not—seen in a session is central to this. As such, the comparison method has implications for research into psychotherapy as well as for the training of child psychotherapists, in which supervision is currently based on the use of process notes alone. Given the power of the comparison method to bring a deeper level of understanding, it would be interesting, indeed important, to incorporate it into the training of psychotherapists. Given that all the patients in the IMPACT study were adolescents with moderate to severe depression, it would also be interesting to undertake further comparison studies using data from other contexts, such as adult and child patients, more intensive therapies, and longer durations of analysis.

This study indicates that there are significant limits to the data captured by process notes on their own. This has implications for the large body of psychotherapy research based solely on process notes. The sessions studied were not presented as part of a wider clinical paper and had, therefore, not undergone the further process of reflection and analysis that process notes in psychotherapy research papers typically have had. It may be that this later stage of reflection could bring to light some of the dynamics indicated in this study, but that would require further exploration. In the light of the study's findings and the lack of clarity about how much the process of writing up a case report can uncover, I suggest that the comparison method should also be developed as a key tool for clinical research.

As such, I suggest that the comparison method, with its incident-by-incident coding, should become both a crucial research tool and a regular part of psychotherapy practice, bringing clinical research and practice closer so that as we supervise, self-supervise, and train using the comparative methodology, we consider ourselves not only as therapists, but also as researchers exploring that complex domain of our own minds and their interactions with those of our patients.

Notes

1. In her doctoral research study, Janet Philps (2003, 2009) developed a method for mapping transference, countertransference, and outcome episodes in process recordings of child psychotherapy sessions. This work showed, with cases of two children in the care system, how measures of depressive, paranoid-schizoid, and borderline states of mind could be developed and validated through blind rating procedures that showed a high degree of concurrence.

2. This chapter identified, in total, eight categories of differences between process notes and audio recordings: emotional nuances of summarizing; the impact of being in a research study; differences in how therapists represent themselves in process notes from how they are in recordings; difference in how therapists represent the patients in process notes from how they are in the recordings; influence of aspects of the transference and countertransference; relationship between the external parents and the transference; evidence of the workings of over-valued ideas; and the nature and function of process notes.

PART II

MAINLY PRACTICE: CONTRIBUTIONS TO SERVICE DEVELOPMENT

CHAPTER SIX

What do babies know? An exploration of the experience of Bangladeshi mothers and their infants

Ferelyth Watt

This chapter is a selective account of a research journey that takes us into the lived experience of a group of Bangladeshi parents, mostly mothers, reflecting on their beliefs about what they know about their babies, including *in utero*, and young children. The research project was entitled "Crossing the Threshold: An inquiry into the lived experience of Bangladeshi parents with young children; their worries and sources of support". I describe the setting for the research, which took place in selected Children's Centres in the East London Borough of Tower Hamlets, and the rationale behind this. I intend to show how the use of interpretative phenomenological analysis (IPA), underpinned by a psychoanalytic conceptual framework, enabled me to access the "lifeworld" of the participants (Smith & Osborn, 2008, p. 53), generating a wealth of rich data, showing the reflexive interplay between the data and the analysis of it and some unexpected findings. I then move on to identifying two of the key findings from the research, the first being the shared beliefs among the mothers about infancy and mothering, and the second about the interesting parallels between their beliefs and the understanding derived from research, notably that by Maiello (1995), Piontelli (1992), and Raphael-Leff (2003). I conclude by reflecting on the value that the psychoanalytic perspective and receptive practice of child psychotherapists can bring to the research process and the research community.

Setting

The research took place in the north-eastern part of Tower Hamlets, where the community was predominantly Bangladeshi, mostly originating from the rural Sylhet region. They were largely Sunni Muslims. At that time, 2005–12, the borough had the highest rate of income poverty across all local authorities in England and Wales and double the national average (22%) At the start the area was bounded by a sprawling industrial estate and major trunk road. The council housing was old, run-down, and in poor repair. During this period, the area changed, as new housing stock with play areas replaced the run-down blocks of council housing and Children's Centres were developed.

Parents with young children often have concerns about some aspect of their parenting, or about a feature of their child's behaviour, and may seek support from family or local support services about this. Bangladeshi parents with young children living in Tower Hamlets were considered a vulnerable group that did not readily take up health services, such as services for under 5s. This had begun to change with the advent of Sure Start and locally based Children's Centres; however, the local Senior Health Visitor and the GPs from a local successful Health and Community Centre were aware of many parents of children under 5 years who did not readily access any health services—for example, ante- and post-natal clinics—and did not consider approaching CAMHS for help. They wanted to know why this was the case.

This question was interesting, and the author, together with another child psychotherapist colleague, decided that CAMHS needed to investigate further. A recent CAMHS survey had identified that mothers with young children preferred to access services within "buggy pushing distance from their homes" (Dawson, 2005; Urwin, 2003, p. 378). Taking this into account, and in collaboration with the health visitor, family support workers, and staff at a key Children's Centre, they developed Help at Hand, a service designed to be more accessible and responsive to the needs of this group of parents. In the course of developing and running this service, the author was keen to explore what kinds of concerns might lead Bangladeshi parents to seek help, and to whom or where they turned for such help.

Research

Through the development of Help at Hand and drawing from research findings related to making health and mental health services accessible to black and minority ethnic communities, we learnt a number of lessons about making such services more accessible to the Bangladeshi population in Tower Hamlets in general and, specifically, to parents with young children. On this basis, Children Centres were selected as the most appropriate venue for the research to take place. It was considered that these centres provided a familiar, ordinary, non-stigmatizing setting for parents to meet and to consider their young children. It was a place where parents, especially women, could talk and mingle with each other, watch their own children, and also watch other mothers with theirs, pick up tips about how to do things, and get help when things were not going well. One key finding of the research was the high value given by the women to Children's Centres as places that they found supportive and which provided them with an important psycho-social space where they could begin to establish their identity as women and mothers in the UK.

A purposive sample of Bangladeshi parents, mostly mothers, took part in one or more focus groups and semi-structured interviews. A focus group is a form of group interview, where the interaction among the participants during the discussion of the focus set by the researcher is the key source of data collection (Morgan, 1997). The transcripts need to be parsed "once for the group pattern and dynamics and subsequently, for the ideographic accounts" (Smith, 2009, p. 71). The study highlights the complex and intuitive understanding that the participants had of their babies *in utero* and as infants and how they valued the opportunity to articulate the complexities of their lived experience. This linked to the finding about the centrality of the Children's Centre as a place where they could share their experience. In contrast, the individual interviews provided women with a chance to further develop in a more richly descriptive and personal way, some of the themes that emerged during the focus group.

The research method involved six focus groups and three individual semi-structured interviews to generate the data. Each group took place in a Children's Centre; the interviews took place in the women's home, and all were tape-recorded. I transcribed the tapes because I found that doing so provided me with a "feel" for the material, and in the groups for the flow of the conversation. In terms of the transcription, I have remained faithful to what I heard and understood. It was evident that each group had a distinctive dynamic, which seemed to emerge right from the start of the group. For example, one group was preoccupied by issues arising from their children's relationships with non-Bangladeshi people, another was responding to issues of normal development raised by one member of the group with a child with developmental delay. While being receptive to each new group and the group pattern, I was also looking at it in the context of previously gathered data. In tandem, I wrote an account of each group, using a process recording style, which provided a more reflexive and psychoanalytically informed description of each group. My understanding during the research was built in an incremental and reflexive way across the groups and further developed through the semi-structured interviews.

Some comments on method: interpretive phenomenological analysis

I want to emphasize some aspects of this research method that were particularly important to me, as they served to bridge my clinical and research perspectives.

Emotion

"Correctly grasped, the emotional factor is an indispensable tool to be used in the service of understanding" (2004, p. 40). Within psychoanalytic epistemology, this capacity is referred to as countertransference (Heimann, 1950). Countertransference lies also at the heart of the infant observation method (Bick, 1964), but it has become increasingly recognized as an invaluable asset for the qualitative researcher, where reflexivity is an essential component of the hermeneutic approach (Hollway & Jefferson, 2000; Hollway, 2011). This direction pointed to my choosing a qualitative research method. Willig offers a helpful account of the qualitative research approach. I quote:

> Qualitative researchers tend to be concerned with meaning. That is, they are interested in how people make sense of their world and how they experience events. They aim to understand "what it is like" to experience particular conditions … and how people manage certain situations. … Qualitative researchers tend, therefore, to be concerned with the quality and texture of experience, rather than with the identification of cause-effect relationships. [Willig, 2001, p. 9]

Phenomenological view

The phenomenological view is essentially intersubjective, so that we view the world through our engagement in it and derive our meaning of it from our relationship with it. Phenomenology is not one thing: it is a dynamic "movement" comprising "parallel currents that are related but not homogenous". These currents do, however, agree "on the fundamental task: the descriptive investigation of the phenomena, both objective and subjective, in their fullest breadth and depth" (Spiegelberg, cited in Davidsen, 2013, p. 320). For example, what is the process by which someone comes to accurately know what his/her experience of a phenomenon is? What is the experience of being a Bangladeshi mother in Tower Hamlets?

In addition, Husserl's conceptualization of "bracketing off" as a way to transcend the personal and contextual in order to identify the universal essence of a phenomenon is similar to Bion's stance that the analyst's state of reverie, when s/he is most open to the experience of being with the patient, is achieved "by the suspension of memory, desire, understanding" (Bion, 1970, p. 46).

The ideographic

In addition, IPA is also focused on the idiographic, or the particular. This focus means fine attention to detail and employing "thick description" (Geertz, 1973), or inscription, to the task of setting down events as they occur, and, through systematic analysis, of understanding how a participant has understood an event or an experience. This idea is important because ideographic should not be taken to mean concerned only with the individual but, rather, that the meaning of a phenomenon is understood through the individual's "unique perspective on their relationship to, or involvement in, various phenomena of interest" (Smith, Flowers, & Larkin, 2009, p. 29) "with an emphasis in the convergence and divergence between participants" (p. 202). In the course of getting the "insider's view", the IPA method is also committed to understanding the "first-person perspective from the third person position, so far as is possible, through inter subjective enquiry and analysis" (Smith, 1996 p. 262), much like the position taken up by the observer during an infant observation.

Reflexivity

The participant involved in a qualitative research project is encouraged to reflect on the issues being discussed and, through this process of reflection, come to make sense of their experience. Smith, Flowers, and Larkin (2009, p. 3) consider that the researcher "is engaged in a double hermeneutic", engaging with the material and needing to be responsive to it, yet remaining outside it. This aspect of the model was particularly interesting to me as it linked with my experience as a child psychotherapist, where I am engaged with and part of the therapeutic process but, importantly, maintaining a separate position that allows me a more reflexive stance from which to try to understand my subjective response as an integral element of the meaning of the therapeutic encounter. This practice derives from Bick's Infant Observation Method (Bick, 1964) which Hollway and Jefferson used in conjunction with the Free Association Narrative Interview (FANI) (Hollway & Jefferson, 2000) in their innovative research project. The Infant Observation Method privileges the observer's subjective response to the observed as a tool for understanding, referred to within the psychoanalytic epistemology as the countertransference response. I made explicit use of this in my interpretation of the material elicited from the focus groups and the individual interviews (Heimann, 1950; Winnicott, 1949b). For example, I noticed that during one group session, while one woman was speaking about the delay in her child's development, the other participants appeared to withdraw their attention, saying little, not joining in as they had done before, and needing to get up to attend to their children. At the same time, I found myself feeling irritated, not wanting to listen to her words, feeling weighed down and exhausted. This information was helpful in understanding more about the speaker's experience and how this informed her perspective of the world. The ideographic component of IPA featured strongly in the semi-structured interviews, and it was also present in the focus groups.

Donald Winnicott, both a paediatrician and psychoanalyst, a wonderful communicator by all accounts, emphasized the importance of play as a means to engage the child in a therapeutic process. While this research was not psychotherapy, I did keep the idea of the therapeutic power of communication in mind while conducting the focus groups and individual interviews. I had also been helpfully advised by Bangladeshi colleagues that providing scenarios or statements about issues would be more fruitful than asking direct questions, and I recalled Balint's caveat that, "If you ask questions you will only receive answers" (Sklar, 2017). The focus groups then had several prompts, setting out scenarios rather than asking direct questions.

So here is the setting: A white woman in her 50s sits at a table, looking at the Bangladeshi mothers who have gathered to be part of one of the focus groups for her research. She is aware of mixed emotions: pleasure at being there and that some women have come; gratitude towards the Centre manager for having responded to her request for help in getting a group together; some uncertainty about the recorder (with the internal refrain "what if it doesn't record?"); excitement and curiosity about what will happen. She is also aware of being there as a white, professional woman using English, and of the differences between her and the other women in the group. She also knows of some similarities, some connection, in our all being mothers and in having become mothers that will, in some way or another, have changed her and each of them profoundly.

The group is meeting to consider and discuss some questions and statements about their experience of being mothers of under 5s, with a particular focus on worries that their children might have and what they would do about this.

Findings

The research generated interesting data with a number of key themes. I have selected one that I have named "Knowledge" to discuss here. This finding was largely unexpected and felt very much a discovery, with exciting consonance with research-derived understanding from the likes of Maiello (1995), Piontelli (1992), and Raphael-Leff (2003), which I describe below.

Knowledge

Two aspects of this theme that I found extremely interesting, moving, and exciting were what I called "transcendental knowledge", which conveyed the awe that the mothers felt about their baby *in utero,* and "relational knowledge", which focused on the way in which the mothers thought and felt about the infant's experience after birth of relationships with others and with their environment. Together, they show how the mother's lived experience of the process of becoming mothers and the foetus's experience of becoming an infant both involve considerable continuity. As Freud stated (1926d): "There is much more continuity between intra-uterine life and earliest infancy than the impressive caesura of the act of birth would have us believe" (p. 138).

Transcendental knowledge

"When the mum walks in beauty the baby, will know this." What follows is a snapshot of some Bangladeshi mothers talking about what they think their foetus knows.

I asked the groups the following question: "Some people think that babies and children can feel and understand many things; what do you think about that from your experience?" The women responded in a profoundly touching way about their feeling of awe in relation to becoming mothers. The word "awe" captures the element of the ineffable that accompanies the process of becoming a parent and being one, especially at the start.

> *Woman:* We think that children are very intelligent. They are very smart children. Children understand everything. They understand everything. But we don't understand everything.

[*The woman spoke forcefully, many nodded as if to provide additional emphasis.*]

> *HB:* I think is baby know mummy.
>
> *MK:* And understand what happen outside.
>
> *HB:* Outside. Everything.
>
> *MK:* People said children see everything.
>
> *MB:* Yeah everything. Like mummy book reading, like baby listening, everything.

Later, in the individual interview, there was the opportunity to ask MK to develop her view about what she thought babies knew, as follows:

> *MK:* Yes. (*Pause.*) But I understand, I believe, baby everything know.
>
> *FW:* (*author*): I think I remember you said that, yes. So, when do you think that they start to know things?
>
> *MK:* I believe that when babies newborn, they know everything. It's not talk but it know everything what happens here, everything he know.

In another group, one woman said:

> *SK:* When you hear, when you talk to the babies, quiet and calm, they switch on and hear you. And it is a power, some power in the world.

I was reminded of the following stanzas from Tagore's (1913) evocative poem, "The Beginning", which also conveys the crucial element of awe that emerged from the respondents.

> As I gaze on your face, mystery overwhelms me; you who belong to all have become mine. [p. 11]

The idea that babies know everything imbued them with a nature and power over and above physical laws and what could be fully understood by the human mind. In this sense, the baby's knowledge provided a link to their view of God's nature and power, something unknowable and transcendent.

The idea of the baby and mother connecting in a miraculous and spiritual way that appeared to transcend rational understanding was also seen in the following comments, where one of the women is trying to account for the way in which a Hindu woman's child uses language reminiscent of the Qu'uran. It may also be that the Hindu woman is a reference to me, as someone outside their religion and culture, who nevertheless was also able to appreciate this sense of awe.

> *Woman:* Some lady is pregnant, I don't know if, er one is Hindu, but I don't know if he's read my religion. But when the baby is born, she speak like you know, my Qur'an, she speaks that. I don't know if mum reads that, she is Hindu. Born baby, how many months he's talk, like Qur'an I forgot. I think mum like some time go to Muslim house. I don't know why God is happening like this.

When the mother said: *I don't know why God is happening like this,* I understood that she was trying to find a way of explaining something that seemed to transcend culture and religion—perhaps a more universal communication between mother and foetus. I also took it as a reference to her feeling understood in a profoundly existential way by the group and by me. This next passage elaborated this further:

> *Woman:* … when mum is pregnant, he listened to like Islamic things and read the Qur'an, then baby listening and some time when he is born and they are crying he can get quiet, listening Qur'an.
>
> *FW:* The baby recognizes the things that the mother listened to when she was pregnant?
>
> *MK:* You read, or something like phone or new play Islamic or … (*tails off*).
>
> *FW:* Music?
>
> *MK:* No music. (*Laugh.*) If you listen music then baby is listening music. You listen like Islamic thing then baby …

NS: Peacefully, like baby.

NK: Yes

FW: … And you talked about going to restful places, didn't you? You know, when you were pregnant?

NS: Yeah. Like, you know a garden with beautiful flowers and a place, err, calm and restful. When the mum walks in beauty, ehmm, the baby will know this.

FW: Mmm so a calm, peaceful place is good for the baby.

NS: Yeah, yeah.

This Mum thinks that the quality of the baby's external environment affects it even *in utero,* and we then talked about the baby being in amniotic fluid.

NS: Yeah and moving around there's no difficulty, I am enjoying this place inside they can feel it.

NS talked poetically about her perception of the uterine world that the foetus inhabited. It was free, easy, and without difficulty; there was mutual pleasure between mother and baby. Here the women conveyed the way in which the baby became imbued with qualities associated with spirituality, such as peacefulness, tranquillity, and calmness, beauty and joy. The latter part of this conversation heralded the recognition that the way the mother behaved, as well as how she felt, crossed the threshold from mother to baby and from outside to inside.

Interestingly, this was also connected to the idea that this kind of experience was a feature of a child who was well raised and that because the child was relaxed, with "no fear", he would be well behaved. This conveyed the idea that the mothers experience the foetus as being capable of differentiating between good and bad sounds and emotional experiences.

This idea might be a means for some women, as Muslims, to connect to their belief in the Unseen that lies beyond human perception and is central to the message of the Qur'an and a mainstay of Islamic civilization (Allawi, 2009). In addition, within the conceptualization of life stages for Bangladeshis, there is the idea that Ruh or the soul is sent from Allah into a foetus *in utero,* where it gives the foetus life. There is a further connection to the transcendental as the *hadith,* or the accounts of the sayings, deeds, and tacit approvals of the Messenger of Allah, considers "every newborn in *fitrah*" or, the natural condition of the human being, that is innocent, clean, and without sin.

Furthermore, this early experience of taking in good things was seen to result in better behaviour in children and increase the likelihood of their being successful in life. This, in turn, was inextricably linked with the child being educated as the backdrop to success. The following quote demonstrated this link beautifully:

> *Woman:* … the more they are good, then, that is the more successful in life. That is scientific. In our country they say, children who do reads more and nourishes, then they will be more successful in their lives. That is recently that they have been teaching about this. They say, they were talking about it in the news actually, they say that people who have more knowledge … (*she tails off*).

This woman linked her assertion that people who read more were more successful in life to current understanding, presented as *"in the news actually"*. "In the news" suggested something informative, up-to-date, and accessible and "actually" served to convey a sense of authority. This excerpt moved the material in this group away from things that were hard to explain into the realm of rational knowledge, with a nudge towards something more identifiably "scientific".

> *Woman:* Some mums, when they listen to music, when they listen to it, the baby was relaxed. But I think in our country, I think our religion is more interest, is more interesting to read Qur'an, and they become more relaxed. They say the child will be good and raised good because he has no fear, so he will be really good.
>
> *Woman:* A pregnant mum will do the good thing, read the Qur'an, read nice things, then that will go to the baby.

Here the women conveyed the way in which the baby became imbued with spiritual qualities such as peacefulness, tranquillity and calmness, beauty, and joy. The mothers also recognized the more negative counterpoint of this, acknowledging that the foetus would also hear nasty sounds, arguing, and harsh words, and these were not good for the foetus. The women did not want to explore this area any further, perhaps both to protect their more idealized idea of the mother–foetus experience, as well as themselves in what is a relatively small community, where, at that time, domestic violence was a worrying feature but kept very hidden.

Relational knowledge

There was the idea that as the foetus grew, it would be influenced by the external environment and in particular through relationships, especially with the mother. Across all the groups and in each individual interview, the women revealed a consensual view that in their experience the foetus experienced the world outside the womb through its senses. They thought that the mother shaped this experience, in the ways described above, but she also did so through the relationships she had with others, like father and siblings, the extended family, who then also had a relationship with the foetus. This kind of knowledge seemed to bridge the more transcendental, unqualified knowledge described earlier, with knowledge that could be understood cognitively and learnt about.

One aspect that was particularly illuminating and compelling to listen to was the women's experience of the significance of sound during the prenatal period, with all its aspects of tonality, pitch, and rhythm. They were also emphatic about the importance, for the baby's life course, of the emotional quality of the sounds as well as the mother's emotional state during pregnancy. As the narratives emerged, the researcher experienced excitement and a sense of marvel as the discoveries of a number of researchers came to mind, as described below.

Raphael-Leff (2003) sees the period of pregnancy as hugely significant for the subsequent relationship between the mother and her neonate. She considers the mother functioning as a container while the foetus is *in utero*, both in relation to the physiological functions that she performs, and for the symbolic correlates this might have for the mother (p. 59). How each woman conceptualises this interaction is determined by her inner reality, and, in turn, affects her experience of pregnancy (p. 59). Raphael-Leff goes on to put forward her thesis that the bio-psychological exchange between mother and foetus can be conceptualized as a "placental paradigm" (2003, pp. 58–61). The women respondents here fitted into her conceptualization, as shown in Table 6.1.

The women were also emphatic about the importance of the emotional quality of the sounds, as well as of the mother's emotional state for the

Table 6.1 Placental paradigm

Mother	*Baby*	*Placental activity*
+Safe /good (processing/nourishing)	+ Safe/good (sustaining)	Mutual communion

baby's life course. The women in this sample believe that the move from the baby's uterine world inside the mother's body, to the world outside her body is bridged by sound. The following quote shows this:

> Yeah they do. (*Pause.*) Yeah when baby they would know, they hear voice, maybe we can't hear them, but they can hear us from inside. You can't feel it, but they can hear voice.

This comment links well with Piontelli's observations that "Foetuses respond to acoustic stimulations by twenty-two to twenty-four weeks gestational age" (1992). For example, their awareness of the mother's own physiological activity, such as eating and drinking, but also to her "vocalizations and from the attenuated environmental noise" (Piontelli, 1992, p. 35). She also mentioned the "preference shown by the infant for listening to the sound of familiar stories which had been read to them by their mother before birth" (Piontelli, 1992, p. 35).

Additional studies by Feijo (Piontelli, 1992, p. 35) and others have also found that the foetus will become habituated to music played during the pregnancy, and where this music has a relaxing effect on the mother, it will induce the same effect on the infant post-natally.

In turn, the data affirmed Maiello's idea of the prenatal auditory experience of the mother and baby being laid down as a body memory and an early introject, which she has conceptualized as a "sound object" (1995, p. 28). Maiello later developed her original proposition and proposed that "The voice does not represent feelings, but is itself the representative of emotional states" (Maiello, 1997). Here she was suggesting that the existence of the "sound object" could be seen as marking the threshold of the differentiation between me and not-me for the baby (p. 159).

I think the significance of the auditory experience of the foetus, as well as other sensory experience that the women thought was laid down prenatally, was clearly identified in the exchange below:

> *FW:* Okay, so imagine your baby. So, what do you think they feel is mum?
>
> [*Women call out, "Smell."*]
>
> *FW:* Okay, so smell.
> *FS:* The way you hold.
> *Woman:* Breast-feeding.

Woman: Your voice.

FS: Yes. I: I think it is before that that time when they are born. When they are in [*points to her tummy*].

FW: *In utero.*

Women together: Yes. [*Child calls out very loudly.*]

T: [*translating*]: When they are inside. She is saying after five months of pregnancy. [*Talking loudly over a little boy.*]

FW: So I, you're saying that it is not when they are born, but when they are inside when you are pregnant.

[*Women nod and say "Ji, Ji." They will hear that.*]

FW: So yeah, so if they are picking up your voice, they will be picking up other voices, eh?

[*Women nod, actively amplifying their previous affirmation.*]

A: Sometimes voice that babies hear are not happy voices, they might be cross voices.

FW: So they will hear voices that are happy and cross voices, maybe if there is an argument going on.

[*Women around table nod, but this is not taken further. There is a feeling that this comment had touched a sensitive "no-entry" area.*]

This extract shows how a woman (FW) offered an account of her own experience and understanding, which was then shared by the other women in the group, who came together over this. The researcher inquired about the view the women shared about the foetus being able to discern voices, and another woman related to this, offering her experience. Then there was a reference to the foetus's recognition of the father's voice. Another woman, A, then developed this idea further, referring to a more negative affect resulting from "cross voices". Again, the implication being that the foetus is recognized to have the capacity to differentiate between qualities of sound.

A did not embellish this, nor did the group; perhaps my line of inquiry did not readily allow it, or perhaps because it may have been harder for the mothers to think about less positive and possibly painful issues. My countertransference in the silence that followed A's comment was one of almost physical discomfort and a wish to wriggle away from something unpleasant. This suggested to me that this issue may have had personal resonance with some of the women, or that it was considered to be too sensitive to talk about in the context of a new group. We could also speculate that some of the women may have been exposed to arguments or domestic violence in their own homes, their in-laws' home, or in their family of origin.

The process of getting to know the baby was considered hugely important by the mothers and central to the task of motherhood. There was also the idea that this process was often difficult and necessarily took time, changing as the infant developed and became better able to express itself. In the following group, a mother talked about the confusion she felt, as a first time mother, when she recognized her feelings of uncertainty and not knowing as a part of the maternal task of getting to know her new baby:

> *SB:* How do I feel? When I was looking after my baby, when a little one, I was confused. She was the first baby. I am confused. I try my best, but I do not know where I take them, but sometimes he loves me and he knows me. He follows me with his eyes, so clearly when he is in his basket or there is someone there, he is looking for me, his mum. When they are older they know their aunties and uncles and they smile at them.

This mother's openness to her feelings and the lingering question of *"does he love me?"* was hinted at further when she said, *"but sometimes he loves me"*. Despite her doubts, she spoke in an assured way about her baby following her with his gaze and knowing her as mum.

In the following group, the women had responded to my question about what the babies know with reference to themselves. I offered the following prompt, to try to bring the baby back into focus:

> *FW:* But what about the baby? What do the babies feel, what do the babies know? Some people say when babies are born, they don't know anything, they are just babies and they just feed and …
>
> *NS and F:* No, no!
>
> *Women [in unison]:* No, no, Babies know lots of things.
>
> *F:* No, babies know lots of things.
>
> *NS:* Yeah, because the baby know who is her mum or dad.
>
> *Woman:* When the baby is born, newborns do not understand, but slowly, slowly, they are learning to understand.

> *Woman:* I think that the baby can understand. If you slam the door, he hears and he jumps. He can understand if he sees your face, if the baby is three months, he smiles, and I think he does understand.

In this group, the women are very definitely talking about the baby as a separate entity who is responsive to his external environment.

The idea that the baby might be negatively affected by things in its environment was further articulated by F, who moved the conversation away from negative things, to thinking about the importance of mothers being happy during their pregnancy and enjoying this time, as she herself had:

> *FW:* It is very interesting about when baby is inside and starts to pick up on things, sounds, what the mother is feeling, stress, …
>
> *F:* When the mother yeah, lady mum is stressed it affect also the baby. [*Shakes her head, other women also nod and say, "Ji ji" (yes, yes).*]

Here, F took up the more abstract concept of "stress" that I had introduced in passing. She clearly linked stress in the mother to a negative effect on the baby, by shaking her head and other woman agreed both through gesture and verbalizing, "*Ji, ji.*"

It was interesting that there was no reference to any negativity when the mothers were talking earlier about influences on the foetus. This suggested that the more mysterious aspects of pregnancy and the subtleties of the intra-uterine period of a baby's development were seen in an idealized way. There appeared to be no room for allowing any thoughts about anything negative. This prompted the question of why not? Raphael-Leff (2003) suggests that some mothers idealize the foetus and their relationship with it, as a means of managing, through denial, any ambivalent feelings they might have. While I can only speculate about this, I am reminded of a comment that NK made during her interview, which, I think, had a bearing on this issue:

> [*We have been talking about her concerns about her son.*]
>
> *NK:* One thing, you told me. Yes, our brains do not like to do anything imagine if this will happen but … [*Laughs.*]
>
> *FW:* Okay, so you don't like to think like that?
>
> *NK:* No, we are not used to. But, er, you are right, because sometimes thinking, if you are not thinking, then you will not be worried. If you

> are not worried, you will not be ... Sometimes, sometimes worried is, I think, good, because if you are not worried, then there is no sense. If there is no sense, then there is no worries, like children. Children has no sense of what will be good, what will be not good.

I understood that NK was telling me that she—and Bangladeshi people in general—were not accustomed to thinking in a speculative way about things, lest they became worried. She also conveyed the idea that "sense" meant knowing about a situation from different perspectives, in order to be able to weigh up different factors and establish what was meaningful. She compared this to a more childish view, where worry could not be countenanced.

The women then intuitively and collectively arrived at the understanding that intra-uterine life is very much connected to the external world of relationships, mediated through the mother. These experiences then shape the developing foetus, and positive and negative aspects of these experiences can be manifest in the behaviour of the infant and child, as well during adolescence.

Cultural factors

Cultural influence is a powerful organizing thread that runs through any research process, as it does through all our lives. It was evident in many ways during my research undertaking, both in relation to the cultural differences between the respondents and myself as a white immigrant, and in the context of learning about research. There were many times when these emerged—for example, over how best to recruit parents to the research, and how they might experience being invited to participate. Would people feel able to refuse, or might they feel that had to agree to fit in, be seen to be participating? What were the ethical implications of this research, and what were the relevant "rules" about ethics? How would I manage the issue of communication with people, some of whom had little English, when my Sylheti was even more minimal? Would the research be worth while, or even valid, if I worked without an interpreter? How would the women feel, being part of a group of women, some of whom they had not met before? Would they feel free to talk, or would the conversation need a lot of prompting? How did this fit in with the need in IPA to explore the ideographic element? Would the women feel that I would understand their concerns and really value what they had to say?

In fact, the women I worked with were all pleased to be involved in the research. They described feeling positive about the opportunity, and they valued the fact that their opinions and ideas were being sought. I felt that as I was not going in as an "expert", this might have lessened any feelings of inequality. The women also wanted to speak English, even if they were not yet very fluent. I understood this as a way of their being able to identify themselves with the more obvious educational aspects of my research, but also to connect with the more robust aspects of their identity and their perception of themselves as people with something of value to offer to society in England, hence enhancing their sense of self-agency.

The individual and the group

In the context of the research methodology, one of the central issues was the use of focus groups, which had not so far been much used within IPA analyses. Palmer, Larkin, De Visser, and Fadden (2010) take up this debate to develop an approach to using focus-group data in an IPA study. Tomkins and Eatough (2010) follow this seminal paper with a look at some of the emerging theoretical challenges, and the advantages and disadvantages of using focus groups. For example, Tomkins and Eatough (2010) raise the epistemological question of whether it is possible to maintain an ideographic and psychological construction of experience in the context of a group discourse. During the data gathering, I was conscious of the pull to be drawn into the dynamics of the group, but I also found that the narrative of each woman had a coherent thread, which ran through the group and was identifiable within the wider discourse. In the smaller groups (4–6 participants) each woman's account built up a picture of her experience of the issues under discussion. Some of these were extremely evocative and conveyed a powerful affect resonant with what I understand "lived experience" to mean. I thought that it was possible to move from part to whole, from individual to group, and to take up the ideographic element, while being sensitive to the interrelational element of the group. I note that Tomkins and Eatough refer to "phenomenology's foundational concern with the interrelational nature of experience and of our reflections on it" (Tomkins & Eatough, 2010, p. 245). The exception to this was in the single large group (13 participants), where the ideographic component of some of the women was lost. This strongly suggests that small group sizes of up to six are advisable.

I suggest that the movement between the part and the whole—the "hermeneutic circle"—is similar to an analytic stance, where the analyst is listening to the story as it appears but also listening with a different ear to the unconscious meaning that runs along with it, as well as being attuned to their own subjective responses to the material. The capacity to bear both the group and the individual in mind seemed familiar in this respect.

Conclusion

My research set out with a question concerning the lived experience of a cohort of Bangladeshi parents with young children. In this chapter I have drawn attention to the importance of the context for the research project, the use of IPA as a research methodology, and the emergence of my discovery about the shared beliefs of the mothers about their infants, including *in utero*, and the links that I made between these and the understanding about infants drawn from researchers such as Maiello, Piontelli, and Raphael-Leff.

I think my research has yielded interesting findings, some, like "*knowledge*", that were unexpected, especially those aspects of parental experiences and perceptions about their babies *in utero*, which I had not anticipated, and the relative absence of concerns about children's worries. Those they did mention were about behaviour in the form of "not listening", co-sleeping, and feeding problems. These were seen by them as part of the expected picture of a young child's development, and in this study the view that children will "grow out" of things prevailed.

The research demonstrated that all the parents had a complex psychological understanding about their child(ren). This understanding was built up from a mixture of sources. These ranged from the mothers' experience of being pregnant; the experience of becoming and being parents, for both mother and father, as well as that of being parented themselves; conversation with "experienced" women, especially sisters, aunts, and friends; for a few, advice from GPs, and, finally, information in the form of leaflets and hand-outs from a Children's Centre, the Internet and, in one case, a book on parenting.

The women's experience of their babies *in utero* highlighted the significance of Maiello's (1995) concept of the prenatal "sound object" as the corollary of the containing function of hearing for the foetus. It was clear that the women experienced the emotional quality of their voices or other sounds as being significant for the baby post-natally, with ideas that uterine experience was a determining factor for the child across the life span. The women were intuitively aware of the impact of other external stimuli on the foetus and made efforts to provide a calm and aesthetic environment for themselves during the pregnancy. They were also aware of the damaging effects on the foetus of any stressful or frightening experiences experienced by the mother during this period. They spoke of this time being important in shaping the child's temperament and behaviour in the future, with better outcomes for children whose mothers had been calm and in relaxing environments during pregnancy. Conversely, children exposed *in utero* to external impingement would be more likely to show overactive behaviour and a poorer prognosis for their future. This data contributes the views of a group of mothers to the increasing contemporary interest in uterine development and the psycho-biological relationship between the mother and the foetus, as well as the impact that environment has upon the developing foetus.

The setting of Children's Centres was an important feature of the research project, because it allowed the women to be in a setting where they felt comfortable and also because it offered the researcher a pool of women who could be invited to join the research project. As an unfamiliar person in most of the centres, it was very important for me to be seen to have the support of the Children's Centre staff, whom the women already knew and trusted. Furthermore, the Children's Centres are places where parents go to discuss their children and to get help if needed, so to be asked to contribute to a project to think more about their children fitted well. In addition, the women in the centres were familiar with the idea of meeting in groups to discuss issues to do with parenting or their children. It also emerged that this kind of psychosocial and educational group was a feature of the lives of women in rural Sylhet, so the focus groups offered a culturally consonant approach to data gathering.

The research process itself was illuminating and instructive. Early on in the data gathering, I was uncertain about how to manage the tension that I felt between the need to be simultaneously part of the research process in a self-reflexive way and getting to know the data from the inside, while also holding a more objective position, looking at the material from the outside. At this point I felt that I wanted to resolve the tension, either by assuming a clinical position and interpreting the data from a psychoanalytic perspective or striking out for coding prematurely. Taking up the clinician's stance left me feeling that I had become lost in a kind of psychological enclave; the alternative position left me feeling deadened, as if the life of the material had been killed off. I found that the remedy was to return to the data and use it as the springboard for the interpretative element of the analysis, just as, as a clinician, I return to the material of a session in order to understand it.

My experience of the focus groups was that they supported but also inhibited certain kinds of conversation. On the one hand, I think that my transcript commentaries show that the women in each group were able to articulate and learn about their own perspective through their discussion with others about the phenomena in question. It was as if the women learnt what they thought as their thinking unfolded during the to and fro with others. I saw the group as being a very important way for the women to talk to and learn from each other. A group can also inhibit certain kinds of discussion; this was evident in one group during a discussion about aggression in the home. The awkward silence at this point, combined with my countertransference, which had a strong flavour of "whoah, back off", strongly suggested that this was not a subject easily talked about in this group context. I am aware that there is an issue, within this community, about the dangers of "gossip", and this may have contributed to some areas of inhibition in the groups.

I understood the group as representing elements of this community's socio-economic and cultural discourse, alongside the unique perspectives of the individuals within it. In this way I saw the groups as representing the wider social context of which these women were a part and through which they shaped their lived experience.

The individual expressions of women's lived experiences could then also be seen as similar to, or different from, the views offered in the group. The use of individual interviews was highly illustrative of the ideographic component of the study and could have been further developed to be rich enough as the sole basis for the study, as is usually the case in IPA research. The interviews allowed the women to talk in greater depth about particular elements and to explore some of the more personal meanings that they might have felt too exposing to be mentioned in the group context.

Griffith (2009) and Loshak (2003) both identified the importance of considering individual experience and personal narrative as an effective way to understand "the complexity of the formation of individualized opinions" (Griffith, 2009, p. 289). This study also recognizes that the complexity of lived experience required an approach that allowed the opportunity for women to offer individual personalized accounts. In addition, the group context gave the women an opportunity to talk with and listen to other women, which had, I think, the advantage of illuminating similarities and differences within a group that provided further information about key questions. In extension, Atkins and Chattoo (2007) identified the need for the "reflexive practitioner" and reflexive services. By this, they mean practitioners and services that take into account individual narratives as a way of coming to better understand the needs of individuals and groups, and then developing services that meet these needs.

With regard to the issue of the psychological element of this analysis, in my view each woman's account made psychological sense in the context of the psychoanalytic framework that I had in mind. In addition, I used my countertransference as a guide to the unconscious elements of an individual's commentary; this use of my own psychological sensibility provided further evidence of the psychological component of the data-gathering process in groups as well as within the individual interviews. I think that there is a good argument for using the researcher's subjectivity in this way, as an element of an IPA analysis. Smith (2004; Smith, Flowers, & Larkin, 2009) reminds the IPA researcher that interpretation "should be clearly developed from the phenomenological core": they should "come from within, rather than from without". In my view, the use of the researcher's subjectivity, particularly when it is rooted in clinical psychoanalytic skills, is a helpful adjunct to the task of illuminating meaning. The need for patience and allowing a pattern to emerge within the research framework was fundamental to the way this study was conducted.

In my view, one of the most important aspects of the methodology was the iterative nature of the research process and being observant, noticing the way that one thing leads to another; also, at times, how difficult it was to find a clear path through a wealth of data. Another key element is my absolute conviction that research is an activity with a high level of subjectivity that manages a degree of objectivity by situating it within a research framework of one kind or another. In undertaking a piece of qualitative research, I think researchers must be open to the possibility that they will influence the research process—for example, in the subtleties of communication involved in setting up and running a focus group, or entering someone's home and finding a way to put them at ease, and yet be able to do what is required to further the research. It seems that the more researchers want to approach the subjective experience of the participant, the more they will need to be aware of their subjective response to the participant and to the data that emerge. The research methodology and its conventions are important in providing a disciplined framework that allows for a degree of objectivity, reliability, and standardization. In these respects, I found that the research process had significant features consonant with the psychoanalytic endeavour.

The discovery about what I have called relational knowledge was enriching and largely unanticipated. The prenatal auditory experiences between mother and baby, and the mother's experience of her infant post-natally in relation to sound, provide interesting correspondence with Maiello's idea of the "sound-object" (1995, p. 28). In addition, the data also suggested that this prenatal experience and the body memory laid down during this period have other sensory aspects that are evident in the post-natal mother–baby experience.

While the psychoanalytic research conducted by Maiello, Piontelli, and Raphael-Leff provides us with a scientific window into the experience of the infant *in utero*, the mothers here consider the infant experience *in utero* through their own subjective lens, in identification with their baby, and informed by shared beliefs. The researchers have employed disciplined research protocols and also used modern technology to assist them in their data gathering, allowing for replicability and a greater degree of objectivity. However, what is fascinating is that despite these different perspectives, there are definite areas of agreement: for example, the age at which a foetus can hear sounds outside the womb, especially voices, and the importance of these in the development of the infant.

It seems that it is at this point the bases for what is being claimed diverge, as Maiello, Piontelli, and Raphael-Leff lead the reader to an understanding informed by a body of scientific knowledge, whereas, in contrast, the women draw on their shared beliefs, which are largely uninformed by current scientific knowledge. It would be interesting to undertake further research exploring the lived experience of several groups of mothers from different cultural groups—such as young white British mothers, Chinese mothers, and Somali mothers. This might yield some interesting information that might link to contemporary understanding of the lives of mothers and their infants.

The research presented in this chapter has been informed by a psychoanalytic perspective, and it is my view that this conceptual framework, along with the receptive practice of child psychotherapists, can bring valuable understanding as well as new tools to the process of research and of understanding complex and rich data.

CHAPTER SEVEN

Breaks and sibling figures in child psychotherapy

Liselotte Grünbaum

The intended aims of this study were: (1) systematic exploration of core themes in child psychotherapy with children who have suffered early abuse and neglect; (2) investigation of possible links between breaks in the time structure of therapy and such core themes; and (3) the development of a transparent and systematic methodology for the psychoanalytic case study by application of a rigorous qualitative research method.

This chapter focuses on an unexpected, yet important, windfall of the investigation: the linking of breaks to hostile sibling figures in a child's mind. A more complete description of findings related to breaks appears in Grünbaum (2014)[1] and Grünbaum and Mortensen (2017).

First, some essential definitions:

» *Breaks:* Any time-limited interruption of the scheduled structuring of therapy sessions—planned or unexpected—no matter who decided the break, for what reason or duration, provided that therapy was resumed at some later point.

» *Core object relationships* (Hinshelwood, 1991): An unconscious core of object relationships, corresponding phantasies, and behavioural tendencies which give rise to repetition of certain relational themes, running like a common thread through the child's relationships in three domains:

a. *The therapeutic relationship,* whether communicated verbally, in play, or through behaviour, and whether in manifest content dealing with the transference or other relationships.
b. *The relationships of current daily life*—for instance, foster parents, birth parents, teachers, birth siblings, foster siblings, school mates, and playmates.
c. *The early relationships* to birth parents and other caregivers, as reported in case files, by parental figures, or in memories.

» *Parental figures in mind*: any communication concerning figures that on a generational basis are given a vertical, adult position, attributed with parent-like authority, good or bad; external, internal; phantasy or transference-related.
» *Sibling figures in mind:* Any communication concerning figures that on a generational basis are given a horizontal position of the same standing as the children themselves.
» *Relationship episode:* A single interaction between child and therapist, understood as a communication made by the child (whether words, play, action, or silence); the therapist's subsequent intervention (words, actions); and the child's response.

Previous studies: breaks and sibling figures in mind

Breaks

Although most textbooks on psychodynamic child psychotherapy offer guidelines concerning the management of breaks, a few studies focus directly on this, among these being Klein's famous work with 10-year-old Richard, in which she grounded his responses to breaks in his subjective experiences of his internal object as good, bad, or integrated (1945, pp. 375, 377–378; 1961[2]). O'Shaughnessy linked the impact of the therapist's external absence to the child's ability to keep in mind the good therapist, even while struggling to contain the pain of parting (O'Shaughnessy, 1964, 1989).

A review of studies in which breaks were not the intended focus nevertheless showed these in evocative ways to impact and suffuse the therapeutic process and relationship. Thus, around breaks, *re-enactment of concrete behavioural fragments of known early trauma* occurred. Furthermore, breaks might kindle potentially *self-harming states*, endangering the child's safety; *sadistic mocking* of the therapist; or reactions outside the therapy that *undermined the therapist's* credibility, threatening the survival of therapy (Grünbaum, 2014).

Some studies differentiated before-break from after-break reactions, among these Labastida (1976) who compared the reactions of four children. *Before the break* reactions tended to annul the parting: for especially vulnerable children, primarily through confused mental states, and ordinary cognitive-emotional functioning falling apart (Houzel, 2004; Tustin, 1986b); for deprived and traumatized children, more often as omnipotent denial, missing the last before-break session, devaluing the therapist, idealizing other events and people. Such evasive devaluation might spread to parents and network, endangering the survival of therapy (Hughes, 1988; M. E. Rustin, 1989, 1998, 2008). *After a break* reactions included confusion, ambivalence, and/or avoidance. Children who had suffered *early neglect or abuse* seemed especially liable to return with fortified defences, in denial of dependence (Kronengold, 2010; Rosenbluth, 1970).

Sibling figures in mind

Contemporary discussions of the status of sibling relationships in psychoanalytic theory seem to hold two major positions:

1. *The vertical position*, formulated by Anna Freud (1955) and Melanie Klein (1932, 1955), assumes parental relationships to constitute an emotional template, inside which develop the attachments between siblings. If care relationships and the parental couple are dominated by aggression, most likely sibling relationships will also be problematic—for instance, one weaker sibling at the receiving end of scapegoating or sadistic assaults, and/or the siblings forming a tight, possibly antisocial gang, excluding parental care and authority. The position does not exclude the influence of real-life sibling relationships, but emphasizes the influence of parental care. This point of view is probably now taken by most child and adolescent psychotherapists—for instance, by M. E. Rustin (2007) and Magagna (2014).
2. *The second, more recently developed, lateral position* was advocated by, for instance, Sharpe and Rosenblatt (1994), Coles (2003), and Mitchell (2003). This claims that sibling relationships develop along their own developmental path relatively independent of the quality of parental care. Supporters of this position are inclined to assume that sibling relationships can compensate for flaws in parental care relationships. This point of view is probably more common among psychotherapists working with adults.

3. *A third position may be under development*, growing from a discussion of possible relationships between the vertical and lateral perspectives (Cohen, Mitchell, & Britton, 2009).

Klein was convinced that during ordinary early oedipal development frustrated, hateful, and envious feelings inevitably lead to imaginary attacks on the "good" inner mother and her babies. If the internal balance between love and hate is severely askew, envious phantasies of the mother´s internal space as preoccupied by a nest of hostile sibling figures may develop. By projection, this phantasy formation may compromise the child's everyday relationships to siblings and peers; in Klein's words: "I have repeatedly found that fear and suspicion of … other children were linked with phantasies that the unborn brothers and sisters had … come to life … represented by any children who appeared to be hostile" (1955, pp. 169–170).

As phrased by Canham (2002), such an export of hostility is liable to "return to sender" in the form of paranoia, henceforth regarding external siblings and peers as dangerous, dehumanized things—in Klein's words, they are "to be hated, envied and destroyed" (Klein, 1932, pp. 197–198). In the further course of development, an evil circle of depressive guilt and increased persecutory fear of retaliation may ensue, creating ever more disturbed sibling and peer relationships. Commensurately, academic research has consistently documented that children who early in their life have suffered deprivation and complex trauma are at high risk of persistent socio-emotional difficulties, especially in relation to peers (Gunnar, 2010; Hodges & Tizard, 1989; Tizard & Hodges, 1978; Zeanah & Boris, 2000).

Taken at its face value, Anna Freud and Dann's study (1951) of a small group of children, who, by sticking closely together, had survived a concentration camp during World War II, apparently contradicts this point of view. Thus, after deliverance, and for a time cared for as a group, conflicts and competition between the children were practically non-existent. But the children's mutual solidarity came at a high price, since they responded to any adult invitation with cold indifference or active hostility. Attempts at individual care bounced off, and the staff were unable to reach out to any individual child. In time, specific links between individual children and teachers slowly developed, possessiveness increased, and envy and jealousy broke out between the children. Anna Freud (1955, p. 147) accordingly concluded:

> The behaviour of these children … confirms … that jealousy between brothers and sisters is not a direct envy of what the other possesses but … is an envy based on their relationship with the parents. The children are jealous of each other, with the figure of the parent in their minds.

Contemporary psychoanalytic sibling studies relating to early neglect and abuse are relatively few. Hindle found young siblings taken into care enacting benign experience of their older siblings (Hindle, 2007, 2014). Conversely, in group psychotherapy with psychosocially deprived children, Canham and Emanuel (2000) found behaviours evocative of vicious sibling-rivals primarily linked together by destructive ganging-up against weaker group members or preoccupied, narcissistic adults.

Anna Freud understood this kind of gang-like behaviour as primarily defensive, building on "identification with the aggressor" (1936). Klein considered conflicts between group and gang tendencies part of ordinary development, the resolution decisive for the child's further emotional and ethical development (Klein, 1926, 1927a, 1927b, 1932). As a fixed defensive structure, gang-like tendencies mean trouble to come, especially during adolescence, signifying that the child's needs for dependent relationships have become subordinate to aggressive inner figures (Blessing, 2007; Canham, 2002; Magagna, 2007; Meltzer & Harris, 1976; Waddell & Williams, 1991).

A clinical case: Samantha aged 5

To ensure that this case is being reported in an ethically responsible way, consent was obtained from birth and foster parents and individuals have been anonymized through thick disguise (Gabbard, 1997, 2000). Although I did my best not thereby to misrepresent psychodynamic processes and characteristics, one cannot be completely sure that disguise does not distort important clinical facts.

Samantha was referred to therapy at the age of 4½ years because her general development and ability to communicate had faltered. Among worries were her lack of reaction to pain, her withdrawal from closeness, and her episodes of non-communicative speech—she mindlessly parroted the aggressive language of an older foster child, 8-year-old Dennis. The foster parents' two adolescent birth children also lived in the foster family.

She was born as the third of three girls. At the ages of 1½, 3½, and 5 years she and her older sisters were placed together at a residential institution because of neglect and maltreatment related to parental alcohol abuse and domestic violence. At placement, Samantha was emotionally shut-down, retarded in most areas, stressed and panicked by tender physical care. She was said to have been roughly treated by her older sisters, who, after placement, were liable to continue this if they were not closely supervised. At the age of 3½, Samantha had caught up developmentally, and the three sisters were placed in separate foster families for permanent care,[3] with future contact maintained through twice yearly sibling get-togethers.

I saw Samantha for psychoanalytic psychotherapy twice weekly from the age of five to nine and a half years old. Parallel work with her foster parents was offered by a community psychologist. Twice yearly network meetings included the foster parents, their supervisor, the caseworker from the foster family agency, and the child psychotherapist.

An applied qualitative methodology

In this study, consistent with the paradigm of psychoanalytic case research, the therapist was also the researcher, her case-notes constituting some of my research data. While acknowledging the subjectivity of this approach, I gave special attention to the development of transparent principles of strategic selection of case material and qualitative analysis, systematically informed by the inductive–deductive principles of Interpretative Phenomenological Analysis (Smith, Flowers, & Larkin, 2009).

The case notes were supplemented by independent case-files covering Samantha's life from birth to end of therapy, written by child care workers, teachers, and institutional staff. Included were also the therapist's notes of parent consultations during therapy and transcripts from taped, semi-structured interviews with birth and foster parents, conducted two years and nine months after the end of therapy (Box 7.1). The role of research supervisors in the research process furthered the necessary role transformation of the therapist-in-the-therapy to the researcher-after-the-therapy.

The case material was analysed in two steps, at each of which principles for transparent data selection and analytic strategies were developed:

1. *An inductive analysis of process notes from the first 24 therapy sessions* to ascertain central themes of the therapeutic process and relationship.

Box 7.1 Samantha's case notes

a. Primary data level: Therapist-in-therapy recording her own experience

Process notes of 188 sessions
Four years, two weekly sessions of 45 minutes (Samantha, age 5–9½ years).
Total number: 220 therapy sessions

Attrition: Missing notes of 32 sessions (i.e., attrition rate 15%). Reasons for data loss: Technical problems (24 sessions); other reasons (8 sessions). Missing sessions nos: 104–119, 142–147, 166–167, 172, 184, 188, 190, 193, 200, 212, 218.

Therapist's recordings of information from external sources during psychotherapy:

a. 10 network meetings with foster parents, their supervisor, community caseworker, and child psychotherapist.
b. 17 consultations with foster parents, face-to-face or by phone.
c. Two consultations with birth mother and child-care worker in legal charge of the placement (the two together).

b. Secondary data level: Researcher-after-therapy exploring participants' experience

Semi-structured interviews two and three-quarter years after the end of psychotherapy:

a. Written notes from a phone conversation with the case worker from the foster family agency.
b. Transcribed tape recording of semi-structured interview with the foster parents.
c. Transcribed tape recording of semi-structured interview with the birth mother.

c. Tertiary data level: Information recorded by independent informants

a. *At referral:* Casefiles of referring agency on early family background, relationships, events, and development to date.
b. *Diary of residential institution:* Day-to-day descriptions by staff (Samantha, age 1½ –3½ years).
c. *Before placement at age 1½ years:* Descriptions by day care teachers, support teacher at home, support family in weekends, psycho-educative parent-guidance therapists.
d. *Clinical assessments by child psychiatrist and clinical psychologist* (Samantha, age 1 year 2 months, & 4 years 9 months).
e. *Court orders*: enforced custody placement at residential institution (age 1½–3½ years); placement in permanent foster care (age 3½ years); restrictions of birth mother's access (age 5 years).

2. Subsequently, *core themes were studied deductively in three different kinds of material*:

   a. *Strategically selected process notes* from *four consecutive Christmas break-sets* (i.e., the last two sessions before the break, the first two sessions after the break, and two no-break sessions). Christmas breaks were chosen as the potentially most agonizing break of the year for children in care. This material was supplemented with reports of twice-yearly network meetings during therapy (age 5–9½ years).
   b. *Independent case-file reports* from child care community workers, teachers of nursery, kindergarten, residential institution (age 1½–5 years).
   c. *Transcribed follow-up interviews* with birth mother and foster parents (age 12 years).

The findings

The analysis elucidated an inner world organized around a persecuted, endangered self on guard against hostile, often allied objects. This comprised four aspects:

1. A *characteristic pattern of hostile family relationships in mind*, with aggressive alliances between poorly differentiated parental and sibling figures prevailing.
2. The emotional quality of *parental figures seemed highly decisive* for the emotional quality of *sibling figures*—but not the other way around.
3. Samantha's ability for *cognitive-emotional exploration and coping appeared highly dependent on the emotional quality of family relationships in mind*. Thus, a combination of hostile family relationships in mind and a brittle capacity for differentiating internal and external reality frequently gave rise to flooded and paranoid states of mind.
4. *The therapist-in-the-therapy experienced fierce distance–closeness dilemmas and complex splitting processes*, quite difficult to contain. At times, this contributed to an escalation of Samantha's violence, yet it also served to enrich my understanding of Samantha's inner world.

The preoccupation with hostile collusions between poorly differentiated parental and sibling figures in mind was a quite unexpected find. This pattern was systematically detailed by a sequential analysis of Samantha's communication throughout therapy of friendly, mixed (i.e., ambivalent), and hostile parental and sibling figures in mind (see Figure 7.1).

	The first 24 sessions																							
	1	2	3	4	5	6	7	8	9	10	11	12	13	14	15	16	17	18	19	20	21	22	23	24
RE 1	M	M	H	M f	H h	F	H h	m	M h	m	M	M	M	H	H	h H	H	H	M	M	M m	H	H	M
RE 2	M m	H	H h	H m	H h	H h	H h	H h	m M	F f	H h	H	H		H	H h	H h	H		M	H h	H	M	H
RE 3	M m	h H	m M	H	H f	F f	H h	H h	H	H h	H h	H	H h		H	H h	H	H h	M	H h	H h	H	H	
RE 4	H h		M	M	H h	H h	M m		H	H h	H	M	H h		M	M		H h	M	H h	M f	M	H h	M
RE 5	M				M m	H h			M	H h	M	H	M		M	M		H		H H	M	M	H	
RE 6									M	H					H	M		h H		H		H		
RE 7										H										M				
RE 8																				F f				
RE 9																				M				

Figure 7.1 Mapping chart: systematic analysis of change. Emotional quality of parental and sibling figures in mind.

	Through 4 Christmas breaks (24 sessions)																						
	10	11	25	26	27	28	64	65	85	86	87	88	120	121	135	136	137	138	178	179	185	192	194	195
RE 1	m	M	H	H	H h	H	H h	H h	H	H	H	H	H	H	H	F	H	H	H	H	H	H h	H	H
RE 2	F f	H H		H	H h	H h	H	H		H	M	H	H	H	H h	F	M m	H	H	H	H h	M	H	H
RE 3	H h	H h	H	M	H	H	M	H	M	H	F	H h	H	H	H	F	M m	M m	M	H	M	M	M h	H
RE 4	H h	H		H m	H	H h	H	M	M	M		M f	H	M h	H	F m		M	H	H		M	H	H
RE 5	H h	M		H				M		F		H		H	H			M	M	M			M	H
RE 6	H																	M	M				M	H m
RE 7	H																	M	M h					
RE 8																		H						

Parental figures: Friendly=F; Hostile= H; Mixed=M
Sibling figures: Friendly=f; Hostile=h; Mixed= m
RE = Relationship Episode[i]. RE 1 = Relationship episode 1; etc. Relationship episodes appear white.
Light Grey = No-session areas **Bold print session number = No-break session**
If none of the above letters are specified it means that neither parental or sibling themes was found in this relationship episode.
Episodes in which parental figures occur together with friendly or mixed sibling figures are marked by Grey colour
Episodes in which parental figures occur together with hostile siblings are marked by dark Grey/White

Figure 7.1 (*Continued*)

> In the first years of therapy, Samantha repeated a play scenario in which a hungry, freezing baby got in the way of sadistic parental and sibling figures, who locked her into deadly dangerous spaces—for instance, icy, burning hot, suffocating, and so forth. Sometimes, the baby was by chance forgotten, excluded from riches enjoyed by sibling rivals, all on its own, indiscriminately going astray with strangers.
>
> At session beginnings, Samantha often rushed eagerly into the therapy room, but was hyper-sensitive to minute traces of other children or the therapist's other activities, moments later distancing herself, for instance, by moving away, arrogant rejection, hostile passivity, literally leaving, and then refusing to re-enter the room, or exploding in fury. Even minor changes fed suspicions that, during her absence, she had been pushed out of the therapist's mind by hostile sibling rivals (or sibling-like parental rivals).

Despite descriptions of considerable progress in affect regulation, mastery, and social relationships, similar relational preoccupations and difficulties ran through caregivers' descriptions from infancy to the end of therapy. Even at follow-up, two and three-quarter years later, despite further reported progress caregivers' descriptions still evinced lingering relational vulnerabilities in relation to siblings and peers (see Box 7.2).

Breaks as a window to fundamental relational theme

As the intensity of hostile communication increased around breaks, Samantha most often experienced any longing for dependence as a sign of weakness, placing her survival in mortal danger. Hence, breaks acted as an intensifier of core relationship themes, the fundamental phantasies of hostile parent–sibling conspiracies and tendencies to complex splitting forcefully brought home in the transference relationship.

An especially puzzling feature of *before-break sessions* was the presence of a few, highly idealized parental figures, which did not appear at other times, while hostile parental–sibling collusions were largely absent as compared to no-break and after-break sessions (see Figure 7.1). In general, apart from the first half year of therapy, very few sibling figures (of whatever emotional quality) appeared in before-break sessions. This indicates a collapse of symbol formation at the brink of parting. Samantha was unable to transform paranoid feelings into images of hostile sibling figures, let alone to link these together with the ubiquitous hostile parental figures. Where it occurred, the later reappearance

Box 7.2 Described core conflict relationships: two polarities

Motivation	Early relations (age 0–5 years)	Daily relations concurrent therapy (age 5–9 years)	At follow-up (age 12 years)	
Longs for dependence ↔ Fears abuse/ rejection	Eager joy at first sight PF ↔ Hostile, impassive, withdrawn • Bodily stressed • Splitting	Eager joy at first sight PF ↔ Hostile, impassive, withdrawn • Bodily stressed • Complex splitting all over ↓ FP: Relate differentiated couple BM: No real change	FP: Tender differentiated couple ↔ FP: Enduring vulnerabilities • Bodily stress • Some splitting	BM: Eager joy at first sight ↔ BM: Anxious rejection • Able to protect self by mobilizing FP & network
Strives autonomy/ identity ↔ Avoids separateness	PF available: joyful roleplay ↔ PF not: dejected, tearful rage • At bedtime: wide awake & self-harming • Denial of partings	PF available: some ability learning and relating ↔ PF not: furious-defiant, withdrawn • At bedtime: wide awake & self-harm • Denial of partings ↓ Academically: middle of class Participate in group work Protection self • Breaks off visit to BM	Academic achievement up to abilities, skills still developing ↔ Enduring vulnerabilities: • Traumatic relapse, fear loss of FP • Stone face • Difficulties speaking up own mind	

Note: PF = parental figure; FP = foster parents; BM = birth mother. Double-headed arrow (↔): alternating states of mind; single-headed arrow (↓): development from the above to new capabilities. *Compatible theory:* Blass & Blatt (1992); Blatt & Luyten (2009).

in before-break sessions of siblings-linked-to-parents (whether in hostile collusion or ordinarily mixed relationship) may have signified decreased splitting and an improved stability of depressive emotional-cognitive functioning.

At *session-end,* Samantha in action demonstrated fierce dilemmas concerning separateness-dependence by encircling the door, triumphantly threatening to leave before time, but at session-end fiercely refusing to leave. At session-end, later in therapy, Samantha might produce a host of drawings, most often keeping these hidden, destroying them before leaving. One, rescued by the therapist from the bin, depicted an austere female figure, as dark-haired as the therapist, throwing a muffled-up infant into a raging stream, signifying that in Samantha's mind being left equalled drowning, flooded by feelings.

Around the middle of therapy, intense approach-avoidance conflicts permeated the *beginnings of after-break sessions.* Samantha might still brighten up at first sight of the therapist, but then immediately backed off, in a panicky state of mind rejecting any form of contact. Sometimes, she was literally stuck at the threshold of the therapy room, in a confused state, neither able to enter nor stay out. While sitting there, she droningly shouted threats of leaving or raised havoc in the therapy room. In the same period, the therapist, in her reverie, experienced inner visual and auditory imagery of an alarmingly violent family life and, outside therapy, developed a slight, but still bothersome, hypersensitivity to noise.

The *subjectivity of the therapist* seemed especially important around breaks, the therapist experiencing intense problems with finding the right geographical and emotional distance from Samantha, sometimes feeling caught up in a negative spiral:

» Samantha, possessed by a suspicion that other children had better toys, with all her might tried to beat her way into a locked cupboard. When this proved impossible, for a time she calmed down by drawing beautiful, cool-looking female figures jointly excluding smaller, slightly disjointed, fragmented, or muzzy figures.
» Samantha had a real talent for drawing, but, especially before breaks, she might fill up sheet after sheet with disjointed, incomplete faces and human beings with haphazardly placed body parts.
» Within split seconds, her mood might change to a fierce dissociated state of mind, in which she appeared totally identified with a sadistic parental or big-sibling figure, without mercy aggressively persecuting the therapist, kicking and shouting, calmed down neither by words nor increased physical distance. In these situations, the therapist-in-the-therapy often felt a naïve sucker, unable to prevent sudden violence. Most often, the only way to stop the assault was use of physical force, taking hold of her, at which violence subsided, Samantha's facial expression going blank, while she rhythmically rocked her body or banged her head against the wall. In the mind of the therapist-in-the-therapy, these episodes resonated as painful reminders of case-file descriptions of an 18-months-old Samantha.

In the last one and a half years of therapy, the intensity of Samantha's reaction to breaks decreased. It was, shortly, however, to increase after the last Christmas break, when the foster parents by agreement told her that therapy would end next summer.

Preoccupying sibling figures in mind

Samantha's preoccupation with sibling figures was conceptualized under four main headings:

1. Am I the first child to come?
2. Hostile parents usher in hostile siblings
3. Oscillations between gang and group states of mind
4. The capacity to pine loss ushers in triangular relationships

In this section, these main themes are delineated as they appear in the process notes of therapy and from the point of view of caregiver descriptions. An overview of development along these themes appears in Box 7.3.

Am I the first child to come?

A fierce longing to be someone's special apple-of-the-eye child was salient both inside Samantha's therapy and in the caregiver's descriptions. If not recognized, it caused unbearable frustration, sudden assaults, or withdrawal.

From early infancy, even before placement (age 1–3½ years), birth mother, day-nursery, and residential institution alike described an easily victimized, anxious-aggressive child, roughly treated by siblings and peers, her fragile social abilities fluctuating with the availability of her special teacher. She would fiercely fight other children for adult attention, but when crowded out or watching her special teacher caring for other children, she collapsed, falling apart in dissociated, sometimes self-stimulating or self-harming states of mind.

Inside therapy, Samantha became acutely suspicious at even the slightest traces of other children in the playroom, as shown below in sections from two early, consecutive sessions:

> (*Session 10*): "… Samantha paints herself as a … happily smiling figure, but soon … covers the figure's mouth with black paint. (I suggest this is confusing, Samantha in the painting smiles, but her mouth is all black.) … Samantha points to the painting:" Something bad came into her mouth" … (I … mention it is 5 days since we last saw each other.) Samantha says: "Yes, she gets

Box 7.3 Overview of central theme: sibling figures (as told by caregivers)

Core Themes	*Early (age 0–5 years)*	*Concurrent therapy (age 5–9 years)*	*Follow-up (age 12 years)*
Am I the first?	» Fierce rivalryfor attention » Crowded out= collapse	» Fierce rivalry » Persecuted suspicion » Crowded out = collapse or violence	» Manages peers & siblings on her own » Skills are still improving » Lingering vulnerabilities
Hostile parents → hostile siblings	» ST gone = persecuted/ victimized unable play/ learning » ST available = somegroup play/learning	» ST gone = victimized/ violentunable play/ learning » ST available = some group play/learning » Unsupervised visits BM's place = breakdown peer relations	» In Foster Family = tender relations to Foster Sibs » At visitation BM: active teasing of weaker Birth Sib
Gang or group?	» Imitation of aggressivepeers » Parroting aggressive Foster Sib	Fierce split: » Inside therapy = gang » Outside therapy= group	Lingering tendency splitting: » Gender-specific learning FP's grown-up Birth Children » Protection of self against Foster Brother-sib » Ganging up Birth Sibs against BM
Pining loss ushers in triangulation	» On ST's lap: pines Birth Family & Birth Dad	» On FM's lap: pines Birth Dad & tells rescue phantasy	» Survivor's guilt Foster Brother-sib bars mourning » Lingering vulnerability at loss

Note: ST = support teacher; FP= foster parents; FM = foster mother; BM = birth mother.

> fire." She looks towards the furniture in the doll's house, which since last session was moved, and asks: "Was someone in here?"
>
> *(Session 11):* "... Samantha ... paints a number of paintings picturing me, ... attacking these with the painting brush, ... in a flat voice threatens to soil and stab me. ... Gradually her messing with the paint gives way to an intense activity, scooping up all paint in one container. (... I suggest that she wants to use up all my paint, preventing other children getting anything at all.) She looks intently into my eyes, asking: "Am I the first child to come? Because if so, you are not stupid, but if not, I will cut your throat." She makes a cutthroat movement at her own throat."

During the first part of therapy, foster parents reported increasingly fierce rivalry with peers for adult attention. If crowded out, Samantha (5–7 years old) now tended to become violent—for instance, throwing stones at another child. However, she also got a bosom-friend, a girl just as liable as Samantha to stand up for her rights.

At the end of therapy, Samantha reportedly managed group work without support, and her foster parents and teachers felt that her relationship to peers had improved considerably.

At follow up, she was managing wholly without support in school and at after-school club, and, according to the foster parents, her social skills were still improving. However, a lingering vulnerability in relation to peers was described, especially a tendency to wear out preferred friends.

Hostile parents usher in hostile siblings

As shown in the relational mapping chart (Figure 7.1) the emotional quality of parental figures seemed decisive for the emotional quality of sibling figures. Thus, throughout therapy, hostile parental figures in mind often appeared alone or together with an equally hostile sibling figure, but, by contrast, sibling figures, no matter what their emotional quality, practically never occurred alone.

> (*Session 6*): [*Samantha is playing*] A family is at a restaurant, ... the nurse doll takes down ... orders. ... Baby in her high chair suddenly falls ... onto the floor. Mum takes up baby, [but is] increasingly explosive and verbally abusive ... Big brother picks up baby, ... handling her roughly. Samantha, in an aside, tells: "He crushes her." Mum intervenes, ... falsely sweet ... to baby: "You are better locked up, so big brother can't crush you." She locks the crying baby up inside the freezer."

Parental and sibling figures practically always had the same emotional quality and often appeared enmeshed, closely allied, and difficult to tell apart. This finding is commensurate with results from an independent clinical-psychological examination performed at the age of 4 years, showing an incomplete differentiation between sibling and parental figures.

From the age of 1 year and through most of the therapy, Samantha's carers uniformly described her experience of parental attention or neglect as immediately colouring her relation to peers and, in addition, affecting her social abilities and cognitive-emotional competence. This tendency appeared especially persistent, not substantially giving way until she was around 8½ years old.

After three and a half years of therapy, a legal decision ordered unsupervised visits to the birth mother's home. Shortly after the first of these visits, the school reported peer relationships to break down in confused violence towards peers and suicidal risk-taking behaviour—Samantha running away, climbing so high up a tree that she was unable to climb down and had to be rescued. The visits ended abruptly, when Samantha and the birth mum in unison broke off a visit, seeking out the foster mother, who was waiting in a park nearby, and asking her to take Samantha home. Thereafter, visits to the birth mother came to an end.

Oscillations between gang and group states of mind

Within her therapy, Samantha oscillated between benign identifications and tendencies towards anxious identification with aggressor—often in the form of phantasies in which an enmeshed, omnipotent, sometimes frankly antisocial, gang of like-minded siblings or peers was a persistent feature.

Early on (Samantha, age 1½ to 3½ years), the residential institution described similar inclinations, Samantha imitating aggressive older peers, pilfering toys from weaker children, spoiling their play on purpose, and showing no sympathy for crying peers. After placement in foster care (at age 3½ years), now fraught by mindless survival anxiety, she took to mechanical parroting of the older foster brother Dennis's aggressive language.

In an early session, the terror bound up with this identification became evident through projective identification:

> (*Session 13*): Samantha mocks me: "You are ... stupid and small, ... so picky with your food, you won't eat it, you fancy it to be poison, don't

> you? ... You don't at all belong here, you better watch out or else ... if you don't do, what I tell you to do, I'll beat you up and bully you and kill your family ... You are ... too small, you won't last long."

During the first six months of therapy, the foster parents reported her relationship to foster brother Dennis had deteriorated into angry, envious rivalry, but, at the same time, her copy-cat behaviour disappeared, and ordinary communicative abilities were restored.

Around the age of 8 years, an increasing split between Samantha's everyday life and her behaviour in therapy developed. Thus, at home and in school, her relationships, her ability to learn, and her general behaviour improved considerably. The foster parents experienced a much more genuine Samantha, less rejecting towards the foster dad, doing better at school with better relationships to peers. Yet, inside therapy, she became increasingly violent and abusive. At some point, I confronted her directly with this split, hoping to bring to her awareness the fact that she had an existential choice to consider, both within her therapy and in everyday life. Samantha reacted to this confrontation with a mixture of surprise and denial, but, nevertheless, in her play a determined policeman appeared to re-establish law and order, and, during the following months, her acting out declined. One of the last—and less trying—displays of the tendency to gang up was this:

> (*Session 185, a before-break session*): ... [*Samantha plays*] ... a ferocious tiger breaks out of Zoo, threatening to gulp down everybody. (I suggest ... this hungry tiger ... broke out because of the break to come.) She doesn't hear me out, shouts a torrent of abuse ... threatens to call in all her friends to duff me up.

This moment probably reflected not only the tendency to gang up in denial of dependence, but also a developmentally derived struggle to bear ordinary separateness. Thus, it seems likely that Samantha also told me (and herself) something like: "What do I care about all this old parental stuff of hungry tigers—I have my own pals to relate to".

At follow up (age 12 years), Samantha seemed affectionately integrated in the foster family, relating well to foster siblings and classmates, but still vulnerable to rejection from peers. In relation to her birth mum and sisters, slight tendencies for splitting and ganging up were still discernible.

The capacity to pine for lost objects ushers in triangular relationships

At the age of 2 to 3 years, Samantha was described by the residential institution as snuggling securely in the lap of her special teacher, crying longingly for her birth parents, and, at times, wishfully imagining her mum around, playing at phoning her. Sadly, her beloved first special teacher left the institution, but, after a backlash, Samantha transferred her confidence to her next special teacher, crying in her lap, now for both her first teacher and her birth mum, sometimes playing a wishful phantasy of birth family together inside a castle.

According to reports by the foster parents, throughout development, Samantha kept up this important depressive ability to seek out a preferred parental figure together with whom she was able to mourn her lost objects:

» (*Six months into therapy, during a break*): Samantha was told that her birth mum had moved out of a boyfriend's apartment. This led her to cry lengthily, pining for her birth dad, while securely snuggling in foster mum's lap. The foster mum experienced this crying as heartfelt, very different from Samantha's ordinary angry screaming, and described this event as greatly strengthening their mutual attachment.
» (*At age 6½ years, after a year and a half of therapy*): Again, in foster mum's lap, Samantha told as a memory the phantasy that she and her birth sisters at the residential institutions in unison had rescued their daddy from drowning.
» (*After two and a half years of therapy, immediately after the second Christmas break*): Samantha said to foster mum: "I am sorry for Dad, he can't come to see me."

This important ability to pine in foster mum's lap occurred during a break in the therapy—greatly strengthening their mutual attachment. Splitting apparently did play a role, since, in the same period, Samantha fiercely rejected the foster dad, pointedly turning her back and moving away when he got near.

Before the second Christmas break, Samantha suffered nightmares in which the therapist turned into a frightful monster. The start of sessions became increasingly difficult, Samantha anxiously expecting to find this monster of her dreams inside the playroom:

> (*Session 86, before-break session*): Samantha loudly protests against entering the therapy room, but ... eventually settles down. ... She makes seven drawings ... the same woman moving away, going upstairs, going downstairs, in riding clothes, on a horse, etc. The last drawings are made in manic haste, ... the motive falling apart ... Every time I open my mouth, she shouts, "shut up" with great force. ... (In the end, I decide to keep quiet) ... Suddenly ... Samantha ... shouts: "And don't you dare say I am going to miss you—because I am not. On the contrary, I will hate you most and forget you." (I say that I know she wishes this, ... however, the closer ... the Christmas break, the worse the Liselotte-monster in her mind grows.) Samantha is quiet for a while, then asks, "Who invented the nightmare?" (I say: Probably, she will find it hard to believe, but, in fact, she herself is the one to invent her nightmares.) She sighs heavily a couple of times: "I know that well."

Immediately before the end of therapy, the now 15-year-old Dennis convinced his child-care worker that he was ready to move in with his birth mum again. At follow-up, the foster mum reported that after he had left the family, Samantha developed an anxious panic-stricken submissiveness, as if she believed the foster parents had kicked him out. They were unable to convince her that the removal of Dennis was against their wishes, and, in the end, they had to get Samantha's child-care worker to tell her that she was "not going anywhere, but is staying here for good". Then she calmed down.

Nonetheless, the loss of Dennis kept bothering Samantha, and, even at follow-up, she would still ask the foster parents why he couldn't come back to stay and as before, join them at Christmas and vacations. Simultaneously, she displayed a dawning awareness that Dennis had changed, hardened into a streetwise bully. For instance, she no longer felt comfortable being alone with him, and during his visits to the foster family backed off their earlier, mutual candy-seeking forays to the petrol station.

Samantha's submissive, terrified identification with Dennis at the age of 5 years was the original reason for referral, and, probably, she was unconsciously worried that, by projection of her bad parts, she had got Dennis kicked out. Hence, her submissive reaction when he left possibly derived from survivor's guilt, related to a phantasy that, like a cuckoo in the nest, she had pushed Dennis out of the family, herself to become "the first foster child to come". This mixture of fright, compassion, and guilt may have created a prolonged sibling solidarity, preventing Samantha from realizing that the good old Dennis she first knew when the two children lived together in the foster family no longer existed.

All in all, regardless of an immense improvement in motivation, skills, and social relationships, the submissive reaction at the removal of the older foster brother and her difficulties in coming to terms with the loss indicates a lingering tendency towards a traumatic relapse of reality orientation, when feeling at risk of losing parental protection.

Summary, discussion, and conclusion

A main finding of the study was a characteristic pattern of subjective core themes running as a red thread through all Samantha's relationships, not only inside the therapy, but also in early infancy and her daily life concurrent to therapy. This result is in accordance with psychotherapy research concerning adults and strongly corroborates Hinshelwood's assumption that core themes found in the transference relationship likewise permeate infantile and current relationships (Hinshelwood, 1991; Luborsky, 1997; Luborsky & Luborsky, 2006).

The specific pattern of core themes noted above probably reflects the fact that Samantha early in her life had suffered severe neglect and maltreatment. However, comparison of core themes in the therapeutic process with children with similar and different early relationship experience is needed to test out this hypothesis.

Furthermore, the results indicate that *reactions before and after breaks, especially the presence/absence of hostile siblings in mind,* are an *important indicator of change*. Thus, a few, highly idealized parental figures appeared before breaks, while hostile parent–sibling collusions primarily appeared in no-break and after-break sessions. This combination indicates that in before-break sessions, symbol formation collapsed, and thus transformation of the overwhelming feelings related to abandonment, jealousy, and envy into symbolic imagos of sibling figures became impossible. The appearance later in therapy of sibling figures in before-break sessions accordingly may indicate improvement of affect regulation and cognitive-emotional functioning. In accordance with this observation, Houzel (2004, 2008) and M. E. Rustin (1998) presented clinical data suggesting that a planned ending of therapy may be within reach when the child continues to make progress even during breaks.

Although foster parents and the birth mother reported considerable progress at the end of therapy—and even more so at follow-up—*lingering vulnerabilities* in relation to loss and tendencies for splitting and ganging up in relation to the birth mother and birth sisters were discernible in descriptions. Thus, as found also by Gaensbauer (1994, 1995), the residues of severe early neglect and maltreatment seem especially resistant to change in relation to the persons with whom this experience originated.

Development of a capacity to mourn lost objects worked hand-in-glove with *early triangulation*, ushering in phantasies of longing for a good daddy figure. However, *complex splitting* also was part of this since, in the same period, Samantha fiercely rejected the foster dad. This recalls Green's concept of "*bi-triangulation*", referring to a projection of the bad part of a primary split maternal object into the paternal object, the child circumventing both an integration of the split maternal object and the acceptance of separateness (1975, 1977). One may speculate whether a certain degree of this kind of splitting may ordinarily be part and parcel of the very early Oedipus complex—or whether this is, rather, related to severe pathology in early processes of splitting caused by early deprivation and maltreatment.

Especially at the beginning of after-break sessions, Samantha seemed caught in fierce approach-avoidance conflicts. The frozen state was probably caused by Samantha's growing ability at session start to remember the pain of parting, which literally kept her stuck on the threshold to the playroom, neither able to embrace her longing for closeness nor to state her separateness and leave the therapist.

Rey described such frozen states of mind as related to *claustro-agoraphobic dilemmas*, the subject caught midways due to the equation of separateness with terrifying isolation and dependency with suffocation (1994). Green metaphorically referred to "sitting on the fence", unable to say either no or yes to separateness, therefore unable to move (1975, 1977). Steiner linked the stuck-ness to avoidance of paranoid-schizoid and depressive anxiety alike, the subject in a state of *psychic retreat* (1993). The evasion of separateness–dependency dilemmas prevents change, since change is equated with pain and catastrophe.

The nest of babies phantasy and foster care of siblings

The findings suggest that severe early neglect and maltreatment in its wake may leave a subjective (largely unconscious) composite phantasy formation of hostile alliances between aggressive parental and sibling figures. This structure, reminiscent of Klein's "nest of hostile babies" phantasy (1932), seems extraordinarily resistant to change, only slowly to be mitigated, giving way to more benign, mixed figures. In this respect, there are striking similarities to Houzel's case research with autistic children (2001, 2008).

This finding touches on a difficult question concerning siblings going into care—namely, when ought they be placed together and when apart? Legislation and psychosocial policy, both in the UK and in Denmark, state that, in general, family ties should be preserved and siblings placed together, provided that it is feasible and consonant with the children's individual parenting needs. Thus, as shown by Hindle (2007) and Wakelyn (2007), when assessing siblings for care, it is not enough to assess the care relationships and attachment to the parents: the emotional quality of sibling relationships in mind and in everyday life must also be considered.

There seems to be a huge schism between reality and the intentions of legislation, since, according to a review of the fostering system in England, in 2011, 70% of those children who had siblings were separated from them at placement (Baginsky, Gorin, & Sands, 2017; Ofsted, 2012). This is probably also the case in Denmark (Egelund & Hestbaek, 2003; Mehlbye, Bonfils, & Andersen, 2011).

Existing research on sibling placements is sparse and the results uncertain, but pointers may be:

1. Possibilities of a benign outcome increase if siblings are close in age, same sex, and enter care at the same time and/or are taken into kinship care (Jones, 2016; Silverstone, 2006).
2. Risk of placement breakdown increases if the siblings share highly traumatic early experiences—for example, chronic neglect/deprivation, prolonged maltreatment, and sexual abuse (Burnell, Castell, & Cousins, 2009; Lord & Borthwick, 2008; Rushton, Dance, Quinton, & Mayes, 2001).

This case study, about a child who early in her life had suffered severe neglect and maltreatment, found an inner structure of hostile, colluding parental and sibling figures in mind. This seemed highly resistant to change and posed special difficulties for re-parenting. It seems likely that this inner situation entails an especially high risk of sibling placement breakdown. Hence, this case study accentuates the importance of a meticulous assessment of sibling relationships being undertaken before deciding whether to place siblings apart or together.

A comment on applied qualitative research methodology

The findings linking breaks to hostile sibling figures in mind were quite unexpected—the therapist-in-the-therapy had not been able to recognize the importance of sibling figures as a decisive focus in the therapy. In addition, the systematic principles imported from qualitative research regarding strategic selection, defining the units of analysis, and the analytic procedures made possible a sequential analysis and a step-by-step comparison of events inside therapy with descriptions provided by caretakers throughout development, thus in a systematic way highlighting relational core themes in the life of this child.

This confirms the value of systematic integration into the psychoanalytic single-case study of inductive–deductive analytic principles from qualitative research methodology, in this specific case IPA. The unexpected findings concerning sibling figures demonstrate the great usability and potential strength of this as an exploratory tool in clinical case research. The combination of methods led to unexpectedly rich insights; it may be of special importance in the development of psychoanalytic and psychotherapeutic theory through single-case studies.

Notes

1. PhD dissertation, the Tavistock Clinic/University of East London. The work was supervised by Margaret Rustin and Nicholas Midgley.

2. References to breaks: Session 7/ loc. 822 & 888; Sessions 35–40/ loc. 3745, 3885, 3967, 4280–4293, 4304.

3. In Denmark, legislation concerning custody is founded on the belief that it is in the best interests of most children taken into care that contact with birth parents and family is maintained; in general, legal adoption to foster parents is not allowed.

CHAPTER EIGHT

What can I tell you? An exploration of child psychotherapy assessment using grounded theory

Marie Bradley

The study

The small-scale study in which I used grounded theory to analyse my primary data (the individual assessment sessions of four children) is a detailed analysis of what can be learned from child psychotherapy assessment, undertaken as part of a wide-ranging multi-professional assessment process. Assessment is always the place where direct work with children begins. It may be undertaken for a range of reasons, some of which are very specific, but a child psychotherapy assessment is always embedded in the broader and deeper context of understanding the child himself (or herself), making sense of who he is and how he comes to be who he is at this time and in this place and in the light of his life experiences. The study assessments were part of my ordinary clinical work and also part of the broader, overarching assessment process concerned with planning the future for these children in alternative family placements. The assessments followed standard child psychotherapy practice, although the presence of the child psychotherapist as researcher was directly raised with two of the children, aged 8 and 10 years.

There is also some difference in the extent of confidentiality to bear in mind. While there are limitations to the extent of confidentiality in most assessments, since some information will go to referrer(s), in this particular situation the information was to be available to many. Explicit reference to the connection between the therapist and other professionals in the network is necessary and can be helpful in giving the child a sense of "joined-up" thinking by those looking after him. The contextual work around the assessments was more extensive than usual: social workers and foster carers were consulted in extensive semi-structured interviews before and after the assessment sessions, and schoolteachers completed Strength and Difficulties questionnaires and most, in addition, contributed detailed thoughts and observations.

The children

The study children are described as "children in transition". They were children in transition through the care system, following the permanent breakdown of care in their families of origin, usually after long periods of difficulty and instability in their lives. The children had suffered much trauma and many losses—loss of family, home, locality, and stability and of an ordinary sense of the future. In each case, there had been ongoing, sometimes extensive attempts to support parents and families, though none of the children had been offered individual support. Three of the four children had received substantial practical and emotional support from teachers at their primary schools. The children (not their real names) were Danny aged 10, Sophie aged 8, Milly aged 6, and Ollie aged 3. Danny and Ollie were black British children; Milly and Sophie were of mixed heritage. All of the children were living in foster care or kinship care, and, at the time of assessment, only Milly had any direct contact with her birth mother.

The context

The title of the study became "No Man's Land? Making a Map: The Contribution of Child Psychotherapy to Decision-Making for Looked-After Children in Transition", and I shall say a little about how this came about. Far-reaching and permanent ideas were being explored for the children's future placement and care. This was taking place in the context of the legal process that would allow and define future plans for the children. These social work processes were pivotal for the decision-making process but lacked a sense of connection to the children and their ongoing daily lives. I came to think of the difficult task of bringing together what often felt like very disparate parts of the whole process going on around the children, sometimes without seeming to touch them, as "making a map". I was attempting to bring together a wide range of sometimes disparate professional knowledge and opinion about the children and their needs. Then, in an attempt to capture the absence of certainty and the particular quality of knowing and not knowing what was happening in the children's lives, I turned to the phrase "No man's land" in an effort to capture the sense of not belonging to either "side"—that is, not firmly rooted in the past nor yet having a place in the future, but living in disputed territory where the outcome is as yet unknown. In this, I drew on what Janet Philps (2009) describes as the "borderline" state of being (Rey, 1994) that is evident in children in transition, characterized by the absence of conscious connection between powerful and potentially overwhelming aspects of thinking about ongoing experience. In the face of the extreme uncertainty and emotional conflict inherent in the children's lives during this transitional time, this can be seen as a profound, but necessary, unconscious strategy for survival. There were no plans for the rehabilitation of the children to their birth families. They were legally now in the care of the state, and alternative permanent family placements were sought for each of them. Many such children find a way of living "as if" life is ordinary when, in fact, they are in such a strange position. They make relationships with their foster carers, go to school, may see birth parents at "contact", quite putting out of mind the inevitably temporary nature of all this. Very often, so do their carers and professionals around them—not to do so seems "unthinkable".

Assessment

Assessments in the service of such momentous decisions are necessarily multi-disciplinary. The needs of children are complex, and the lives and needs of these children are particularly so. The children will be assessed by social workers, doctors, teachers, legal representatives, foster carers, and other specialist workers—so why add a child psychotherapy assessment? What may be missing from the extensive information already available, and what can a child psychotherapist usefully add?

In the inner-city Child and Adolescent Mental Health team where I worked (before the advent of specialist looked-after children's teams in CAMHS), we noted a small, steady number of requests for a child psychotherapy assessment to assist social workers in understanding the future needs of children in transition. We wondered why there were not more, and from this began the idea of the study. An initial, lengthy period of discussion with social work managers and social workers was valuable in helping me understand why this might be. Those who sought a child psychotherapy assessment essentially wanted to know more about the child himself, as directly as possible. Referrals began with this kind of request: "This child puzzles me; I'm struggling to know what makes him tick and what will give him a decent chance in life. Help!" Talking together, this then became a series of questions, like:

> What sort of boy/girl is this child? What does he/she make of what has happened to him/her? Has he/she been deeply damaged by his/her experiences? What might help with this? What sort of family should we be looking for? What sort of support would that family need?

Questions such as this were characteristic of these social workers' thoughts about referral. At that time, they were much in the minority and, interestingly, had in various ways some experience of knowing about psychotherapy, from personal experience or from further training. Therefore, "child psychotherapy" did not suggest to them something disconnected from the ordinary reality of children's experience. It meant something ordinary and useful. Other social workers were less convinced. Already weighed down by the responsibility and complexity of understanding and planning for the future lives of traumatized children, child psychotherapy assessment seemed to threaten the "opening of a can of worms", further traumatizing children. There is much to think about here, not least the need for a shared language and a capacity to know about the demands on those who are closest to the children through this time, to find ways of understanding and supporting those in direct contact with the children so that they, too, are less likely to be thrown back on similar "borderline" ways of surviving transition.

What can a child psychotherapy assessment say?

To the child psychotherapist, it can feel both necessary and potentially limiting to meet a child with a list of the information required by the professional network in the front of one's mind. It also seems unhelpful and discouraging not to offer some idea of what might be learned from the intervention, to justify engaging the child in yet another professional relationship, and a brief one at that. The impingement of the external "task" may risk reducing the therapist's sensitivity to feeling, seeing, and hearing the patterns and quality of unconscious communication between therapist and child, observed in the processes of transference and countertransference between them. I thought the social workers' questions were often spot on. These questions really were about the very specific emotional impact of their experiences on the children, the consequences for the children's ongoing growth and development, and the implications for their future care. However, from the ongoing, systematic attention to the clinical material that grounded theory methodology afforded, there gradually emerged a clearer sense of the unconscious meaning and connections of what happened in the room.

I worked at finding a way to talk about the aims of my child psychotherapy assessments which reasonably clearly said what I hoped to explore and describe, and which related meaningfully to the questions posed by the social workers. This was surprisingly straightforward, and the fit felt genuine. It is true that the social workers connected to the study were essentially "psychologically minded" in wanting to know more about the child, from the child, as it were. Nevertheless, the task of finding a valid common language that did justice to wider professional concerns and a child psychotherapy perspective was an important step in talking to and working with the multi-disciplinary network, with its particular stresses and conflicts that at times closely reflect the tensions and stresses in the child's world.

This is what I proposed to explore and discuss with the social workers:

» personality—what kind of boy/girl?
» state of mind
» vulnerability and resilience/strengths
» child's ideas about him/herself
» developmental levels
» engagement—attachment
» anxieties and conflicts
» defences—available to thought?
» hopes and wishes
» child's understanding of the assessment?
» what it feels like to be with the child (countertransference)

Before, beyond, and around the assessment sessions

Assessments that contribute to a multi-agency, multidisciplinary process are somewhat different both from the starting point of the clinician and the extent to which the work of the session will be shared with others. The child psychotherapist knows more than usual about the child and his experiences in the external world and is in direct communication with more people in the child's external world than is usually the case.

Not infrequently, the child psychotherapist knows more about what is "going on" or ongoing than the child himself does, creating a curious "Alice in Wonderland" sense in the psychotherapist's mind and in the capacity to attend to the child in the session in the moment.

Around the sessions and the setting up of the research, there was a great deal to be done beyond exploring the viability of the study, requiring as it did the informed cooperation and consent of other professionals, including ethical approval in the formal sense from the NHS Trust and less formal but essential agreement from the wider professional network that the work was ethical and justified in terms of the child's needs. Alongside the direct work with the children as noted above, I carried out semi-structured interviews with each child's social worker and foster carer before and after the intervention, and Strengths and Difficulties questionnaires were completed by teachers.

Standard child psychotherapy technique

The research assessment sessions, four for each child, followed the framework for a standard child psychotherapy assessment. Each child came to four sessions of 50 minutes with me, at weekly intervals where possible, at the same time of day, in the same room, with the same play materials available. This ordinary, rigorous framework helps the therapist to be more certain that what happens in the sessions and what is experienced by the child and the therapist is to do with the child himself and what he brings to the encounter. This standard psychoanalytic framework creates a space where it is more possible to experience and think about being with the child, to engage with the complex interplay of his unconscious mind, his internal world, evident in what he says and does and how he does it, and his communication—or absence of communication—about experiences of people and events in the external world which makes each child and his view of himself and the world unique. (The child is referred to as "he" since the child I discuss in further detail is a boy.) It is also good research practice, as far as possible to hold extraneous variables constant, allowing confidence in the validity of what holds centre stage—the encounter between two specific individuals (M. J. Rustin, 1997).

Assessment and its vicissitudes

Assessment is a pivotal part of the child psychotherapist's work—nothing begins without assessment. It is fundamental, elementary, and immensely complex. "Doing an assessment" is often spoken of, but the process of doing so is less frequently explored in depth in our day-to-day work. In addition to what I think of as the ordinary anxiety associated with anticipation of the as-yet unknown complexity and demands of the experience to come, it always carries for me an additional anxiety that I can best describe as, "What can I tell you?" Not the "This is what I can tell you" implied above but the "How can I really tell you anything", a free-floating anxiety about finding myself unable to understand what I experience, of having nothing "to tell", or, worse still, of missing something crucially important. Thinking about this with some distance from the task of assessment, this particular kind of anxiety seems inherent and crucial to the task. In psychoanalysis, it is axiomatic, as well as often deeply unnerving, to approach an encounter with another in a state of "not knowing" and to be able to withstand or bear it "without any irritable reaching after fact and reason", as the poet Keats described it. It can be thought of, too, as a response to the likely state of mind of the child himself, and such experiences can have much to say to others who will meet the as-yet unknown child in different, as-yet unknown circumstances. Finding the balance between the experience of "negative capability" described above and what feels like an imperative to come up with fact and reason is, I think, always daunting. It felt, in these assessments, that the enormity of the task leaned towards an emphasis on what can be reliably called a fact, with a tendency then to split fact from feeling. Added to this was a justified anxiety about undertaking a brief psychoanalytic intervention with very vulnerable children who were often, one way or another, managing to "go on living".

Grounded theory

On first encountering grounded theory, it was with a rather heavy sense of having to find a way of "analysing primary data" in a way I could understand and which did not distort the clinical material too greatly. Thus I approached it with caution and suspicion, although it was not until I began to read more contemporary accounts (Anderson, 2006; Charmaz, 2006) of the method and its application that I began to breathe more easily. Grounded theory is a qualitative method of discourse analysis that categorizes primary data into themes or patterns of increasing abstraction. The theory emerges from the data—as simple and as complex as that.

In my study, the primary research data are the process recordings of the children's assessment sessions. These recordings are rich in detailed information about what was done and said, though, on closer observation, they include a great deal more than this. What gradually emerges through the ongoing process of data analysis is a finely detailed picture of the child's emotional state of mind throughout the time he is with the therapist. In the context of the psychoanalytic setting, and in the therapist's trained and responsive use of psychoanalytic understanding, the underlying unconscious thoughts and feelings begin to be perceived and to shape what is seen and heard in the moment, and the relationship between these is also then perceived. This took place with particular emphasis on the therapist's exploration and use of her countertransference feelings, a crucial aspect of unconscious communication between child and therapist and one that I was particularly anxious to demonstrate meaningfully.

Constant perusal of the data, coupled with ongoing comparison of what was happening with what had already happened, with the child in the room and, in time, between the other children in my sample over many moments in the assessment sessions, began to show me a sense of pattern(s) of integration, or of unintegration or disintegration, and these patterns began to make sense of the unconscious communication between us. In time, I was able to cluster categories into concepts that reflected my psychoanalytic child psychotherapy theoretical and clinical orientation. As the work progressed from case to case, I was both implicitly and explicitly using this constant comparative methodology, thinking about what was happening with the child in relation to what I had already learned from being with him and then, as I moved on to the other children, reflecting on and comparing this with these subsequent experiences.

Grounded theory was first proposed by Glaser and Strauss (1967), who emphasized the need to explore the data without preconceptions about its meaning. The child psychotherapist Jan Anderson (2006) observed that this rather closely resembles the way psychoanalytic understanding of the meaning of a psychoanalytic session, or part of it, emerges. She notes that this does not happen in a naïve framework but in the context of the sophisticated theoretical framework of psychoanalysis and the framework of the mind of a highly trained professional. Charmaz (2006), building on the work of Glaser and Strauss, believed that emphasis on the data as the sole basis from which meaning and interpretation can be drawn is neither possible nor desirable. She diverges significantly here, asserting that "we are part of the world we study and the data we collect. We *construct* our grounded theories through our past and present involvements and interactions with people, perspectives, and research practices" (p. 10). Charmaz explicitly assumes that any emerging theory offers "an *interpretive* portrayal of the studied world, not an exact picture of it" (p. 10). It does seem more useful to be rigorously aware of the theoretical framework of one's research, with its strengths and weaknesses, rather than attempt to divest oneself of it. This development—that data would, could, and should be analysed and understood in the context of the pre-existing theoretical framework of the mind examining it—is the sense in which grounded theory is often now used in qualitative research, notably in the field of child psychotherapy. I endeavoured to do this in my study.

An unexpected bonus

As I grew more confident about the validity of the methodology, so it seemed to provide me with some containment for the anxiety I referred to earlier: that I would understand nothing of the experience of the child, I would have nothing to usefully contribute. Bion's (1970) advice to "eschew memory and desire" asserts the benefits of complete open-mindedness. But how was I to achieve something of this stance in the face of my anxieties about coming away empty-handed? Bion's advice seems a way of ensuring, as far as possible, that elusive unconscious phenomena are not hidden by screens of pre-conceptions and conscious aims for the patient, rather than an argument that one can do without theory. I began to trust that "it—understanding—would emerge from the data" and to allow myself "open-mindedness". This may seem a curious use of research methodology, but in time it assumed a helpful internal presence in my mind, a kind of internal supervisor, which has continued on into my practice, long after the research.

The children in context

The children were selected from the weekly referral meeting, the only inclusion criteria being age (between 3 and 10 years), legal status (in the care of the Local Authority without plans for rehabilitation to families of origin), and the request for a contribution to assessment for permanent placement in alternative families.

The place the children came from, a generally vibrant inner-city area with an unusual mix of wealthy and working-class families, has a very culturally and ethnically diverse population. There is a significant number of multi-generational black British families, and many younger members of these families are of mixed ethnic heritage. It is an area where social deprivation is widespread for some groups, but it can be difficult to see this in the context of a more superficially upbeat atmosphere. There are many immigrant families, some now second and third generation, who in some respects maintain their separate identity within the mainstream population.

The children—Danny, Sophie, Milly, and Oliver—all came, as it happened, from the area's group of long-standing families of mixed cultural heritage and, with the exception of Milly, were children whose deprivation seemed to have been unseen in the vulnerabilities of their families and thus for some considerable time seemed to slip between the gaps in health and welfare services. The children were strongly representative of these aspects of the local population, aspects not easily seen in a culturally and economically diverse population. They were, however, highly representative of the CAMHS clinic population in this area. The clinic had strong, accessible links with many other local services, statutory and voluntary, which proved of great value in ongoing work with the children after the assessments.

Substance misuse, largely Class A drugs, with associated mental health problems, was significant in the breakdown of all of the children's families. The mothers of two of the children, Danny and Milly, suffered from severe and enduring mental health problems that predated and were exacerbated by drug abuse. All of the families were poor, all parents were unemployed. Violence, including domestic violence, was a significant occurrence in the children's families, with parents being both perpetrators and victims.

For some of the children, the extended family had tried to help but failed. Thereafter, they withdrew, perhaps from a sense of helplessness, but also of shame. This seemed to preclude seeking outside help until it could no longer be avoided.

School (or nursery) played an enormous part in supporting each child. The older children were at times being fed, clothed, washed, and loved at school. Sometimes referrals had been made to statutory services without intervention taking place, and school support continued sometimes for years. There is much to think about here: the input of the teachers was enormous and gave the children some important sense of being held thoughtfully and lovingly in mind, and yet the teachers felt powerless to get help for the serious underlying problems in the children's lives.

The children: brief accounts

Danny, age 10, was the oldest child in the study. His mother suffers from a severe and enduring mental illness, while his father, a transient and longed-for presence in Danny's life, had frequently been imprisoned for crimes of a violent and sexual nature. Danny appeared to be a very tough small boy, dauntingly self-reliant.

Sophie, age 8, was a slender, aloof, and seemingly fragile girl, with great difficulty in showing anyone her vulnerability or needs. In the sessions, she "ebbed and flowed" with a "Cheshire Cat" quality, like her mother who came and went in her life but to whom Sophie remained determinedly and hopelessly devoted.

Milly, age 6, was a beautiful, delicate mixed-race child. At the time of assessment, Milly had contact with her birth mother and struggled desperately to be the daughter she thought her mother wanted. Feeling sure her different skin colour was the reason her mother failed to love her, she scrubbed at her skin to make it white. Being with Milly felt sometimes unbearable, as if she "got under one's skin" in a profoundly painful way.

Oliver, age 3, was so withdrawn and silent he was thought autistic or brain damaged. Cared for by his grandmother, meetings with her revealed how traumatized she was following the death of her daughter, Oliver's mother, after years of alternating hope and despair about her. She agreed to help for herself, with her loss and her grief. Oliver slowly came to life. He played vigorously, with anger and sometimes with laughter. His grandmother took on his permanent care.

Meetings with Danny

All of the children surprised and touched me but Danny was the first of the children I assessed, and he brought such unexpected aspects of himself. I try to capture something of this in the excerpts from work with him included here. Danny's unfolding story, internal and external, grew in depth and complexity, as did the experience of being with him.

In the first session, the tough and daunting boy looked around the room and shrugged. "I like to play, sometimes." I note his guardedness about "playing", as if it were an indulgence in one so worldly weary. I asked what he liked to do, and he told me, "I like the World Wrestling Federation, and the Hulk, and Spiderman and Superman." I replied that he liked some tough characters, by the sound of it. He agreed and told me "Spiderman and Superman are actually human beings who can change to become very powerful and then save people." He spoke in a way that takes the validity of this observation for granted, as a younger child might do, and this was touchingly at odds with his appearance. He added, "Superman often looked quite weak and not many people knew he could be so strong." A reference to himself, I thought. I asked about the others. Danny said, "The Hulk isn't one who saves people. He gets angry … "; he paused: "… and love is his weakness." I was entirely taken by surprise, quite unable to gather myself for a moment. Then I wondered about that and he told me: "Loving people took the Hulk's strength away." The feeling in the room was poignant with longing and sadness. I thought how easily this part of Danny might not have been seen.

He then began to play with the people and wild animals, who were quickly embroiled in a terrible fight. He turned to me with a hard, frightening smile, and the fighting became cruel and murderous. Quite suddenly then, he turned to the doll's house, gently, even tenderly looking in. He found a baby and quietly placed it in a cot.

After the session I felt sorrowful and neglectful, as if I were guilty of failing to see beyond his tough street-kid front, and I was reminded of my initial sense of hopelessness when I met him. I was also curious and hopeful. Here began the "unexpected bonus" of the research methodology, grounded theory. Subtle, sometimes seemingly disparate aspects of the experience of being with Danny emerged and took shape in the process of repeatedly revisiting the sessions, finding ways to describe and name the experiences between him and me. Making the experience more abstract also gave, paradoxically, growing emotional depth and substance to my understanding of Danny.

Through the following sessions, Danny moved rapidly between enacting ferocious scenes in which animals and people were tortured cruelly while he seemed sadistically untouched, then suddenly turning to the small animals and doll children with what felt, at moments, unbearable tenderness. He seemed at first unaware of the extremes in what he did and said, and he was extremely sensitive to any premature attempt on my part to speak to the vulnerability and tenderness in him, shutting me down and drawing away from me, angry and hurt.

By the third session, however, he began to be curious about this idea of "him and me", something quite different from me as onlooker/commentator, and quite unexpected. He picked up a doctor's bag and took out the things inside, looking closely. Then he found the stethoscope and asked me what it was for. I told him it was for listening to a person's heart and breathing. He put it into his ears and quite gently placed it on his chest. "Here?" he asked, tentatively. I helped him find the place, then he clearly heard his heart beating, and he looked pleased and thrilled. He took the stethoscope away and looked at me. "Did you always want to be a psychotherapist?" I smiled and asked what he thought. He paused then replied, "Yes, I think you did." (It felt as if the idea of a live connection between two hearts, two minds, had meaning for him.)

The doll's house featured in much of his play, both ferocious and tender. Towards the end of the assessment Danny asked me "Where did you get this house? Did you make it?" We thought together about his interest in the house, and he added, "Can people buy that house off you? Could you sell me the house?" The house seemed to stand for the experience in the sessions of exploring both himself, his internal world, and his internal objects, good and bad. I said we had thought about so much in these sessions, with the house often in the middle of it all. Nevertheless, there was more to be said about the house. I said he'd shown me all sorts of things about himself and his life here in his sessions, and the house, which he liked, was still there just the same. I wondered if the house was a bit like the house and the family he hoped for? He didn't say yes or no, but he smiled.

The boy towards whom I first felt despair and hopelessness seemed to know of the possibility of real, live, and even loving interest and connectedness with another, and I came to feel he had known something of this before his mother became so ill. In the brief intervention of assessment, he had come to know something of a house/relationship that could countenance and contain the extremes of his emotional and lived experience. I came to understand why some people went "the extra mile" for him (perhaps the basis for the request we had received for assessment), while he also showed me the risks he took in letting himself look and be seen beyond the fearsome defences of his identification with tough, perverse characters, including the father he longed for.

The contribution to the multidisciplinary network

The primary aim of child psychotherapy assessment of children for whom decisions are to be made about their future permanent care is to make available to the professional network information and understanding that is significantly different from that which comes from other professionals, including social workers, foster carers, teachers, and other specialist professionals or from birth families. It is only on this basis that an additional, brief intervention that aims to reach deeply into children's thoughts and feelings about their lives and themselves can be justified.

So what is the difference? If you look back to the framework I proposed to give social workers an idea of what they might expect from such an intervention, you find a fairly comprehensive list of things, which will tell you something about what kind of boy this is, what has happened to him, how he makes sense of it all and of himself, and what this says about his future needs."

In some ways, some of what I learned about Danny was held by different parts of the network—though often networks, however good, are less than the sum of their parts. The nature of the work may militate against too much connected thought (Menzies Lyth, 1988). So with Danny. What spoke most eloquently to the network was the child himself, the experience of hearing from him, particularly when I was able to show the connections between different unseen parts of him and to speak directly about the process of finding out with him and from him about who he was and how he was that boy. My assessment report concludes:

> Danny is a boy whose tough, self-reliant presentation can be misleading. He has idealized the toughness and cruelty he has experienced in his earlier life as a way of surviving the very real possibility that his emotional needs would not be recognized or met. Danny is an emotionally alive, sensitive, and passionate boy who shows the potential to engage fully in a new family where he can go on to develop to the fullest of his potential.

In fact, it was two years before Danny joined what became his permanent family, a family of two parents whose children were already "grown". In the time between, he was fairly settled in foster care, separately from his sister, though with frequent direct and indirect contact between them. Danny began twice-weekly psychoanalytic psychotherapy, he began to mourn the life he could not have with his parents, and he began to have an idea of a future of his own.

Life in his new family was sometimes turbulent, but he thrived. His new family stood squarely beside him through trials and tribulations at school, with friends and in relation to his birth parents. When I last heard, he was nearly 16 and doing well.

Conclusions

The assessment of children in transition brings sharply into relief the potential benefits against the potential risks inherent in all brief psychoanalytic interventions: such children are exposed to another short-term relationship in a plethora of transient encounters. The nature of the task for the child and the therapist, looking beyond what can be seen on the surface, inherently raises anxieties about re-traumatizing the child in an encounter that will explore the internal as well as the external uncertainty in that child's life. Concerns include questions about what the child will make of the intervention. What is he to do with what it raises? What will others do with what assessment may bring to light? These are ethical concerns of profound importance, and they are also at the heart of the dilemma of how to help children manage through an indeterminate time of great uncertainty without relying too heavily on the need to live "as if" life were reliable and ordinary. This should not be, and was not, taken lightly by the therapist and the professional network.

For the daunting multidisciplinary task of planning for the children's long-term futures, in addition to the considerable body of knowledge about the important facts of the children's outside lives, what the child psychotherapy assessments contributed was the piece of the jigsaw often missing—the rich complexity of the child's deeply individual and personal inside, emotional self, from the perspective of the child him/herself. When the assessments were discussed in the context of the overarching process of assessing and planning, the sense of the child came alive, and the picture became multidimensional.

For each child, the assessment had a different significance. For two (including Danny), it opened up something hopeful. For Sophie and Milly, it led to the recognition of their need to grieve deeply before moving forward. I think it is right to say that each of the children found him/herself feeling carefully thought about and heard, not simply by me but by the people most closely involved in their care and with whom I had worked most closely: their social workers and foster carers. Space precludes deeper discussion of the building of relationships with these professionals in setting up and supporting the assessments, or the talking, thinking, and struggling to make sense of what the children had revealed. The depth and complexity of the children and their external and internal worlds was strikingly revealed in new and compelling detail. What emerged in these brief interventions seemed to me clearly enabled by the closeness of scrutiny afforded by the process of grounded theory, gradually supporting a move towards confidence in the integrity of what became known of the child. This offered an internal framework for me from which it became possible, in studying this small group of children, to be more open to the subtle, nuanced communications in the sessions. It also added much richness to the meaning of the encounters with the children.

I was able, more informally, to follow the children's progress for some years. Each of the assessments proved, in time, highly relevant in shaping both short- and long-term provision for the children, on many fronts. Beyond the choice of placement—that is, the choice of family—these included the provision of ongoing therapeutic support for the children and for their new families, provision for the needs of children to have contact with their birth families, and acknowledgement of their need for time and space to mourn the losses suffered in the breakdown of their first families. The permanent placements for the children eventually included both kinship care and placement in "atypical" families, decisions strongly shaped by hearing from the children. This raises the need to be open to a multifaceted range of alternative family options relating to the scope and depth of the children's needs and wishes.

The child psychotherapy assessments, with careful, psychoanalytic attention to the fine detail of conversations and communications between children and child psychotherapist, added an important dimension to arriving at decisions that might weather the ongoing developmental challenges and achievements ahead. The study strongly validated the inclusion of child psychotherapy for the study children, and it is worthy of a regular, ordinary place in the multidisciplinary process of planning for the future of children who are in transition.

CHAPTER NINE

Focusing on the carer of the traumatized child: on the benefits of psychoanalytic short-term parent work

Kristine Tiltina

The research project described in this chapter explored the contribution made by the psychoanalytic child psychotherapist in supporting the placement of looked-after children with foster carers, with a particular focus on the benefits of psychoanalytically informed short-term parent work with the foster carers. It took place at the Family Trauma Centre in Belfast, a specialist CAMHS facility that provides treatment for children and their families suffering from the effects of severe trauma.

Each day, across the UK, over 65,000 children live with almost 55,000 foster families. The Fostering Network estimates that a further 8,100 foster carer families are needed in the next 12 months (Lawson & Cann, 2018). Foster carer families are a scarce resource, and the sustainability of the placements of looked-after children (LAC)—that is, doing everything possible to prevent their breakdown—has more than ever become a priority.

Data was gathered from five foster families seen for four sessions each. The research project sought to contribute to our understanding of the defensive responses aroused in the foster carer when faced with the intense, distressing affect associated with the child's early trauma, and the impact of this legacy of trauma on the child, on the carer, and on the wider social services system.

In the psychoanalytic literature, the phenomenon of psychic trauma is understood as encompassing the effects of severely traumatizing events in the child's external environment, as well as the distressing, yet more ordinary, life events of an infant and young child that shape its internal world (Garland, 2002, *passim*). Freud conceptualized the mind as a "psychic apparatus" that has developed a "protective shield", which enables the mind to be highly selective in its reception of stimuli from the external environment via the senses. In *Beyond the Pleasure Principle* (1920g), he describes as "traumatic" any "excitations" from outside that are powerful enough to break through the protective shield and overwhelm the fragile mind (p. 31).

Shifts in meaning and usage of the concept of trauma continued after Freud. Ronald Fairbairn suggested that the danger of "trauma" is ever-present in the life of every child:

> The greatest need of a child is to obtain conclusive assurance (a) that he is genuinely loved as a person by his parents, and (b) that his parents genuinely accept his love. ... Frustration of this desire to be loved as a person and to have love accepted is the greatest trauma a child can experience. [Fairbairn, 1952, pp. 39–40]

In contemporary psychoanalytic thinking, clinicians understand more than ever that the internal world of the child is largely shaped by and dependent upon external events and circumstances; and this is especially pertinent to the emotional development of looked-after children. Furthermore, the early and pre-birth experiences of children in care often have a particularly damaging quality that is more significant and more enduring than any ordinary impingement. The emotional patterns created by traumatic experiences in the pre-verbal stage of development, or primal repetitions, are exceptionally difficult to put into words, as they will most likely have their roots in experiences that were not only pre-verbal, but also "pre-imagistic" (Wilson & Malatesta, 1989, p. 296). When foster carers are subjected to the full force of the child's distress and trauma-fuelled communication, the exchange between them may well be experienced by the carer as traumatizing and can trigger defensively unthinking responses, thereby narrowing the carer's cognitive or emotional awareness of the child or both. Caroline Garland (2002) describes the impact of trauma (in this case, in the carer) as follows:

> However well any individual feels he is normally able to take care of what he feels to be his own well-being, some events will overwhelm

> that capacity, will knock out ordinary functioning and throw the individual into extreme disarray. [Garland, 2002, p. 9]

"Parent work" has become a common practice among child psychotherapists, whereby child psychotherapists support each other in offering psychoanalytically informed sessions to parents, in parallel to the child's psychotherapy. This parent work takes several forms, including, for example, various parenting programmes, or training for foster carers and kinship carers. The emphases of these programmes are on providing information, teaching coping strategies, or providing therapeutic input. Margaret Rustin highlights the significance of shame and envy in parenting:

> The experience of shame among parents who need help with their children is a significant clinical problem—their sense of failure and incompetence, and their dread of being despised and humiliated by those felt to be more successful at being grown-up is a severe hindrance in parent work. Linked to this is unconscious envy, with its corrosive impact on relationships which stir up a sense of need. [M. E. Rustin, 1999, p. 210]

Martha Harris and Helen Carr (1966) describe a type of brief "therapeutic consultation", in which the "containing" role of the therapist is similar to that of the observer in baby observation. "A genuine interest, conveyed without any claim to 'magical expertise'", Harris believes, "can aid in restoring the parents' own creativity, putting them back in touch with their own unique knowledge of themselves and their child" (Harris & Bick, 2011, p. 304).

Even within a strictly psychoanalytic framework, parent support includes a wide spectrum of work, with different emphases depending on the child's developmental stage, family constellations and dynamics, the child's presenting difficulties, and so on. In this research, the investigation explored the nature and benefits of the support provided by a psychoanalytic child psychotherapist to long-term foster carers, who routinely experience a uniquely daunting set of challenges when they assume the care of a child who has suffered adverse and traumatizing experiences while in the birth parents' care, has been removed from the birth family, and therefore has lost birth mother and father, and who almost certainly has subsequently experienced several losses of carers before reaching his or her long-term foster carer(s).

Initially the research study explored two research questions:

» **"What is the nature of short-term psychoanalytically informed parent/carer work?"**
» **"What impact does short-term psychoanalytically informed parent/carer work have on the foster placement?"**

When the research data were analysed, in accordance with grounded theory and the principles of psychoanalytic listening, one of the significant factors (or themes) that emerged was the carer's capacity to remain focused on the child's emotional needs, which, in turn, was linked to the direction of the therapist's focus during the parent work. Repeated analysis of the data culminated in the hypothesis that the more the therapist focused on the carer and the carer's emotional states in the course of the parent work, the more the carer was enabled to focus on the child's emotional needs.

As the system of categories emerged according to the themes exemplified in the sessions, a particular focus of analysis became the concept of psychological-mindedness (in the carer), considered under several sub-categories: voicing insightful comments; awareness of the child's bodily states; awareness of the child's affect; the carer's ability to recognize the child's defences; and the carer's ability to make links between the child's current difficulties and the child's past experiences. Through this analysis, it became apparent that degree of psychological-mindedness was closely linked to the individual carer's capacity to metabolize the child's distressed and distressing communication. This, in turn, led to a deeper exploration (again, in line with grounded theory methodology) of situations that were particularly challenging for the carers—such as instances when the child was compelled to repeat past traumatic emotional states and was, as a result, communicating intense distress.

This exploration eventually generated the second hypothesis: that in response to the child's distress, the reaction of each carer could be plotted somewhere along a spectrum from distancing themselves from the child's emotional state to seeking excessive closeness with the child (merging). The final stage of the analysis developed four new categories of carer responses to the distressed child: identification and distancing from the child; identification and merging with the child; the category that describes the carer's psychological-mindedness as being "impaired'; and "good-enough" caring.

This research clearly demonstrates that, even within the short space of four sessions of weekly psychoanalytic parent work, it is possible to achieve significant improvement in a foster carer's capacity to bear the child's compulsion to repeat early traumas, and to help the carer to become more emotionally available to the child, in order to provide the child with effective psychological parenting at such difficult and challenging times.

The research participant selection criterion was: an individual foster carer or foster carer couple currently parenting a looked-after child (age 4–11 years) in a (non-kinship) long-term placement. This criterion was chosen to minimize as far as possible the variables among the children, such as major developmental milestones, transition to secondary school, or the circumstances of the placement—that is, short or long, kinship or non-kinship.

The referrals were made by social services' LAC team and consisted of the carers of three boys and two girls, aged from 6 to 11 years. All the children's birth mothers had either diagnosed (4) or undiagnosed (1) significant mental health difficulties, which were, in some cases, trans-generational, and included psychotic episodes, suicide attempts, and substance abuse that precipitated physical and/or emotional abuse and neglect of their children. None of the children knew their birth father. On average, the children had remained in their birth mother's care up until the age of 6. At the time of assessment, all of them had regular contact with their birth family. All five foster families consisted of a foster mother and a foster father; five foster mothers and only two foster fathers attended the sessions.

Following an initial meeting involving the carers, the referring social worker and the researcher, a state of mind assessment of each child (i.e., a detailed description of the child's internal emotional world, main patterns of relating to others, and level of development) was carried out by the researcher over a period of three individual weekly sessions. This was followed by four weekly psychoanalytically informed parent support sessions with each set of carers. These sessions were audio-recorded and later transcribed in full. The sequence was concluded by a feedback meeting with each carer or carer couple and their referrer. A written State of Mind Assessment Report was provided in relation to each child; and in some cases a recommendation was made for further therapeutic work.

Data analysis and findings

My first encounter was with a 7-year-old girl I shall call "Anna" and her foster mother, Mrs Morgan). (All names have been changed for reasons of confidentiality.) Anna's birth mother suffers from long-term mental illness that manifests as suicidal ideation, psychotic episodes, and substance misuse, with the result that Anna and her siblings suffered chronic and extreme neglect, including starvation. Anna's birth father's name and whereabouts are unknown. Anna was initially placed with the Morgan family at the age of 5 years. Her placement became long-term a year later. The referral described Anna as a child who assumes an adult role during her contact with her birth mother: for example, defusing conflict situations and being anxious about her mother's ability to cope, with Anna being in care. Normally a placid and happy child, Anna was also described by her social worker, and by Mrs Morgan, as showing some "out-of-character behaviour"—such as mood swings and being emotional, angry and tearful—following contact with her mother. My first impression of Anna was one of an eloquent, cautious, compliant little girl. I also observed that outside my consulting room, in her interaction with Mrs Morgan, Anna tended to display a strong sense of rivalry, evidence of her struggle with child–adult relationships. To an outsider, Anna could convincingly give the impression of an intelligent, imaginative, and easy-to-care-for child, who is doing well and needs no help from others. However, it became evident that she struggled to seek support in an age-appropriate way. Mrs Morgan's social worker described Mrs Morgan as someone who is "happy to attend any trainings". Mr Morgan chose not to take part in the study and seemed to have minimal or no involvement with social services.

The initial data analysis began by reading through the transcripts of each of the sessions held with Mrs Morgan (FM1, the first of five sets of foster carers), noting and reflecting on themes as they emerged paragraph by paragraph, as is commonly practised by psychoanalytic child psychotherapists. In this case, however, the data consisted of full transcriptions of audio recordings of the sessions, not the usual process notes. This provided immensely detailed content, including some distressing accounts of the child's early experiences (some of which might well have been unconsciously filtered out by the researcher if process notes had been written up after the sessions); and at times this made the transcripts very difficult reading material. One possible disadvantage of using audio recordings was the dilution in the transcripts of the researcher's immediate countertransference experiences and observations in the room; however, some of that countertransference experience was captured in the words of the researcher that form part of the recording of the sessions (and thus part of the research data).

A psychoanalytic analysis of the session between carer and researcher produced the following psycho-dynamic elements for further consideration:

» the dynamics in the room—that is, transference and countertransference experiences between the therapist/researcher and the carer(s)
» the dynamics of the foster carer couple
» the dynamics of the carer's internal world
» the dynamics of the child's presentation as it was re-presented by the carer: for example, representation of the child's internal world, affect regulation issues, defences, interpersonal relationships, the child's view of self, etc.

This initial analysis also resulted in a basic framework of research "themes":

» How the carer(s) viewed their role in relation to the child in their care.
» How the carer(s) described the child.
» How the carer(s) viewed the system around them: for example, how social services or the therapist are seen and used by the carers.
» How the carer(s) viewed the child's contact with birth parents and siblings.
» More specific themes that carers wanted to think about in the session, such as how to deal with special occasions, such as Christmas and birthdays, or related to food, or how to deal with the child's worries that the carer has forgotten about them, etc.
» How the therapist experienced and responded to the presented material.

These themes could then be tested against the rest of the research participants (see Charmaz, 1995).

Figure 9.1, a schematic representation of these complex dynamics, illustrates the intricate interplay of multiple objects and multiple internal worlds. Particular attention had to be paid to the challenge of bearing in mind various points of view—the foster mother's (FM); the foster father's (FF); the therapist's (T); the child's—simultaneously as reported by the carers (CH); the birth family's (BF); siblings (SI); and

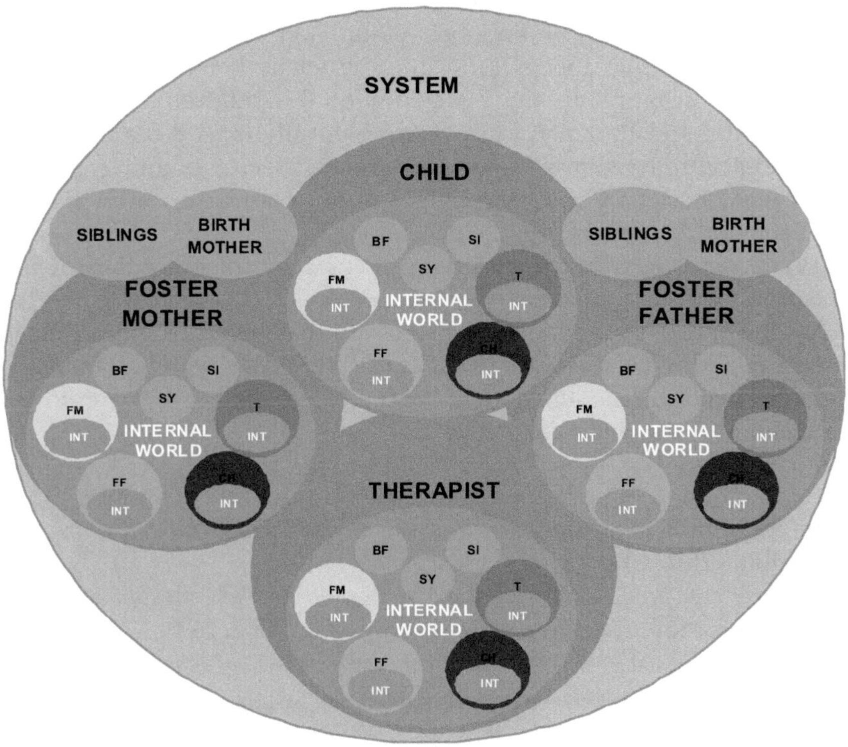

Figure 9.1 Interpsychic and intrapsychic dynamics.

the perspective of the wider network (SY); also bearing in mind the intrapsychic, or internal, psychodynamics.

From the analysis of the material presented by Mrs Morgan (FM1), the significant category of "psychological-mindedness" began to emerge, where she demonstrated some insights and empathy with respect to the child but, at other times, a marked absence of those qualities. And so, a third research question then emerged, which created a core category for the research:

» **What is the quality and depth of psychological-mindedness the carer or carers display in relation to the child in their care?**

Stephen Appelbaum (1973) offers a useful definition of psychological-mindedness: "a person's ability to see relationships among thoughts, feelings, and actions, with the goal of learning the meanings and causes of his experiences and behaviour" (Appelbaum, 1973, p. 36). However, given that the present study crucially considers the carers' capacity for insight into the behaviour of the children in their care, Conte, Ratto, and Byram Karusa (1996) helpfully extend the concept of psychological-mindedness beyond simple self-focus, pointing out that it involves "both self-understanding and an interest in the motivation and behaviour of others" (p. 251).

When tested against the material presented by the other participants, it became apparent that there were several ways ("two sub-categories") in which the carers were able to demonstrate their psychological-mindedness in relation to the child in their care. There may well be others, but the sub-categories identified (and tabulated) as being relevant to this research project were the following:

» an insightful comment—or, conversely, an absence of insight—about the child, indicating the carer's *ability to make links and empathize* with the child (2E & 3E)
» the carer's *awareness (or lack of awareness) of the child's bodily states* and communication through physical expression (2F & 3F)
» the carer's *awareness (or lack of awareness) of the child's affect* (2G & 3G)
» the carer's awareness of the child's ways of coping—that is, references made by the carer to *the child's defence mechanisms,* including occasions when the carer is not aware of making such references to defences (2H & 3H)
» the carer's ability (or absence of ability) to make *links between the child's past experiences and presenting difficulties* (2I & 3I).

The findings from the collated data were then presented in the form of graphs. The example of Mrs Morgan, Session 1, is shown in Figure 9.2.

Figure 9.2 demonstrates how Mrs Morgan (FM1), in her first parent support session (S1), shifts from struggling to be psychologically minded (statements below the horizontal axis) to becoming more available to feeling and thinking about the child (above the horizontal axis). The numbers on the horizontal axis in the graph represent a paragraph of the data, making it possible to trace each rise and fall in this variable. The following example from Paragraph 113 (the grey dot below the axis) scored three negative categories of psychological-mindedness

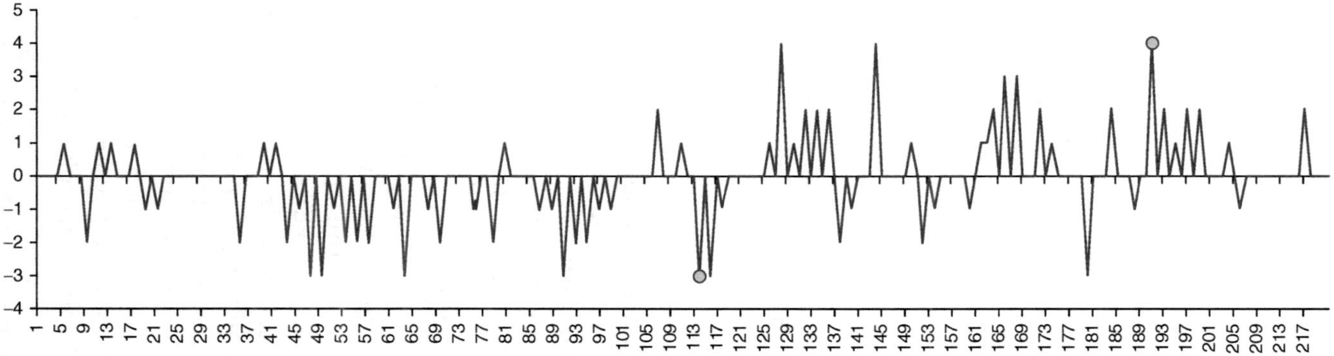

Figure 9.2 Levels of psychological-mindedness, FM1 S1.

(–2G, –2H, –2I): in other words, it indicated a significant absence of psychological-mindedness.

> *Mrs Morgan* (S1, Paragraph 113):
>
> And I just say, "Ach, I know, you do miss your mum, but this is just the way it is at the minute, I'm just here to look after you".

It has to be acknowledged that a foster child's personal narrative—already gravely fragmented because of their early life experiences—is often further complicated by the fact that these children usually experience several moves, and at different stages of their development.

> At each stage of development ... family members have the task of adjusting to the ... emotional climate within the family, boundaries, patterns of interaction and communication. The foster child is faced with the task of adjusting to these normative tasks while transitioning to a new home environment. ... The foster child is unsure of his or her future and lives in a world of uncertainty. [Craven & Lee, 2006, p. 288]

For many of these children, their life experiences have been so unbearable and so fragmented that the passage of time has no meaning. Their experience of life becomes a cluster or a jumble of moments, with a "confused sense of past, present, and future, where past experiences remain undifferentiated from the present and where an idea of the future is of something just like the past" (Canham, 1999, p. 160).

This captures the essence of the "flashback" experience, a consequence of severe trauma that is widely associated with the sudden and unexpected "reliving" of the past in the present. O'Callaghan, Storey, and Rafferty (2012) refer to the ways in which former child soldiers retell their traumatic narrative in such a way that it becomes less threatening to their psychic survival. Thus, the incoherent narrative becomes an essential defence against breakdown. This is particularly significant when considering the foster carer's task of providing a foster child with an alternative set of family experiences to the traumatizing experiences that had brought the child into care in the first place. On the one hand, the child's ways of being and its distressing ways of remembering the past may stir up such anxiety in the carer that the latter may experience this as a threat to their own psychic equilibrium and may simply demand that the child adopt new roles in its new family; on the other hand, the child's story may be so compelling that the carer may feel unable to question the child's beliefs. Lorne Loxterkamp (2009) suggests:

> What the child needs most of all is help to come to terms with [their] loss and its causes, help to manage knowing and understanding the harrowing information that will explain (with greater sophistication as the child matures) why he had to be removed permanently from the birth family. Without this knowledge it is likely that the child will come to be injuriously convinced, for example, that he is blameworthy because he wasn't good-enough for his birth parents, or that he is being prevented from returning to his birth parents for no good reason. [Loxterkamp, 2009, p. 434]

Despite the endemic fragmentation within Anna, towards the end of this first session, in paragraph 190, one of the highest peaks in the graph (the grey dot above the axis) represents four categories of psychological-mindedness in Mrs Morgan's responses (2E, 2G, 2H, 2I).

> *Mrs Morgan* (S1, Paragraph 190):
>
> There are some times when she would hide her feelings, but there are some times when she would say, "I love you", and I obviously would return back, "I love you too". But she wouldn't say it very often. Maybe I could count it out on my fingers the number of times she has said it to me in the two years she's been with me. I think maybe she's afraid to say it because then she doesn't want to upset her mummy. That's what I think. She has a loyalty towards me and her mummy as well, she's kind of confused a wee bit probably, about where her loyalties lie, but she'll get there eventually. But at the minute, I'm delighted to hear that, it was nice to hear her saying that to me, and I said it back, but I wouldn't hear it too often, if you know what I mean.

This detailed analysis of the material led to a follow-up question: What were the facilitating factors that fostered this psychological-mindedness during the parent support work? From the re-analysed material of Mrs Morgan's sessions, there emerged a hypothesis:

> ***The carer's ability to sustain psychologically minded thinking towards the child was directly correlated with the therapist's attentiveness to the emotional states of the carer.***

The data revealed that the ways in which the carer's psychological-mindedness shifted during the session correlated with the therapist's focus of interest—that is, whether my interpretations and comments were directed towards the carer(s) or towards the foster child.

Data on this theme was then collected from every family in every session.

Several psychoanalytic theories describe processes at play between infant and mother, and correspondingly between a patient and a therapist, that could account for this kind of transformation in the psychological-mindedness of the carer. Since the early days of Freud's practice, a sense of being "held" has been provided through the analytic setting. However, in these early encounters between therapist/researcher and foster carers, Donald Winnicott's idea of a "holding environment" seems the most fitting:

> The term "holding" is used here to denote not only the actual physical holding of the infant, but also the total environmental provision prior to the concept of living with. ... It includes the management of experiences that are inherent in existence, such as the completion (and therefore non-completion) of processes, processes which from the outside may seem to be purely physiological but which belong to infant psychology and take place in a complex psychological field, determined by the awareness and the empathy of the mother. [Winnicott, 1960, pp. 43–44]

To explore these interpsychic processes further, Figure 9.3 was created to demonstrate shifts in the therapist's focus between the child's needs and the carer's needs.

The graph in Figure 9.3 shows that at the start of the session the therapist's focus is primarily on the child (below the horizontal axis), but in the second half of the session more frequent statements are made by the therapist in relation to the carer as well as the child. These two graphs together indicate a correlation between the therapist's focus and the carer's capacity for psychological-mindedness towards the child.

This example of psychological development within the session, and its representation in the graph, offer a good illustration of Wilfred Bion's (1962a) concept of *container–contained*. Bion's theory claims that knowledge of the psychological precedes knowledge of the physical world. In his view, the infant's use of projective identification is its first mode of communication, which, in turn, is (or in many cases is not) internalized by a mother (the container), who then bears the emotional impact of these projections and makes sense of what the infant is transmitting via projective identification (the contained). Bion called this maternal engagement with the infant "reverie" or "alpha-function".

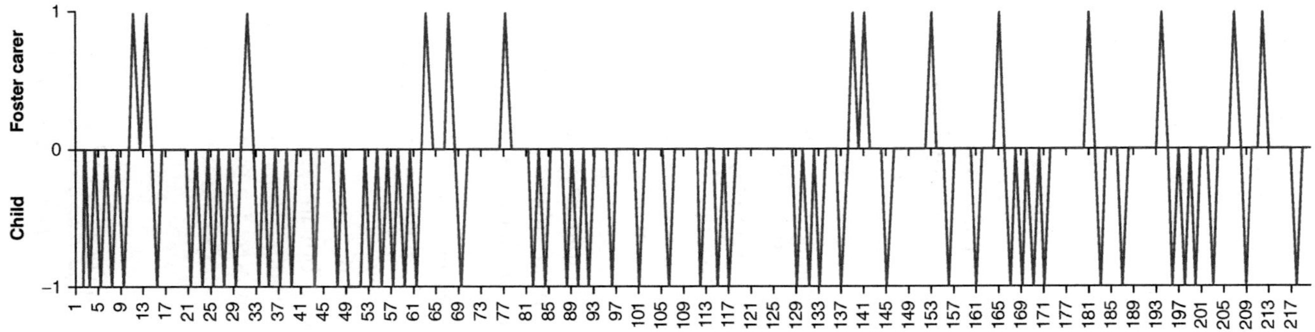

Figure 9.3 Therapist's focus in F1 S1.

Esther Bick (1968) considers the "containing" function of the mother in terms of "the primal function" of her skin and the skin of her baby:

> in its most primitive form the parts of the personality are felt to have no binding force among themselves and must therefore be held together in a way that is experienced by them passively, by the skin functioning as a boundary. [Bick, 1968, p. 484]

This latest finding demonstrates that even within one session of psychoanalytic parent support work, it is possible to bring about an improvement in the extent of the carer's psychological-mindedness.

It is important, however, to acknowledge that each set of carers presented quite differently in showing psychological-mindedness (PM) in Session 1 (S1), as is demonstrated in Table 9.1.

For example, already in Session 1, Mrs Winters (FM3) showed a picture with respect to psychological-mindedness that diverged from the rest of the group, a score of 96 indicating a much higher capacity for psychological-mindedness; whereas, Mrs Morgan's (FM1) score in the first session was –6. However, the overall trajectory of change over the course of four sessions was consistent with the initial finding of the importance of the therapist's attention to the carer's state of mind, as is demonstrated later.

Although the sample of participants in this study is small, it also demonstrates that the gender of the carer is not, in itself, an indicator of level of psychological-mindedness. This might seem obvious, but it is still worth highlighting, especially since it seems to be culturally accepted that the female carer usually bears the main responsibility for fostering liaison with other services. The male carer's role often does not receive adequate attention.

As mentioned earlier, all five foster families consisted of a foster mother and a foster father, but in fact only two foster fathers attended the sessions, and one of them attended only two of the four sessions. Regardless of the physical absence or presence of the foster father, the foster mother's ability to demonstrate her capacity to keep the foster

Table 9.1 Foster carers' "psychological-mindedness" in Session 1

Participant	*FM1*	*FF1*	*FM2*	*FF2*	*FM3*	*FF3*	*FM4*	*FF4*	*FM5*	*FF5*
PM S1	–6	n/a	31	n/a	96	13	11	41	37	n/a

father in mind varied greatly. These dynamics were coded as 3B (FM's view of the FF) and 3C (FF's view of the FM). For example:

- » Mr Morgan was physically absent and was not mentioned by Mrs Morgan until prompted by the therapist.
- » Mr Woods was physically absent and was not mentioned by Mrs Woods until Mr Woods played a part in a story about the child.
- » Mr Winters was physically present, and Mrs Winters made frequent references to Mr Winters, and vice versa.
- » Mr Patterson was sometimes physically present, sometimes absent, and was referred to by Mrs Patterson and vice versa.
- » Mr Stewart was physically absent but was frequently referred to by Mrs Stewart.

Despite this being a small-scale study, this was particularly significant, as four of the children in this study did not know who their birth father was, and one had been told by his birth family (untruthfully) that his birth father was dead. All of them had at some stage shared a household with their birth mother's male partner(s), some of whom were known sex offenders.

Table 9.2 represents the changes in the overall psychological-mindedness score (PM) after the four sessions.

From this data it can be concluded that even short-term psychoanalytically informed parent support for carers can bring about a significant improvement in the foster carers' psychological-mindedness in relation to the child in their care.

Not only had the overall levels of psychological-mindedness increased, there were also significant changes in the ways in which psychological-mindedness was expressed (2E, 2F, 2G, 2H, 2I and 3E, 3F, 3G, 3H, 3I). Figure 9.4 presents some examples of the changes that occurred in the families with the lowest and highest overall score of psychological-mindedness: Mrs Morgan (FM1) & Mrs Winters (FM3).

Table 9.2 Foster carers' "psychological-mindedness" in the first and last session

Participant	*FM1*	*FF1*	*FM2*	*FF2*	*FM3*	*FF3*	*FM4*	*FF4*	*FM5*	*FF5*
PM S1	–6	n/a	31	n/a	96	13	11	41	37	n/a
PM S4	22	n/a	58	n/a	90	29	24	n/a	86	n/a

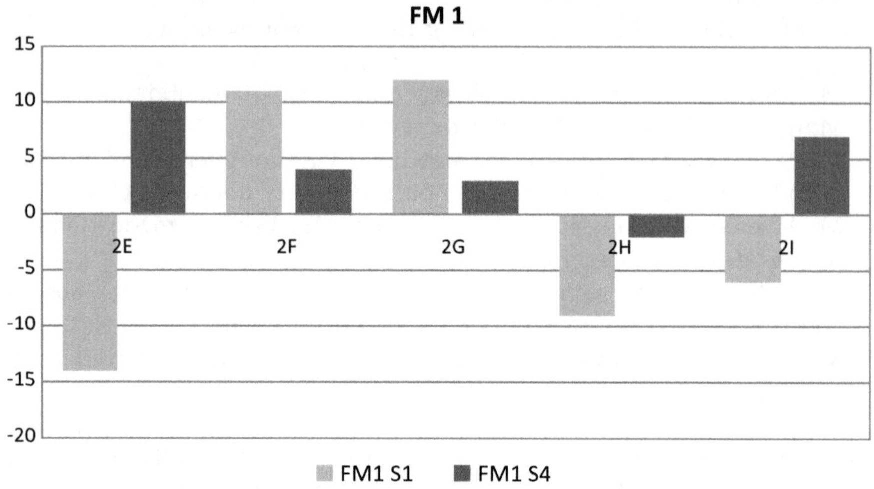

Figure 9.4 Changes achieved in foster carers' "psychological-mindedness": Subcategory Analysis 1.

In this example, it is evident that Mrs Morgan's (FM1) comments that suggest an insight or her empathy regarding Anna have increased significantly (2E); however, her focus on the child's bodily presentation (2F) and her descriptions of the child's affect (2G) have reduced significantly. Instead, more thought is now given to the child's ways of coping (2H) and the impact on Anna of her early experiences (2I).

This suggests a significant shift in the foster mother's thinking about the child, away from a focus on the child's behaviours and towards a focus on the underlying causes of those behaviours. This, in turn, suggests that psychoanalytic parent support is particularly important in fostering the relationship between the internal worlds of the foster carer and the child.

To illustrate the further trajectory of the data analysis, I now briefly introduce "Tony" and Mrs & Mr Winters (FM3 & FF3). Tony was almost 7 years old at the time of the referral. He was the youngest in a family of eight. His family had a complex and turbulent trans-generational history involving violence, drugs, and murders.

Tony was described by his social worker as a boy who has significant developmental delay, particularly where his learning capacity and comprehension are concerned. He suffered from distressing dreams and flashbacks that were also evident in his play, such as memories of being covered in his mother's blood or of his grandmother being resuscitated by paramedics. He also tended to soil and wet his bed. He had developed a particular interest in the subject of death and showed unusual interest in the pain of others. It was noted that Tony struggled to share or to empathize with others. His relationships at school were problematic. He also tended to inflict pain on himself: for example, he would bang his head against hard or sharp surfaces, spontaneously swallow staples, push the leg of a chair into his genitals, and so on.

Mrs & Mr Winters described Tony as a very impulsive child: he tended to lash out, at times with little or no notice, and on occasion this involved knives or scissors. They recalled that for the first few years they caring for him, he screamed in distress for several hours every day, for no apparent external reason. He also had a diagnosis of epilepsy. Nonetheless, it was evident that Tony had warmth about him. He presented as a severely traumatized boy, whose early beginnings had obstructed his development at a fundamental level, so that his perception of the world was fragmented. He gave the impression of a child with no sense of a continuous self, someone who depended on other people around him for his memory.

However, it seemed as if he was also making tentative attempts to build some sense of self. I saw this as a hopeful sign and attributed this potential development to the exceptional quality of care provided by his carers. The approach of Mrs & Mr Winters to Tony's difficulties and needs was thoughtful and compassionate. It was evident that they were committed parents. However, it also became apparent that they seldom reflected on their own responses when encountering the boy's sometimes shocking re-enactments of his earlier life—for example, when Tony stabbed their eldest son in the hand with a knife and threatened to kill his foster father in his sleep.

Figure 9.5 charts the changes observed in the psychological-mindedness of Mrs Winters (FM3) over four sessions.

Mrs Winters showed little change in overall psychological-mindedness over the four sessions in comparison with the rest of the group, but a pattern similar to the others does occur where the carers become more preoccupied with understanding the reasons behind the child's presentation. Although such minor discrepancies are not unusual, they still seemed meaningful. While for the rest of the carers, including Mr Winters, there was a change indicating increased closeness to the child—that is, the carer's level of insight and empathy increased—in the case of Mrs

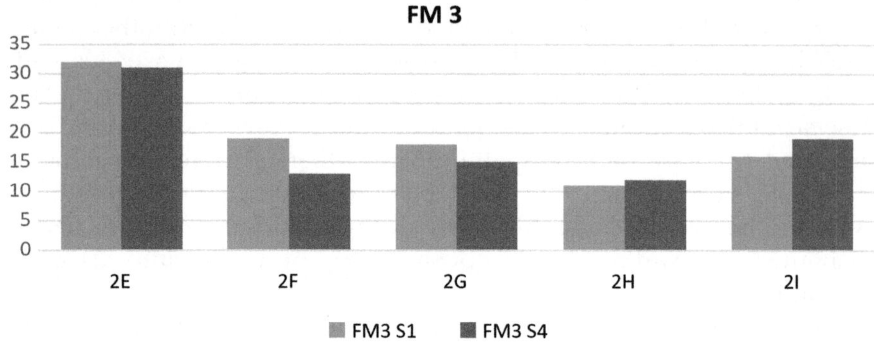

Figure 9.5 Changes achieved in foster carers' "psychological-mindedness: Subcategory Analysis 2.

Winters a slight distance was created over time. This prompted a further hypothesis:

> *There is a continuum, or a spectrum, of distance and closeness between the foster carer and the child. For example, at times the carers felt emotionally closer to the child they were caring for, in a way that an effective parent would; while at other times, they adopted more distant, more "professional'-type stratagems to help them manage the emotional challenges presented by the child. It became evident that there were times when something about the foster child's distress felt unbearably distressing for the carer.*

This observation pointed to a particularly important function of psychoanalytic parent support work: that of regulating this dynamic of closeness and distance, thus supporting the carers with a more balanced, more rounded view of the child, which, in turn, allows the carer to gain appropriate and sufficient understanding of the child's trauma *without becoming overwhelmed by it*. Furthermore, a fuller understanding of these supportive processes at work in the therapeutic setting could potentially play a significant role in facilitating more effective liaison between the carers and the professional system around them, since a parallel process of distancing and closeness was observed to be taking place with respect to the carer's relationship to the wider system.

Following further re-reading of the research material, the following new research question was created:

» **What is the quality of the foster carer's response to the child's communication of distress or trauma?**

Owing to the large quantity of such material, it was necessary to restrict the data for this analysis to the first and last sessions with each family, so as to capture the change that occurred over the four sessions.

The most significant factor in the child's communications—the factor that generated these responses in the carer—was the manifestation of the child's distress. The children's displays of distress ranged from feeling sad and stroppy to re-enacting traumatic past experiences through impulsive, risk-taking behaviour.

This "compulsion to repeat" past experiences, in an attempt to cope with disconcerting archaic affect, was first elaborated by Freud:

> We see that children repeat in their play everything that has made a great impression on them in actual life, that they thereby abreact the strength of the impression and so to speak make themselves masters of the situation. [Freud, 1920g, p. 14]

Many foster carers will recognize this tendency in a child's play, but without some understanding of how these processes relate to infantile and childhood trauma, they will often struggle to make sense of the child's sometimes bizarre, challenging, and frequently self-sabotaging behaviours, especially in what is clearly a good and caring (and new) family situation.

In "Remembering, Repeating, and Working-Through" (1914g), Freud observed that patients tended to repeat their neurotic conflicts during analysis rather than remember those conflicts' traumatic origins: repeating, Freud concluded, is the neurotic's way of remembering. The concept of a "compulsion to repeat" was then introduced by Freud in his seminal *Beyond the Pleasure Principle* (1920g).

Sándor Ferenczi insisted that this compulsive repetition was caused by severe trauma early in the life of the child. He proposed the theory that, if traumatic assault has taken place at an early developmental stage, the ego will respond by a mimetic (or imitative) reproduction of the aggressor's desires, leaving an imprint on the child that Ferenczi called an "alien transplant" (Avello, 1998, p. 229).

In Freud's view, the "excitation" produced by severe trauma can be neither discharged nor psychologically worked through; as a result, it is experienced by the individual as threatening to his or her cohesion and therefore cannot be accessed in the usual (cognitive) way. He suggests that, in attempting to understand the resulting psychic state, "a purely descriptive method of expression" must be replaced by "a systematic or dynamic one". Accordingly, the repetition compulsion must be ascribed to "the repressed element in the unconscious". And the "repressed element" that fuels the compulsion to repeat cannot find expression and emerge from the unconscious until repression is "loosened" in the course of the treatment (Freud, 1920g, p. 19).

Child psychotherapists working with severely traumatized children, as well as with the children's foster carers, often find themselves in a distressing situation with a child that seems to be repeated by the child over and over again. They often feel utterly helpless in their attempts to reason with the child. For Freud, "the repressed memory-traces of his primitive experience" cannot be symbolized in words and expressed in discourse. With his rational (or "binding") functions overwhelmed, the individual can only repeat the traumatic situation in a compulsive fashion, as a way of trying to "bind" the experience (Freud, 1920g, p. 43–44). However, as he had already made clear in his "Little Hans" case study, "a thing which has not been understood inevitably reappears; like an unlaid ghost, it cannot rest until the mystery has been solved and the spell has been broken" (Freud, 1909b, p. 122).

Freud also observed the perplexing fact that the repeated events seemed to violate his cherished pleasure principle: the experiences being repeated tended to be painful and unsatisfying past events and relationships that had never led to pleasure in the first place and "included no possibility of pleasure" (Freud, 1920g, p. 20). He came to the conclusion that the compulsion to repeat is rooted in something "more primitive, more elementary, more instinctual than the pleasure principle which it overrides" (Freud, 1920g, p. 23). He described the driven quality of the compulsion to repeat as "demonic" (Freud, 1920g, p. 21) and attributed it to what he called a "death instinct".

Interestingly, in this research material the specific category of distress-triggered behaviour was not a predictor as to how the carers would respond to the child. What mattered more was the individual carer's capacity to metabolize (or contain) the child's distressed and distressing communication. In other words, the children's trauma-fuelled communications trigger transference responses in their carers. The carer's own childhood experiences are triggered by the child in their care and are then repeated, rather than remembered, in the carer's transference to the child (Freud, 1914g).

Unfortunately, this being a short-duration project, there was insufficient opportunity to explore the carers' own childhood experiences, other than the few that were spontaneously shared in the course of the support sessions. Moreover, whereas some carers seemed to share those memories fairly readily, others were reluctant to explore their own childhood, insisting that they were "here to talk about the child".

In the original report on this research, before listing each carer's responses to the child's distress in the first session, a short introduction was given to that carer's views on fostering in general, in order to establish a context of the carers' expectations and reasons for fostering. This was then followed by lengthy lists of the carers' responses, the extended descriptions conveying the more qualitative and more human quality of the carers' struggles in caring for traumatized children. The data analysis showed that there are times when the child's powerful feelings are acutely felt by the carer, but their own responses are adequately regulated so that they remain psychologically minded. At other times, the carer's psychological equilibrium is rocked and becomes somewhat impaired, or insecure. In some cases, out of their intuitive empathy for the child, carers fully identify with the child's pain. In these latter situations, facing up to the child's distressed and distressing communication becomes so unbearable for the carer that she or he has to turn away from the reality of that pain. Hamish Canham (2004) comments on his clinical experience of what it is like to be on the receiving end of such powerful communications:

> Deprived and abused children bring to the therapy a set of experiences and feelings that are often of a truly terrifying nature. ... When these experiences begin to enter into the transference they can lead to a complicated set of feelings in the therapist: a desire to protect oneself and not hear, to protect the room, to fight back when under attack, overwhelming states of rage, sadness and despair. [Canham, 2004, p. 145]

I now briefly consider each of the above "parenting" stances in turn. Although it has been used in a great variety of ways in the psychoanalytic literature from Freud onwards, the term "identification" is being used in this study to refer to the various ways in which a foster carer, by—largely unconsciously—using the mechanism of empathy, "feels into" the affective experience of a traumatized child in his or her foster care in a particular situation. Freud summarizes the phenomenon as follows:

> A path leads from identification by way of imitation to empathy, that is, to the comprehension of the mechanism by means of which we are enabled to take up any attitude at all towards another mental life. [Freud, 1921c, p. 110]

Below I list several possible response dynamics to the child's distress.

1. ***Carers identify with the child's distress, and in protecting their own psychic equilibrium, they distance themselves from that distress.***

When the child's distressed communication awakens primitive early anxieties of annihilation, the carer may become unable to deflect the destructiveness of the death instinct (however understood) from within, and this, in turn, triggers the carer's early primitive defences. As a result, the carer either expels the unvented emotional states that are stirred up by the child's communication of distress by means of projection (including projective identification) and envy (an attack on the good object), or turns to denial of their own responses to the child's communication and to external reality, or takes flight to the idealized good object, or uses the mechanism of splitting. Thus, part of the carer's ego turns away from the reality of the child's pain, since that pain gives rise to unbearable anxiety in the carer.

2. ***Carers identify with the child's distress and attempt to protect the child by psychically merging with it, often at the cost of threatening their own psychic equilibrium.***

The experience of being confronted by the child's distress can generate powerful anger and aggression towards the child, who has destabilized the carer's equilibrium and capacity to parent. For Melanie Klein, defence mechanisms are primarily activated when anxiety and guilt towards the object are aroused: thus, defence mechanisms defend against one's own angry, even murderous, impulses. In an attempt to "undo" the presumed damage of the anger generated by the child's distress, the carer suddenly becomes in touch with the child's powerful affect, at times "devoting him/herself entirely" to the child; but to an extent that there is no longer any freedom to think about the gravity of the situation: so that, for example, the carer can no longer recognize her or his own urgent need for respite (Hinshelwood, 1994, p. 89).

3. ***Carers identify with the child and switch between merging and distancing.***

In some cases, the carer can switch between merging and distancing in ways that are completely unpredictable for the child, often replicating by identification the child's early care experience. This response is likely to put considerable strain on the stability of the placement. Anna Freud writes about this in terms of identification with the aggressor, as a means of coping with the anxiety (A. Freud, 1936). This dynamic of unpredictable switching between the extremes of merging and distancing is also captured by Mervin Glasser's theory of a "core complex" (Glasser, 1992).

4. ***The carer's psychic equilibrium is somewhat impaired.***

In the relationship between carer and traumatized foster child, the dynamic interplay between distress, anxieties, and defences is always seeking expression, but the carer's responses are not always defensive. This depends on the carer's capacity to bear the anxiety produced by the way the child comes across—both the distressing quality of it and the frequency of its occurrence. In these exchanges, while the carer's own personal trauma is inevitably triggered, the reach of psychological-mindedness becomes extended to encompass the task of protecting the child from what Selma Fraiberg and her colleagues have studied as "transgeneration behavior" (Fraiberg, Adelson, & Shapiro, 1985). They considered the impact on parents and their children of "ghosts in the nursery"—that is, when the ghosts of the parental past are unconsciously inflicted upon the child. The key here is the degree of the parents' repression of the painful experiences of their own childhood, such as anxiety, grief, shame, or self-abasement. What Fraiberg et al. highlight about birth parents applies just as much to the foster carers in this study. If those early experiences had never been fully repressed, or if repressed memories of them had been released and dealt with through psychotherapy, the parents in the Fraiberg study were able to say, "I would never want that to happen to my child":

> For these parents, the pain and suffering have not undergone total repression. In remembering, they are saved from the blind repetition of that morbid past. Through remembering they identify with an injured child (the childhood self), while the parent who does not remember may find himself in an unconscious alliance and identification with the fearsome figures of that past. In this way, the parental past is inflicted upon the child. [Fraiberg, Adelson, & Shapiro, 1985, p. 420]

In situations such as this, the foster carer can often remain merely somewhat impaired, or shaken, by the force of the child's distress, rather than experiencing it as a lethal threat to their ego integrity. Anna Freud describes a kind of denial as a precursor of defence, where the individual simply withdraws her attention from something unpleasant or threatening (Sandler & Freud, 1985, p. 340).

5. *The carer can offer "good-enough" psychological parenting.*

The above range of carer responses encompasses the various degrees of psychological-mindedness that underlie foster carers' responses to the distressed feelings and states of the traumatized children in their care. The various responses illustrate how the impact of the child's past experiences, which are being relived in the present, can be absorbed and metabolized by some carers and not by others—and by some carers some of the time but not all of the time. The "good-enough" carer who is providing a distressed child with a "holding environment" (Winnicott) is, in fact (intuitively and unconsciously) "containing" and detoxifying the child's terrified projections (as outlined by Bion).

It is also worth reflecting that, at times, and especially where severely traumatized children are concerned, it takes more than one carer to make parenting "good-enough". When considering fostering placements, the vital role of foster fathers (or an alternative "third') and other family members is often underplayed.

Summary of the findings

Table 9.3 provides a summary of the impact the dynamics analysed above have on each party in a fostering arrangement, including the impact of these dynamics (traumatized child/foster carers) on the wider system. Owing to the limitations of this study, this finding could not be adequately tested in the data, and it is here presented as a set of hypotheses for further research.

It is important to bear in mind that the carers in this study have all been deemed by social services to be fit to provide adequate care for the children in their home. Also, the four categories above have been applied only to the situations that the carers found most challenging, and not to the carers' overall responses to the child, which might well paint a different, perhaps more hopeful picture. However, this categorization highlights the fact that it is not helpful to take a blanket approach either in selecting foster carers or in preparing a person to become a foster carer; and, furthermore, that the preparation required to produce a good long-term foster placement is not only about

Table 9.3 The impact of the child's trauma on the care provided

Response of the carer	*Child's emotional needs*	*Carer's emotional needs*	*Psychological parenting*	*Relationships with the wider system (item for future research)*
"Good-enough" parenting	met	met	awareness of the interplay between the child's internal and external worlds, between the present and the past	good and reliable communication
"Identifying and distancing"	mostly neglected	mostly over-compensated	carer's emphasis on tasks at the expense of feelings	over-compensated by the system
"Identifying and merging"	mostly over-compensated	mostly neglected	carer's emphasis on feelings at the expense of the real world or others in it	ambivalent commitment by the system (e.g., frequent changes in social worker)
Carer's equilibrium "impaired"	mostly met	mostly met	somewhat impaired but partially functioning, from time to time	carer can be either seeking support or distancing from the system

preparing the child. On the contrary, to provide a "good-enough" long-term parenting experience for a traumatized child, one must become familiar with one's own responses to extreme distress, or at least acknowledge the fact that they play a significant role in how one responds to the child overall, so that additional external resources can be called upon if and when necessary.

It is idealistic to hope that every foster carer would, at some time in their fostering career, consider undertaking some therapeutic self-discovery work themselves. Even those attending parent support sessions are often reluctant (for various reasons) to discuss openly their own negative and difficult-to-bear responses to the child in their care. However, an experienced psychoanalytic psychotherapist can identify reasonably accurately the attunement level of a carer and support them in achieving

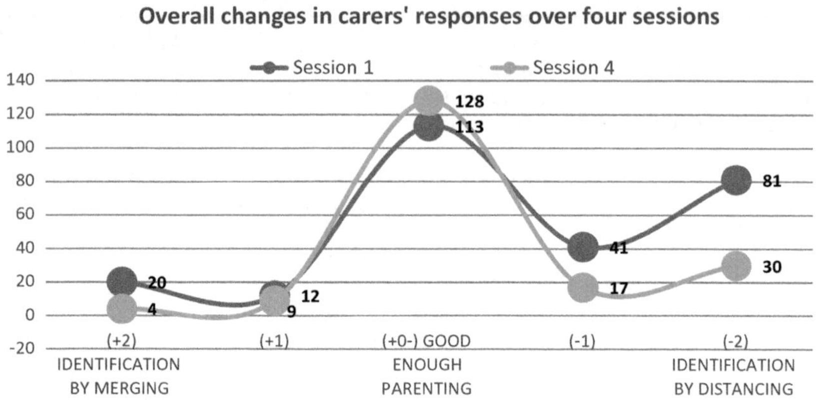

Figure 9.6 Overall changes in carers' responses over four sessions.

a more balanced view of the child in their care; and, as is evident from the data in this study, the most effective parent support work is not always about helping the carer to achieve a closer alignment with the child's affect, but, in fact, the opposite: that is, it is often just as necessary to help the carer to gain sufficient distance from the raw force of the child's affect in order to become a more effective parent.

Figure 9.6 represents the overall changes achieved over four sessions of parent support work in relation to carers' responses to the child's communication of distress: examples of "Identification by merging" decreased from a score of 20 to 4; examples of "Identification by distancing" decreased from a score of 81 to 30; and examples of "Good-enough parenting" increased from a score of 113 to 128. The graph demonstrates clearly that even within the short space of four sessions of weekly psychoanalytic parent work, it is possible to achieve significant change in carers' capacity to bear the child's compulsion to repeat early traumas and to help the carers to become more available to provide the child with effective psychological parenting at these most challenging times.

Conclusions and some recommendations

Although this is a psychoanalytic research study, its conclusions and recommendations are also aimed at our social work colleagues (and their managers) working with looked-after children and their several families. Following careful grounded-theory analysis, the study has produced a series of visual representations of psychoanalytic thinking, with the aim of furthering communication about the nature of psychoanalytically informed carer support and hopefully offering new ways of illustrating, to the wider system, its beneficial outcomes.

These conclusions highlight the contribution that psychoanalytic child psychotherapists can make in supporting foster carers, and through them the children in their care. Although this was a small-scale study, it was able to illuminate various ways in which changes in policy might facilitate the process of recovery for traumatized children, while improving the fostering experience of their carers.

When foster carers are faced with the almost impossible task of caring for a child who has suffered severe trauma in its early life, the child's communication of distress, hopelessness, and despair can often be so powerful that carers are in a position where their natural empathy towards the child (which had usually brought them into the caring job in the first place) makes them feel too acutely their child's intense feelings, often without fully realizing that this is what is happening. Surviving these very difficult emotional states, then, becomes, by necessity, the carer's number one priority. It has become evident from this study that even short-term psychoanalytically informed parent work reduces considerably the levels of the carer's defensive responses to the child's compulsion to repeat its trauma in the form of distressing behaviour and increases the level of "good-enough" parenting responses to the child.

Christine Olden (1953), while acknowledging that "the adult's capacity to empathize with children is rarer than the capacity to empathize with other adults", highlights an aspect of the concept of empathy that seems particularly relevant to this finding of the present study:

> Empathy may be described as a feeling that emerges spontaneously in social contact, that enables the subject instantaneously to sense the object's apparent emotions of shyness, hate, haughtiness, happiness, etc. But empathy goes further. It has the capacity ad libitum to trespass the object's screens of behaviour, behind which the real feelings may hide. [Olden, 1953, p. 115]

Within the short duration of this small-scale research study, carers were enabled to trespass their traumatized child's screens of behaviour, so as to access their deeper feelings of distress.

This study has also demonstrated that, when dealing with children who have suffered severe early trauma, it sometimes takes more than one person to help the child safely bridge the gap between their incoherent sense of their own narrative and a "good-enough" new narrative of self, in which some acknowledgement of the past can take place without feeling too threatened or overwhelmed in the process. To assist a traumatized child in this transition, and to survive the journey themselves, foster carers have to master a delicate balancing act between "distance from" and "closeness to" the intense emotional experiences presented by the child. For a lone carer (whether single or in a couple), this can be an extremely intense and demanding task. A supportive and attentive third (a partner, a social worker, or a therapist) can, while keeping external reality in mind, make this process of metabolizing the impact of the child's trauma much more manageable by breaking it up into discrete episodes of closeness and distance, until a more coherent approach can be developed and managed by all. For example, there may be times when the foster mother will have to experience something similar to what Winnicott referred to as "maternal preoccupation", or what Bion called maternal "reverie", and she may need help from others to ensure that her own needs are not being overlooked, precisely because of her absorption in the child.

It was evident from the nomination of the participants in this study that the role of a father figure was generally underestimated, both in the foster family setting and in the child's early life. In most cases, the child's early experiences had included males who were violent, were substance abusers, and/or were known sex offenders. This early formative experience of men will almost certainly significantly colour the foster child's transference relationship to the foster father—yet this factor did not seem to have any significance in the wider thinking about the placement. Not only can proactively involving foster fathers in the various aspects of fostering strengthen the placement, but the specifically psychoanalytic insight into the typical transference relationships of traumatized children may also shed some helpful light on why some of the foster fathers report that they feel the child might make accusations against them if they set boundaries for the child or show the child affection.

Although it has been impossible to include the relevant research data in this short summary, this study also suggests that there is a significant gulf between the emotional tasks required of short-term and long-term foster care. Although they might not be mutually exclusive, there are certain components that long-term fostering must include, such as giving thought to the child's future trajectory and longer-term care plan. In my experience, the child's future options are not always sufficiently considered or planned for.

One of the other interesting points coming out of this research data is that a carer may not want to "rock the boat", as it were, with either the child or social services, if the placement is expected to last only a year or less. In this case, the role of psychological parenting may be seen as less important than is the task focus of more concrete parenting in the here-and-now (e.g., hygiene, formal education, sports). In contrast, carers who expect the placement to last until the end of the child's teenage years are more likely to invest their energy, time, and emotional resources in addressing the more chronic difficulties presented by the foster child. This likelihood is particularly relevant to carers with a tendency to distance themselves from the child's compulsion to repeat early traumatizing experiences. Thus, the findings of this research may be used in the consideration of whether a particular carer is better suited to providing short-term or long-term care; and in helping to give more thought to whether the particular carer should be encouraged to continue to care for the child long-term, or whether the priority should, instead, become the planning of a good ending to the current short-term placement and transition to the next placement. This research has demonstrated the likely problems associated with what Jane Rowe et al. have characterized as "'drift' into unplanned, long-term placements" (Rowe, Cain, Hundleby, & Keane, 1984, p. 231).

This study has demonstrated that even short-term psychoanalytically informed parent support can significantly increase the level of "good-enough" responses to the child's distress by enabling foster carers to remain psychologically minded towards the child in their care. The data analysis demonstrated that this type of support is able to shift the carer's preoccupations from *what* the child does to *why* the child does it, so helping the carer to view the child's "compulsion to repeat" behaviour as communication and thus gain a better understanding of the links between the child's past experiences and the present disconcerting actions, which, in turn, allows the carer to recognize the challenging behaviours as re-enactments of early traumas rather than as the carer's failure to provide good-enough care or the child's unwillingness to bond, thus reducing the strain on the placement.

Concluding reflections on the unique role of the psychoanalytic child psychotherapist

The key role of the psychoanalytic child psychotherapist as a member of a multi-disciplinary team can be summarized as follows:

- The psychoanalytic training of child psychotherapists allows them to:
  - understand the impact of traumatic early experience on the child's current modes of relating
  - foresee the likely future trajectory of the child's development in his or her later childhood and adolescence
  - assist carers effectively in providing psychological parenting
  - foresee future strains on the placement
  - support a transition to an alternative placement or respite, where necessary, thus avoiding a sudden breakdown of the placement
  - support other professionals in assessing, training and supporting carers.
- Psychoanalytic child psychotherapists trained in infant observation can play a uniquely important role in providing training for health visitors and social workers in the field of infant mental health, and in fostering a deeper understanding of the lasting impact of parental mental ill-health on the wellbeing and future prospects of the child.
- Finally, as this study demonstrates, psychoanalytic child psychotherapists also undertake research, which can inform best practice in child health and social care.

Acknowledgement

I would like to express my thanks to the supervisors of the doctoral research study on which this chapter is based, Biddy Youell and Margaret Rustin.

CHAPTER TEN

An exploration into the impact of a child psychotherapist's pregnancy on her clinical work

Rajni Sharma

One of the most challenging times in my work was during my first pregnancy. I had anticipated the emotional upheaval of this life-changing event, but the impact of this on my work with children and adolescents was quite unexpected. On my return from maternity leave, the priority was to slot back into the clinic and pick up new work that awaited me. There was no space to think about the impact of such a personal event on my clinical practice, and the wish to shelve the experience was strong. Were it not for attending a conference soon after my return from maternity leave, where Jessica Yakeley presented a paper about the pregnant analyst (later published as Yakeley, 2013) I might well have put it all aside. Instead, I was inspired to investigate work that, in my mind, had been obscured, ambiguous, and clouded by my altered state during pregnancy.

I designed a qualitative clinical research project using grounded theory that drew on my direct experience. I broadened this with a series of six interviews with child and adolescent psychotherapists (CAPTs) with recent experiences of work while pregnant and interviewed three consultant CAPTs, who were senior members of the profession with extensive supervisory experience, which included clinical supervision of pregnant CAPTs. This gathered together vivid layered descriptions which I examined through a dynamic employment of grounded theory, a systematic and meticulous process of coding that methodically explored the rich qualitative accounts through a psychoanalytic frame of reference. Triangulating viewpoints emerged from my first-hand experience and that of six clinicians in similar circumstances, as well as the supervisory perspectives from experienced senior clinicians. I have distilled the key findings of my research in a brief survey of the literature and, following one case study of 10-year-old Kyle, I include some discussion of interviews with CAPTs and consultant supervisors.

Brief survey of previous literature

The eclipsing of pregnancy in the early days of psychoanalysis is noteworthy. Balsam (2003, 2012) suggests that there was a defensive erasure of the pregnant mother, rendering her invisible. Freud himself suggested that the taboo of pregnancy was a universal difficulty for men (Freud, 1918a). Pregnancy is dramatic evidence of the difference between men and women and the "for ever incomprehensible and mysterious, strange and therefore apparently hostile" (Freud, 1918a, p. 271) nature of pregnancy, which makes it difficult to think about. Pregnancy would have been an ever-present reality in Freud's own childhood as his mother was in an almost perpetual pregnant state, giving birth to seven more children before he was 10 years old. It is also significant to note that the illness that gripped Freud's attention and facilitated the birth of psychoanalysis was hysteria, a condition said to be particular to women and thought to be caused by disturbances of the uterus (from the Greek ὑστέρα *"hystera"* = uterus). The presumed site of pathogenesis where pregnancy is housed possibly indicates why its creative and vital aspects were so difficult to comprehend.

Pregnancy was also a feature in the first psychoanalytic case study of a child, "Little Hans" (Freud, 1909b). In this case study, Freud focused on Hans's experience of his mother's pregnancy and the birth of his little sister when he was 3 years old. Hans struggled to ascertain the difference between the sexes, with a dawning recognition that girls have something that boys do not have. For Freud, the presence or absence of the penis (the castration complex) took primacy in distinguishing the sexes over the ability to bear children. However, Klein's development of child psychoanalysis highlighted that children's prevailing phantasies were shaped by their response to the maternal body and the mother's ability to create babies. Klein emphasized the importance of female sexuality for girls and for boys: "As in the castration complex of girls, so in the femininity complex of the male, there is at bottom the frustrated desire for a special organ" (Klein, 1932). However, Balsam (2003) states that Klein was not able to locate the state of pregnancy as especially significant among other phantasies about body phenomena, such as the feeding or depriving breasts, the "internal phallus", the vagina, or the conjoined parents. It was subsequent to the development of theories about countertransference phenomena, coupled with an increasing number of women psychoanalysts, that papers on pregnancy and the pregnant psychoanalyst began to be published. The first was Hannett's 1949 paper, which discussed the reaction of her patients when she had to take two weeks' leave after a miscarriage. She showed how personal events in an analyst's life impact on the transference and how such circumstances provide an opportunity for deeper scrutiny of the interpersonal relationship with the analyst. Lax (1969) considered that the pregnant analyst would be more sensitive to the "onslaught of conflict manifestations" in her patients and that there would be an increase in countertransference reactions during the therapist's pregnancy. Lax discussed how the analyst's anonymity and neutrality, which created a "blank projective screen", was compromised, yet opportunities opened up to become an "optimal projective screen" that emphasized the relational aspects of psychoanalysis.

There has recently been a steady flow of literature in the form of case studies and interviews with pregnant psychoanalytic therapists. Repeating themes such as the reactivation of infantile conflict, fears of abandonment, oedipal issues, sibling rivalry, and envy of the therapist are highlighted across an emerging conceptual framework. Along with an intensification in patients' clinical material during a therapist's pregnancy, the pregnant therapist has to manage an intensification of her own primitive anxieties, which can make her feel vulnerable in her clinical work. A special edition of *Psychoanalytic Psychotherapy* in 2004 was dedicated to the therapist's pregnancy. This included a comprehensive literature review (White, 2004) and clinical papers that showed how patients are faced with a non-negotiable fact of life. This symposium suggests that while phantasies of pregnancy could now be explored with relative ease in psychoanalytic treatment, a real pregnancy presented an intrusion that inhibited the freedom to explore phantasy for the patient and the therapist. Primitive envy, hostility, and jealousy were stimulated, which were difficult for the psychotherapist to tolerate as the needs of the unborn baby were prioritized. However, useful and important work could also occur, especially when the therapist returned from maternity leave and the experience of pregnancy could be worked through. The importance of not allowing the patient to express unbridled hostility while also having his feelings of displacement understood and tolerated was highlighted. The idea that a new baby can be born into the world and accommodated along with those already there provided a useful framework for the continuation of therapy.

However, the existing literature predominantly concerns psychoanalytic work with adults. There are some case vignettes of child patients, but these brief accounts of children have quite different clinical presentations from those seen by CAPTs in Britain today. Reviewing my caseload while I was pregnant highlighted how many of the children's histories consisted of massive life catastrophe, complex trauma, transgenerational adversity, and illness of parents and parental figures. Over three quarters of the patients discussed in my interviews with clinicians were either adopted, in foster or kinship care, or had an absent parent. For such children, phantasies of abandonment, rejection, and rivalrous sibling dynamics were very daunting. I and the therapists I interviewed were particularly worried when pregnancy occurred early in the therapy. This was the situation with my 10-year-old patient Kyle as I became pregnant three months into his once-weekly long-term psychotherapy.

My case study: Kyle

Kyle was referred to our CAMHS when he was 6 years old, about four years before I assessed him for psychotherapy. At referral he presented with significant emotional and behavioural difficulties related to separations and traumas in his early years. He was defecating in inappropriate places, smearing his faeces, and masturbating until he was sore. He was 18 months old when his mother left him with his father, and when she did return, after intermittent contact with Kyle, she gave birth to his sister when he was 4 years old. Soon after this, Kyle's mother left again with her infant daughter. Kyle's father described how painfully rejecting and devastating this was for Kyle. At the time that I began working with this family, I experienced how raw the loss remained for both father and son.

CAMHS provided a range of interventions, including play therapy, support for the father, placement in a CAMHS day unit, and ADHD medication to address Kyle's difficult impulsive and fidgety behaviours. While there was some improvement, concerns remained about behavioural outbursts at home and about how sad and ostracized Kyle was from his peers and how much he struggled to learn and settle at school. Tensions between father and son were often at breaking point.

Kyle's father needed the support of his own mother to provide child care while he worked, and Kyle would often stay with her before and after school and for several nights a week. His frail and at times unwell paternal grandmother found this increasingly burdensome, which was also a cause of friction and arguments within the family. An experienced CAMHS clinician, who had been involved with Kyle from the beginning, asked if I could assess this troubled boy with such chronic and entrenched mental health difficulties for psychotherapy.

Looking back at the beginnings of this case, I remember the familiar daunting feeling of embarking on work with such a troubled child mingled with the complicating dimension of my own hopes of becoming pregnant. My apprehension in starting this work was perhaps not dissimilar to Kyle's feelings of reservation and scepticism when I first met him to introduce the assessment process, but this changed in the first assessment session. Although Kyle looked vulnerable and younger than 10 years, there was a playful and light-hearted rapport that reached out to me. He told me that he was a bit like Dennis the Menace. There was an unusual old-fashioned quality in him that made me wonder about the influence of his grandmother. His charm gradually gave way to his being a little boy sitting hunched forward on the couch, as if he had the weight of the world on his shoulders. He picked at his cuticles as he told me about the strain he placed on his dad, who "already had enough on his plate". He explained that he didn't know how to stop being bad: "I don't want to end up in a school for delinquents." I was moved by the burden of his concern and guilt. The emotional quality was of intense sadness and isolation and fear of damaging and losing another parent.

Kyle came to his next assessment session pretending to be a dog crawling and barking, a bundle of instincts rather than the boy in the first session, who could insightfully convey his complex circumstances. I thought about the risk that Kyle was taking in opening up to me and the raw feelings that this could induce. He took out some plasticine from his therapy box and kneaded it aimlessly but as though the malleability provided sensory relief. It gradually formed a shape that Kyle said was a dinosaur, which transformed into Frankenstein's monster (a boy here with some knowledge of the wider culture) and then metamorphosed into a dragon. As I closely observed this evolution, quietly conveying my fascination, Kyle smiled and said that he was making a combination of all three creatures. He then added that he guessed he was making something to do with his feelings! Subdued, Kyle then hollowed out a big hole inside the creature. We thought together about this, and Kyle wondered if the hole needed filling up. It was unclear if this would be with good stuff or bad. I found myself thinking about what Kyle imagined he was filled up with and what he imagined about my internal space, the internal space of his object. As I was thinking this, Kyle asked if I ate curry; he said he loved curry and his dad made a great curry! This correlation between his curiosity about what stuff I took inside me, so linked to my Indian ethnicity, was strikingly congruent with my wonderings about his internal world. There was also a poignant plea for a parental couple, a father who fed a mother, the need for a link between a father and mother, a theme that threaded through the subsequent therapy. In the final assessment session, Kyle set about investigating the boundaries of the room, peeling away at flaky plaster on one wall and picking at the locked drawers.

Through my experience of this assessment, I had a much clearer understanding of my colleagues' long-standing commitment and persistence with this vulnerable family that felt on the edge of breakdown. Despite chronic difficulties within the family and the many interventions that had already been offered, here was a boy accessible and wanting help. In the review meetings after the assessment, I spoke about my experience of Kyle's openness to understand and make sense of his confusion and difficulties and my feeling that there were realistic prospects of meaningful and effective work if the family could invest in this by accepting the necessary parallel parent work. Close multi-agency cooperation was also vital between our service, his school, and social care. Kyle would have benefitted from intensive psychoanalytic work; however, the family could not manage to bring Kyle more than once a week, and securing an intensive resource within the service at that time was also problematic. Once-weekly work with children like Kyle, especially alongside regular parent work and multi-agency liaison, which provides a multi-layered approach, can, however, harness a child's potential, and for Kyle it was agreed to by all parties.

As the sessions began to gain continuity in the early months, Kyle played out scenes of alligators wrestling and a game of tug of war, and he built an erupting volcano. I felt that I was to be impressed and beguiled much like a mother by her little child's potency and fervour. I was taken by how Kyle's expectation that these aspects of him could be received and held on to by someone else. He was curious about me in the gaps between sessions and worried that we would be interrupted during sessions. My detailed notes at this time convey Kyle's intense scanning of me, as if checking that I was not damaged and that I was available to him in the same way I had been in the previous session. There was a hunger for a protected space—something that Winnicott described as the need in the patient to be emotionally held by a mother who is "alive, awake, and ready to make active adaption through the quality of being devoted to her infant" (Winnicott, 1949a, p. 183). Kyle began to take the risk of making more and more mess and told me that he was a "divvy" (a slang insult meaning stupid) and explained, with some shyness/embarrassment, that he could not tell the time. He imagined that I would therefore think he was "thick" (another slang word for stupid).

The impingement of pregnancy

Kyle's family were under considerable strain as we approached the first break. His father was losing his patience with his son's bad behaviour, which he found particularly exhausting as a single parent. He was often depressed in his parent sessions and conveyed how his elderly mother was also finding it hard taking care of Kyle while he worked long hours. I felt concerned about the precariousness of Kyle's psychotherapy and anxious that it would not survive the impending holiday break. My clinical notes captured how closely I observed Kyle, thinking about him in detail during the last session before the break. He responded to my close attention by asking me if I was bored. I was bowled over by this contrast of our experiences in that moment. It was as if Kyle felt it to be too dangerous to think that I cared, unsafe to think about what is in a maternal mind, initially interested and then suddenly not, depressed and absent. I was in the early weeks of pregnancy at this time and did not make this link until I analysed my notes and realized how gripped I had been by morning sickness. In many respects, my close attention and focus on Kyle may have been in response to an anxiety that I was experiencing of being engulfed and distanced from the transference by my pregnant state. Kyle might well have experienced this as boredom. He was unusually restless and resistant in the sessions before the break. He said that he wasn't bothered about having to come any more and complained about why he had to come anyway. He smeared the lid of his box with plasticine, which put me in mind of smearing or marking territory, an impoverished mindless state, which left me feeling detached, and passive. Analysing these notes later when I embarked on my research, I made a strong connection between my own experience of feeling in a mess, with no reduction in nausea and fatigue, and the unconscious dynamics of Kyle's messy communications. I was astonished to read in my notes of the last session before the break that Kyle pretended to be pregnant and then played at giving birth to an alien, represented by some plasticine he had been kneading. (This may be linked with his earlier mention of Frankenstein's monster.) Kyle tipped himself upside down over the couch so that his hair brushed the carpet and his legs rested against the back of the couch. He had a rudimentary lump of plasticine in his hand and explained that it was the birth of an alien. I had the strong impression of him simultaneously giving birth and being born. I made no comment in my notes linking this to my own pregnancy. I think that this may have been because the thought of an alien foetus/infant was too disturbing to register at all.

Wanted and unwanted babies

In the sessions after the break, Kyle talked about difficulties with an after-school football club and how kids at school called him names like "gay boy". He talked about his ADHD medication and how it made him more aggressive and stronger than the other boys. He warned them that they should not mess with him. But then he became uncertain, and there was a profound question about what the medication was for and whether it helped. He said he hated taking the tablets and they tasted disgusting. He decided that the medication made no difference. Instead, it was counterproductive and slowed him down so much he wasn't able to do anything. I took this material up as an uncertainty about the helpfulness of therapy—"it's too slow and has not made any difference." Kyle agreed, saying he didn't know why he had to come. During this time his play became increasingly destructive, stabbing at toys with scissors, making a mess with glue, and spoiling toys and art materials so that some became unusable. He asserted that there wasn't any point in therapy. His spoiling was disturbing and with a quality of defeated relentless inevitability that almost felt impossible to think about. I noted, in rather a broad-brush way, that Kyle was questioning my commitment and was expecting that I would abandon our work. I struggled to think about this in relation to my pregnancy and to acknowledge the part of me that just wanted to leave this disturbing work, and also the likelihood that Kyle would have had an unconscious awareness of this. I resorted to familiar ways of thinking about Kyle's play in terms of post-break dynamics and the emergence of the negative transference in response. I empathized with Kyle and imagined him thinking that it was better to leave than be the one that's left. It was complicated to disentangle this from my preoccupations with my pregnancy and a maternity break on the horizon. The sessions continued to feel very messy and chaotic, an aspect concretely represented by the disordered state of Kyle's box. On occasions he tried to sort out his toy box, but this was an overwhelming task and ultimately just increased his dissatisfaction. There was plasticine and water everywhere, and he tried in vain to stem the spread of detritus and to limit his quite ruthless attacks and denigration of his therapy and me.

Analysing my notes through grounded theory offered a detailed systematic procedure that met well with psychoanalytic close observation. My confidence grew about the meanings that were emerging from the thoroughness of this method, which captured crucial themes through the coding process. I could see more clearly how challenged I had been by chronic and energy-sapping morning sickness, which coloured my experience of the messiness and destructiveness of his play. I never felt utterly repulsed by the mess he created, as I have on occasion with other patients, or threatened by the attacking themes in the play. I noticed that, all the while Kyle was able to create a manageable limit around his destructive impulses, there was some space for us to think together, and there could be some exploration of the negative transference. This was related to whether he felt he had a legitimate place and whether I wanted to be with him. Was I just going through the motions as his therapist, or was I really emotionally engaged with him? My morning sickness and its effects on me leant some reality to his suspicion.

Kyle being brought late and missing some of his sessions compounded this situation, as the support around his therapy became unreliable. With intermittent attendance and the Christmas break now looming, I struggled to gather the reality of my pregnancy together with the themes in Kyle's play. With five weeks left before Christmas, I felt compelled to talk to Kyle about the break and also to tell him at the same time about my pregnancy. I just ploughed on with the news. Kyle steadily listened, and there was a quiet pause, a heavy, pregnant pause. In these moments, I felt as if he had already had some preconscious awareness of the pregnancy. Yet I am not certain why I thought this. Was it his composure and receptivity to the news, or a need in me not to see a response that might be more stunned or troubled? After the pause Kyle said: "If I tell my dad, he would say congratulations." I felt muddled—who was saying/feeling what? On one level, Kyle was letting me know about the social norms and a mature response to such news. I do not know what Kyle made of my perplexed expression. He added, somewhat earnestly and with more emotion, that he just wished me one thing and it was that I didn't have a baby like him. This generated a heartbroken feeling in me. I asked Kyle what he meant, and he replied that he had been a "gross" baby and one time ate his own pooh. Kyle was matter of fact, as if stating a defining, all-encompassing reality. As if Kyle sensed my perturbed state, he added that he had also been told that he was a good baby too. I wondered where he had heard these stories about his infancy, and I felt the absence of his mother. This was an intense session, with so much information. I talked to Kyle about my maternity leave and the possibility of continuing psychotherapy when I returned. Kyle listened thoughtfully and there was almost a gentle quality to him, as if he were containing me in my concern for him. There was a steadier pace for the remainder of the session while Kyle played in an undemanding way with the cars and the plasticine, trying to make propellers.

After this session, I redoubled my efforts to link with the professional network to support Kyle's family in prioritizing the importance of Kyle's psychotherapy. In the remaining sessions before the Christmas break, his attendance improved. He came with more interest and with new play. He played at making propellers, attaching these to the toy cars and making them into hybrid flying vehicles. He brought a small motor from home and spent a session trying to attach this to one of the cars. He seemed to feel more resourceful, talking about how he was now allowed to have lunch at school (an indication of positive development) and how much he preferred this. His play had a more pubertal quality. For the first time, there was some developmental synchrony where he seemed neither regressed nor pseudo-mature. The car play evolved into high-speed chases: daredevils, hidden cops trying to catch the daredevils, who escaped in triumph. But the narrative became confused, and Kyle would lose track in the heady mix of excitement, potency, violence, and power.

Kyle returned after the Christmas break with a game of hide-and-seek in the waiting room. The friendly "peek-a-boo" between us contrasted with the precarious conflicted sessions after the summer break. At six months, my pregnant body was now prominent, and, although Kyle didn't comment on this, he used the holiday chart to count down the number of sessions before my maternity leave—eight in all. In the first session back, Kyle moulded a hammer, treasure chest, and Viking boat out of the plasticine. He wasn't able to say anything about these objects, and I was left with my own musings about masculinity, something less primordial and more human, more latency than pre-latency. As the sessions before my leave played out, I was struck by how undemanding and gracious Kyle was. Although his play was rich and varied, it lacked the challenging raw edge of the sessions prior to the announcement of my pregnancy. He seemed to be taking the position of an older sibling who wanted to show his mummy that he could be caring and thoughtful of a new baby. However, I felt sadness about what was repressed. I gently talked to Kyle about how he was being quieter and undemanding when it was understandable that he might be feeling fed up and annoyed. Kyle denied this, saying that he knew that during pregnancy women needed to relax. He seemed to value the opportunity to demonstrate his capacity to be protective, reparative, and caring as if it was important for him to experience playing a part in the safe arrival of a new baby. This echoed the reparative wishes described by Etchegoyen (1993) when she came to understand her little patient's wish to look after his therapist and the baby as a supportive father would. Yet what a responsibility to take on, so soon. So much on his plate, could he believe that I was strong enough and interested enough to want to hear how he was and also be able to manage the pregnancy? Although I was not as incapacitated by morning sickness as I had been in the first six months of my pregnancy, I thought that my fragility might well have contributed to Kyle's need not to burden me with complex and challenging emotions. I tried to think about this with him, reflecting on how futile it might feel to him to convey what's on his mind when he feels my mind is preoccupied by another baby.

Kyle was quiet and introspective while also seeming to need an opportunity to be more ordinary and undemanding. This was illustrated in one session when he began methodically and purposefully to tidy his box. I found this to be a relieving experience and also difficult. It was as if the work of thinking about complex untidy feelings was being side-stepped so as to spare the challenges of conflicted and painful split-off states of mind. My concern about this clouded the significance of Kyle showing me the thoughtful, caring, and organized parts of him, and it took me a while to notice the importance of these communications. While tidying his box, Kyle was prudent about what he threw away and careful in categorizing the different toys into bags, reminiscent of the way I had given Kyle his toy box when his therapy began. Kyle noted how many sessions remained, and he came to all of them! He would listen to some of my reflections about a longer-than-usual break and the plan to continue after my leave. To begin with, Kyle was reserved about this, which felt like a reasonable position to take. Yet he communicated a strong sense of his capacity to invest in a relationship despite so very many experiences of loss and turmoil. In the penultimate session, Kyle was quieter, undemanding, and slightly detached, polite, friendly, and efficient in playing with the plasticine, making food. Kyle briefly talked about how he sometimes cooked at home with his dad, simple things, and how he also helped with tidying. In the final session, he played with the plasticine, moulding it subconsciously, akin to free association, with abstract shapes forming and folding in his hands. Apparently aimless plasticine-shaping gave rise to two intertwining threads, a double helix—a strand of DNA, which we both simultaneously recognized and were amazed by. He was proud and delighted, and I interpreted the liveliness of creativity and reflected on Kyle's interest and thirst for learning about how things come and work together. I commented on the symbolism of the intertwining strands, and we thought together about the building blocks of life. The session ended with a hope to continue on my return.

Too long—bridging a maternity leave

I wrote to Kyle ten days after the birth of my baby letting him know that we were both well. This is something that I discussed in supervision and with other child psychotherapists who had experience of being pregnant. The letter was to acknowledge the reality of the baby's safe arrival. I also had in mind the more disturbing phantasies that Kyle might have had about the baby. I returned to work on a sessional basis after ten months.

I then heard that Kyle's father had begun a new relationship with a woman in another city. Father and son had moved to be with her and her children, and so, I discovered, they had been discharged from our service. Four months after my return from maternity leave there was news that Kyle had returned with his father, who had made contact with our service to arrange for a prescription for Kyle's ADHD medication. I discussed the situation with CAMHS colleagues and offered an appointment for Kyle, but the family did not attend. I wrote again and heard nothing for another six weeks, until a phone call from Kyle's Nana (paternal grandmother). She wanted an appointment for Kyle as she felt pressured and stressed by Kyle and his father living with her. I offered to meet for a review with Kyle. It had been nearly eighteen months since I had seen him. Kyle was polite and pleasant but somewhat detached and disaffected. He explained the predicament he and his father were in. His Nana had little space in her home for them, and this caused arguments and tension. Kyle was upset about losing his home and wished his dad had rented it out instead of selling it. Kyle was frustrated that the housing needs of other families were prioritized over theirs and talked about an unjust system. He was reluctant to talk about the gap since we last met or the move. There was a general sense of bleak dislocation. At the end of the session, he took up my offer of another review appointment, and I was pleased when he attended this. However, he was in a different mood this time. Although he was outwardly jovial, I experienced him as somewhat hardened and sarcastic. He explained how he wasn't bothered by his situation and subtly mocked my concern. He was not yet properly in the school system, and the housing situation remained stuck. Dad had been visiting the woman whom they had moved to live with. It felt awkward and uncomfortable, both of us aware of the enormity of the mess. Kyle was uncertain about coming to see me again. I offered another appointment, giving him the option to come back, and explained that I would like to see him. However, Kyle did not come, and there was no further response to several letters. I did not see him again.

It would have been a mammoth step for Kyle to return to psychotherapy after my maternity leave and his experience of leaving his home and school to live in a new city and join a new family. His understandable anger about the loss of his home and school place left him with feelings of cynicism and contempt. There were significant, specific external obstacles. I felt I had little fight in me to galvanize systems and fight for support to re-establish Kyle's psychotherapy. With hindsight, I am struck by what a struggle it seemed to get the work going again. I think the significant adjustments I faced on my return from maternity leave were additional factors. For the first time, I was working part-time, adjusting to a timetable and work relationships that were altered. I think this did affect my capacity to advocate for Kyle's psychotherapy and to engage my colleagues, as well as the school and social care services that had supported this work. This linked to the fantasy I had of having abandoned my colleagues during my maternity leave, and their possible ambivalent feelings towards me. I could not expect them to make another concerted effort for this child in the face of all the other pressures and demands on them. It is a peculiar feeling, as a returning professional after maternity leave, of being one of the additional demands and pressures that colleagues have had to shoulder. These blurring organizational dynamics within a shifting professional identity and with a troubled young patient were difficult to process effectively. It put me in mind of Kyle in his first assessment session with me describing with despair that he was a burden, a strain on his father "who had already enough on his plate". In thinking about this further, I can also recognize how daunted I felt at the prospect of working with Kyle and the clinical material that was likely to emerge if Kyle had returned to his therapy.

Discussion of the case

The circumstances that brought Kyle into psychotherapy and the transference dynamics in the early weeks of this work are typical of child psychotherapy in Britain today. A child patient in psychoanalytic treatment experiences this new relationship as one stirring up early feelings towards parental figures but also influenced by current family experiences. Children who have suffered severe deprivation can feel that they are the product of a malignant conception and can feel themselves to be revolting and damaging. Thus, the transference is often infused with early raw and elemental experiences that require containment equivalent to maternal reverie. Close work with parents/carers and the professional networks around the child emphasizes the essential emotional and relational work that families and agencies need to prioritize in order to address the needs of such vulnerable children.

Early in Kyle's therapy, there was a strong theme about the place of fathers. Concerns for his father and the strain he was placing on him were heavy burdens of guilt and anxiety for Kyle. Having lost his mother, he was tormented with a fear that he would lose his father too. Kyle vividly communicated a wish for a parental couple (both internal and external) who could nourish and help each other, as if he fundamentally knew the centrality of this for a child. In his sessions, Kyle would ask who was going to help me retrieve the paper aeroplanes that he had thrown into high, inaccessible places in the therapy room, which he thought I could not reach. I felt that Kyle was full of an irresistible drive to know about the mother's body and its link with the paternal. The transference was infused with oedipal curiosity and an interest in a supportive loving couple. My review of the psychotherapy material highlighted for me that Kyle wasn't just anxious about an intrusive and excluding parental couple, but was more preoccupied with the need for a creative parental couple that could be available for him. I was surprised to see how I had struggled with picking up multiple communications about fathers in his sessions.

In my experience of work with Kyle, I felt strongly that it needed to continue after I returned from maternity leave. I had a sense of how Kyle reined in his aggressive and rejected responses to my pregnancy and repressed more hostile and desperate feelings. Although the pregnancy afforded a space to also communicate aspects of himself that were concerned and understanding, the work was incomplete. It was possible to negotiate with the parent worker to keep in touch with the family from time to time, as a way of maintaining a reasonable link that wasn't too labour intensive, but the family's move away extended and disrupted this opportunity. Had we been able to resume Kyle's psychotherapy, this might well have provided a unique prospect to confront powerful and ingrained internal-object relations to do with his sexual feelings and identity, the shame of abandonment, and justifiable grievance against failed parental objects. Work beyond the maternity break[1] might also have provided space for Kyle to experience an object that can attend to sibling dynamics and a space for more than one baby.

The vividness of Kyle's play was compelling. The communications about mess, stupidity, and the fear of being the destroyer offered early compelling insights, which I experienced through the symbolism of mother–infant dynamics. Not unique to the work with Kyle, my caseload often consisted of play and symbolic communications about interuterine and womb-like places.

For example in my work with another patient, a teenage fostered girl, Gemma, there was a series of sessions of making paper goldfish held in plastic bags of water that turned murky and were precariously balanced or were poked and tormented with being dropped. The jabbing and torturing of the plastic membrane chimed with the ruthless picking of her skin, which was very similar in emotional quality to Kyle's picking his cuticles around his fingernails in the first assessment session. Gemma's unconscious communications were of a conception that happened within a depleted, attacked, and broken maternal object, and she powerfully communicated her feeling that she should never have been born and that her birth was a catastrophe (M. E. Rustin, 2006). These were the dynamics of her psychotherapy before I became pregnant. There was a tyrannical internal object, an internal destructive mother that threatened the infant's very survival creating an atmosphere of fear and peril. There was a terrifying suicidal depth to Gemma's anger and despair, a foreshadowing in my mind of the risks that lay ahead for Kyle.

Interviews with child psychotherapists

The second part of my study consisted of the interviews mentioned earlier. My personal experience and the predominance of maternal themes in the interviews I undertook suggested that the maternal in child psychotherapy is a familiar and comfortable identification and may often shape the child psychotherapist's transference to her professional role. While the importance of the paternal was appreciated, it is striking how limited references to fathers were in the accounts offered by my child psychotherapy colleagues. It is perhaps likely that the pregnant therapist's intense preoccupation with her female body shuts out the masculine. There is quite possibly a strong pull to protect the dyadic over the triadic space. Birksted-Breen's (1996) distinction between the introjection of a penis as a link in contrast to a phallic state of mind is pertinent here. The predominance of the maternal as exemplified in the pregnant state may pull the therapist into a state of mind in which the function of the penis is occluded. This then creates a distorted vision of parental functioning, characterized by female omnipotence, a phantasy of completeness, and exclusivity. I am suggesting that the recognition of the penis as link that promotes thinking and recognizes the full oedipal situation and the interdependence of the sexes may come under considerable strain during a therapist's pregnancy.

As well as not seeing or minimizing the symbolic communications of the paternal, there was also another significant feature when fathers were mentioned by my interviewees. They tended to appear as angry and intrusive—for example, in this extract, which describes a pregnant psychotherapist's experience of telling her 12-year-old patient's adopted mother about her pregnancy and the response of her patient:

Jane: I can remember talking to her mother letting her mother know, her adopted mother, who was very angry with me … erm … who said that she had had a discussion with this girl's father, this girl's adopted father who made a comment that I had left her just like all the other women in her life. I was going to leave her just like all the other women in her life and abandon her. So I felt an awful attack on myself but also an over whelming sense of guilt. When I told the girl she just lay her head down on the table and just cried for about the last 15 minutes of the session which I have never seen before. You know I had never seen her display emotion like that in her previously and I think generally with her and with some of the other patients it really brought up a lot of stuff into the sessions about their birth family and, I mean, with this particular girl there was quite a lot of attacks on me. I can remember a session when she said she knew someone, a woman who … Do you want all this?

RS: *Yes.*

Jane: A woman who ... erm ... , whose husband didn't want her to have a baby so she just took a tablet and got rid of it and I remember saying to her well perhaps there's a part of you that wishes I could take a tablet to get rid of my baby and she turned around and said, "obvious", so I think taking it too, negative transference, was really important for her. Here is the first:

In this very disturbing extract, a father is described as being angry with the pregnant therapist, evidence of yet another woman abandoning his child. The 12-year-old patient (this is a patient in the midst of puberty) is also reported as describing a father/husband who wanted his pregnant wife to abort her baby.

In another interview, a child psychotherapist described how the transference altered significantly in her parent work with a father when she became pregnant. This father had experienced the therapist as a concerned maternal object but now felt her to be sexually irresponsible and abandoning.

The therapist's pregnancy dramatically brings her sexual life into the work. This can stir up transference dynamics suffused with corrupted, denigrated, and violent images of sexual intercourse. The sense of a healthy and creative parental couple is often massively disrupted, and the space to begin to conceive of this is limited. The pregnancy can then become synonymous with attacking or rejecting the therapeutic work. Rather than the pregnancy being a natural and accommodatable reality, it seems that, at times, it becomes an aggressive sexual intrusion in the minds of both patients and therapists.

The interviews brought to the fore a pattern of disturbance both seen in the response of patients and only partly registered in the minds of their therapists. Where the pregnancy occurs at a time when the therapy has run some considerable course, or is working towards an ending, there is potential to experience it as part of the natural order of things. When there is solid supervisory and team support around the therapist, which the pregnant therapist can make use of, the impingement of a pregnancy can be thought about from a range of perspectives, sometimes with the effect of re-establishing a paternal function that can mitigate an enmeshed coupling.

My research interest in this topic began from my belief that my own clinical work was not as rich and detailed during my pregnancy as in my usual practice. The pall of prolonged morning sickness shook my confidence and created a need to triangulate this with clinicians in similar circumstances. I had, however, anticipated fuller clinical accounts from the interviews. Some participants wished they had looked through their clinical notes to refresh their memories before we met. Overall, there was a sense that their pregnancy had obscured recall, and this contrasted with a time when they had felt better able to hold detailed clinical sequences in mind before pregnancy supervened. However the turbulence of the transference dynamics was richly discussed in detail across all the interviews. The countertransference was communicated with an immediacy and honesty that was striking and provided significant insights into the clinical encounter, indicating that pregnancy can make the therapist more porous to transference phenomena due to the experience of shifting identity (particularly during a first pregnancy), increased levels of preoccupation, and a reactivation of inner conflicts and chaotic feelings. Participants' ready agreement to take part in this project seemed to be because of an intensely felt need to make sense of these powerful experiences.

It is unsurprising how daunting bringing a pregnancy into psychoanalytic work can be and natural that it heightens a therapist's concern and anxiety about the clinical work. Here are two examples from interviews with CAPTs who had recent experiences of working while pregnant. Here is the first:

Robin: I think she had very vivid memories of being a baby and I used to feel very, very guilty that I was pregnant when I was with her-very guilty. I felt very bad that I was letting her down and I remember she used to ask me, why, when I had the baby why couldn't I bring the baby to sessions? Why couldn't the baby come and I could still see her and she could help me look after the baby. That was quite a painful piece of work.

Karen: I felt that I was in a position of … em … having a lot of support and help and having this relatively stable life compared to those two patients and that my child, I felt, would not be exposed to these things, I felt the inequality of that and also that I couldn't give them what I felt well this child had; what I hope for this child to have, I couldn't give them that. I certainly felt a lot of guilt anyway thinking about it now.

As already noted, concern was stronger when pregnancy came early in a patient's treatment, in contrast to a pregnancy that came towards the end when a maternity leave would reasonably fit alongside a clinically indicated ending. Feelings of worry and guilt were also less acute when patients were in stable families where parents were available to provide a continuity of experience and the ending was less likely to be emotionally charged by past traumatic loss and severe deprivation.

The interviews with the three clinical supervisors confirmed anxieties about pregnancy impinging upon the clinical setting. The supervisors conveyed how prevalent pregnant CAPTs' concerns were that their pregnancy would precipitate a crisis in the psychotherapy. The importance was conveyed of working with pregnancy as a fact of life, in the same way that supervision is often called on to think about a variety of impingements into an essentially relational experience, while also recognizing the significant symbolic valency of pregnancy. Supervisors described their awareness of their own identification with the patients. One supervisor talked about a gut-response questioning in her own mind—"Why did she let herself get pregnant, why couldn't she wait?"—and her concern about what the pregnant therapist was putting her patient through. This echoed another child psychotherapist's account in her interview with me, about one of her patients when she became pregnant: "[He was] a child who was so deprived and so needy and actually so engaged, so completely attached to me and doing very well, and I could see that the maternity break would be a tremendous gap for my patient to bridge."

In another interview, a supervising consultant psychotherapist wondered if it is these kinds of intense feelings that explain why CAPTs have not written very much about this subject. It is painful to write about setting up a situation that can be experienced and perceived as one where one child's needs are met and another's are not. The possibility of *both* being attended to in a good-enough and developmentally appropriate way is hard to hold on to.

Further themes from the interview material

Five out of the six child psychotherapists described how morning sickness hampered their fuller understanding of the transference. At times it felt like an achievement just to get through a session. One clinician described how absent she felt in the early stages of her pregnancy and reported a vivid experience of a patient saying "hello" in the middle of a session. It was as if the young patient had unconsciously picked up a point when her therapist's nausea was subsiding and she was able to return emotionally to the work. Interviews with clinical supervisors echoed this experience, describing how the pregnancy of a psychoanalytic clinician is complicated because of the very nature of the work being one of attending to primitive and intensely felt internal-world dynamics. This can be difficult to sustain, and there is a propensity to retreat from exploring the unconscious material. The six child psychotherapists all worried that their work in the transference was diminished during their pregnancy, particularly in the early stages, and this echoed my own experience. They feared that their inevitable turn towards their developing baby displaced and excluded their child patients, and this generated anxiety and guilt.

Clinical supervisors described how pregnancy throws up particular complexities in clinical work with very deprived children and adolescents where phantasies can abound of dangerous and perverse intercourse resulting in malignant conception. A pregnancy and the arrival of a new baby provoke conflicts about competitive and needy siblings that further deprive and push aside the compelling needs of the patient. The challenge seems to be one of maintaining an internal world focus in the face of the real pressures of the therapist's changing body. The experience of pregnant therapists is that phantasies can feel akin to concrete external reality. For example, therapists can feel that they are actually doing something cruel or irresponsible in becoming pregnant, rather than this being in the ordinary rhythm of life. The distress is linked to the impingements of pregnancy into a highly rarefied clinical setting. A therapist becoming pregnant forces the personal into the professional in one of the most concrete and evocative ways possible. External reality absolutely intrudes, and striking a balance that attends to both the internal and external is the task. One supervisor put it thus: "There shouldn't be a need to feel incredibly worried that the pregnancy is just a terrible intrusion. It is grist to the mill; it is the food of life—a fact of life that has to be engaged with."

A prominent theme discussed in all the interviews was how the period between the child psychotherapist's becoming aware of her pregnancy and before telling her patients was quite fraught. It was difficult to decipher the patient's unconscious or conscious awareness of the pregnancy before he was actually told of it. With latency and pre-latency children, this seemed linked to their play, which ubiquitously concerns babies, parental figures, and siblings. If this increased at the time of the pregnancy, the dilemma seemed to be whether this was a part of the more usual developments in psychotherapy, a coincidental occurrence unrelated to the pregnancy, or due to the therapist's pregnancy?

Listening to the clinical descriptions in the interviews, and working over the data subsequently, I was convinced that the patient's communications were in some measure linked to the therapist's pregnancy. The interviews indicated, in fact, that patients did have some awareness of their therapist's pregnancy, and this contrasted with clinicians' uncertainty and hesitancy about what was going on. Reviewing my experience of Kyle's psychotherapy, I am struck by how late I left it to tell Kyle of my pregnancy when it was in the material from an early stage. Entangled communications and a complex interplay between internal and external phenomena meant that, like me, other pregnant therapists had experiences of taking longer than they intended to explicitly reference their pregnancy. One child psychotherapist remembered how:

> I noticed with, well, definitely with one of them, that until I told him he became incredibly anxious in our sessions before I told him. And I was very, I really thought he knew. And I think it was a real relief when I did actually say and I think that was a sense for most of them, that once I actually said, we could then start thinking about it. It was better.

In a significant majority of the clinical examples, the parent/carer was told before the child. This was technically similar to telling parents about break dates and changes in sessions in the ordinary clinical process. But there were occasions where the timing was determined by concerns that the parent would be so unsettled and aggrieved by the news that they might not be able to support the frame of their child's treatment, as they had previously done. On one occasion, there was a significant gap between telling the parent of the pregnancy and then telling the child. This was to create a space to support the parent with the news so that the parent could be in a more solid position to support the child when he was told.

The interviews also contained vivid descriptions of the possibilities and openings that the pregnancy afforded. This was often a surprise to the child psychotherapists, who were more readily expecting unhelpful or even harmful effects. One repeated pattern was indeed where children and adolescents were significantly stirred up by the pregnancy. This was communicated in a variety of ways, such as an increase in acting-out behaviours (e.g., running out of the consulting room) and in anxiety, anger, hostility, and sadness. But interviewees then talked about how these responses opened up new ground and felt like a broadening of emotional expression that could be explored and worked with. There were also examples of patients who responded to the news with relief and a lessening of acting-out behaviours. Some young patients responded to the pregnancy with a new, creative curiosity. However, these varied developmental responses to the pregnancy seemed to go against the expectations of the child psychotherapists. In a proportion of the clinical accounts where developments were evident in the interviews, and could indeed be discussed, child psychotherapists were surprised to realize what they had missed.

My grounded theory analysis of these accounts captured substantiated themes created from the work of coding. This highlighted, in particular, significant clinical transformations in psychoanalytic work during a clinician's pregnancy indicative of turning points in treatment. For example there was a description of a 9-year-old boy who began to stay longer in his sessions after he was told about his therapist's pregnancy, "even to the point where he didn't want to leave". This boy began to make rudimentary gifts out of paper for his therapist, and although the work was emotionally painful and complex there was space to express and notice dynamics of care and generosity, interest and concern. Another interview described how the monotonous stripped-down play of a 6-year-old adopted girl became richer during the child psychotherapist's pregnancy. The girl became more curious and creative, making her unconscious more available. One supervisor remembered how a patient's response to his therapist's pregnancy was thoughtful, pleased, and optimistic. It seemed to provide an opportunity to counter the child's phantasy that pregnancy had an unwanted and violent root. For this patient, who had experienced neglect, his therapist's pregnancy enabled a more ordinary consideration of the facts of life in a direct way. There was something reassuring about his therapist's pregnancy, which could occur in the face of his omnipotence, his demands, and his belief that he could exhaust his therapist. Another supervisor gave an example of work with a 17-year-old boy who seemed to be enlivened by the pregnancy of his psychotherapist. He was struggling with "a complete interruption of his … of the, unfolding of his life in developmental terms after his mother died when he was twelve years old, and he just went into a terrible loop and became obsessional". Feelings of rivalry, curiosity, and some urgency and immediacy entered into the psychotherapy, which the supervisor felt were directly linked to the therapist's pregnancy and provided opportunities for progress.

Nevertheless, there was a cautious and careful consideration of these developments across all the interviews, which addressed the tensions and uncertainty of where the patient's response to the pregnancy lies on the continuum of development and defence and the importance of keeping this question open. This is vividly captured in a supervisory experience described of work with an adolescent girl who had a very difficult history, where her mother had an ongoing incestuous relationship with her own father, the patient's maternal grandfather. This young patient struggled to think of herself as a woman, but during the therapist's pregnancy she could feel a positive identification with her therapist as a woman. During the interview, the supervisor acknowledged that this may have been, in part, the patient's psychic manoeuvre to avoid feeling excluded, yet the supervisor had not previously seen it in that way. Instead, there was something very powerful about an example of a mature, non-abusive creative coupling that countered this teenage girl's internalized experience of an incestuous "sordid sexuality". The actual pregnancy of her therapist thus provided an opportunity for her to become interested in a more ordinary sexuality and womanhood. This young person was in late adolescence and had never menstruated. She began her periods during her therapist's pregnancy. "I could see that the interest she took was not just defensive, it was developmental; it was like a way of finding a positive identification", the supervisor asserted.

My findings highlight significant challenges to the continuation of psychotherapy after a maternity leave in public sector CAMHS. This project demonstrated that psychotherapies sometimes come to a reasonable end at the point of maternity leave when there has been a long-enough period of prior work. Yet there were clear examples of work that needed to bridge the maternity break and, instead, were curtailed or transferred to another therapist but where such a transition did not work. There can be understandable resistance and complications for patients and family to tolerate the period of maternity leave, but more significant seems to be the problem in hard-pressed services where it is difficult to provide the holding work that can contain and stabilize the feelings generated by the maternity leave. There was some evidence in my data that there can be an unconscious idea that if the pregnant therapist is leaving the patient, then the clinic will also let go. It can feel to colleagues that they are left holding the clinical baby, in a way that feels burdensome and unfair in face of the needs of all the other patients.

This small project does not capture or represent psychoanalytic work with children that do bridge maternity leave. I am aware that this work does take place, and it would be invaluable to research this.

Conclusion

The use of grounded theory provided me with a thorough and systematic procedure that has fitted well with psychoanalytic approaches to exploring clinical material. The opportunity to explore psychotherapies that were obscured by pregnancy has been important in addressing a gap in the literature and theory of a regularly occurring event in a clinician's life. I suspect that there is considerable experience and knowledge that has not been tapped into. Further exploration into psychotherapies that break down during a CAPTs pregnancy, and those where effective work during pregnancy and beyond maternity leave, would be important in understanding the circumstances that lead to good clinical outcomes. It would also be useful to extend this work to encompass fatherhood and to better understand the experience of male therapists and the impact on their psychoanalytic work with children and adolescents. Most powerful for me was how this research revealed patients' yearning for a creative couple and a capacity to be nurturing and concerned for a therapist and a new baby sibling. Also revealed was the challenge for child psychotherapists of attending to the sexual transference and the pull into dyadic enmeshment that is intensified during pregnancy. And, finally, was that the need for supervision and team support is a vital factor: when these are available, complex dynamics can be attended to and new opportunities for exploration and discovery in treatment can emerge.

Note

1. Retrospectively one wonders whether there may even have been some link between my pregnancy and the interrupted therapy that resulted from it, and what then happened to Kyle's family, with father and Kyle moving away and becoming involved in new relationships. Is it possible that the limited extent to which the issues arising from pregnancy were able to be worked through in Kyle's therapy had some influence on this development?

CHAPTER ELEVEN

Clinical research and practice with babies and young children in care

Jenifer Wakelyn

My role as a child psychotherapist and the under-fives' lead in a mental health service for children in care has provided a fertile context for clinical research with babies and young children in care. Originally a specialist child and adolescent mental health service providing treatment for around a hundred children each year, the service was re-configured three years ago as a screening and assessment service for all children and young people in the care of the commissioning local authority. My colleagues and I work closely with social workers, foster carers, and the children in care paediatricians and nurses who conduct statutory health assessments for children in care. In addition to screening children after they enter care as well as annually if they remain in care and consulting to social workers, the service provides brief intervention where indicated and refers to relevant services for long-term treatment. In the previous service, very few referrals were received for children under 5, and none for children under 2, whereas in the new service over a third of interventions are for infants and young children. Concerns include the cumulative adversities of foetal drug and alcohol exposure, abuse, neglect, and placement moves (Birk Irner, 2012; Needell & Booth, 1998; Schore, 2001; Wade, Biehal, Farrelly, & Sinclair, 2010; Ward, Munro, & Dearden, 2006). Some children show clear signs of emotional, relationship, or behavioural difficulties; in the case of others, social workers, foster carers, or adoptive parents may be concerned about the impact for later development of early trauma and disruption.

This context has provided opportunities to carry out clinical research on the needs and experiences of a particularly vulnerable group of children that has gone on to inform service development and, in turn, further research. In this chapter I outline stages in the research, describe how it has been disseminated within and beyond the local authority, and illustrate a brief intervention model developed to address the particular needs of young children in temporary foster care. Names and identifying details in the clinical vignettes have been changed to protect confidentiality.

Qualitative research on therapeutic observation using grounded theory

Therapeutic observation is an intervention derived from the psychoanalytic model of infant observation introduced to training in child psychotherapy by Esther Bick (Adamo & Rustin, 2014; Bick, 1964; Miller, Rustin, Rustin, & Shuttleworth, 1989). It offers a home-based, non-intrusive approach with minimal disruption to family life and has been applied with infants at risk of autistic spectrum disorder and with young children at psychosocial risk (Houzel, 1999; Rhode, 2007; M. E. Rustin, 2014). In hospital settings, observation-based approaches have been used with premature babies since the 1970s (Negri, 1994), and there are published accounts of the applications of psychoanalytic infant observation in a range of institutional settings, including orphanages and children's homes (Bardyshevsky, 1998; Cardenal, 1999; Mendelsohn, 2005; Tarsoly, 1998; Urwin & Sternberg, 2012).

The therapeutic observer aims to retain the open-ended, naturalistic, receptive approach of an observer in training, while also taking up a more proactive role, often by promoting connections between child and primary caregiver (Houzel, 2010; M. E. Rustin, 2014). Repeated close observations in the consistent setting of the foster home help the observer to notice a signal, a sound, or a fleeting glance that might otherwise go unnoticed and not be responded to.

In medical contexts, where there are high levels of anxiety about an infant's well-being or even their survival, therapeutic observation may be supportive both for parents and medical staff. Anne McFadyen, a child and adolescent psychiatrist in a special care baby unit, describes infant observation as both "an informer of intervention and an intervention in itself".

> At its simplest, an active interest in the baby, no matter how premature, fragile or disabled, provides a model for both parents and staff. The curiosity aroused in those observing the observer often seems to act as a powerful catalyst for a new kind of way of looking at the infant, and consequently a new kind of interaction. ... Parents can then begin to do the job, which they do naturally with older and fitter infants, of acting as an emotional container for their baby. [McFadyen, 1994, p. 164]

Therapeutic observation is a planned intervention that aims to address particular concerns or difficulties, alongside the overall aim of gaining a deeper understanding of the child's relationships, difficulties, and needs. In this way, therapeutic observation differs from a participant observation stance taken up in the course of a training observation during which significant difficulties become apparent for the family (Blessing & Block, 2014). The role of therapeutic observer working with young children in care requires the skills of an experienced clinician with prior training in psychoanalytic observation and the support of an experienced supervisor. The work can be harrowing as well as rewarding, bringing the clinician into closer contact with young children who have been exposed to trauma early in life. Feeding back to and maintaining communication with professional networks to help sustain a focus on the child during complex care proceedings is an aspect of the therapeutic observer's role that requires sensitivity and tact as well as persistence.

Freud highlights two contrasting aspects of attention: the active and the passive. He describes attention as actively "meeting the sense-impressions half-way, instead of awaiting their appearance" (Freud, 1911b) and as a form of "observing thought" that gathers perceptions and looks for patterns of meaning (Freud, 1912e). He also describes a stance of free-floating or "evenly-suspended attention", passively receiving the material rather than selecting from it, which allows the most direct contact with instinctual life (Freud, 1912e, 1923a). In psychoanalytic observation, these aspects of attention are separated in time: the regular visit and the circumscribed role of the observer create the conditions in which as much information as possible can be received, unconscious and emotional as well as the conscious and perceptual. The active aspect of attention, the observing thought that asks "What does this mean?" comes into play later, in the discussion in supervision and the continuing processing and reflection in the clinician's mind that this way of working facilitates.

My clinical research into how this model of therapeutic observation might be applied with an infant in foster care was carried out under the University of East London/Tavistock doctoral research programme. The findings suggest that observation-based ways of working could have a particular value in work with children who have experienced disruption of their early relationships and with the professional networks supporting them. The idea behind the research was to find out more about the early lives of children in care and to see whether an observational approach would be acceptable to foster carers and social workers. When I discussed the project with social workers, it was welcomed: there was a general idea that it would be helpful to understand more about the experiences of babies in care. Relatively little has been written in the research literature about the youngest children in care, and social workers were aware of a lack of practice guidance to support them in work with this particularly vulnerable group. Ethical permission was obtained from the local Research Ethics Committee, and I was able to observe a baby boy, "Rahan", for ten months during his time in the care of his foster mother "Nadira", until he was moved to his adoptive family (Wakelyn, 2011, 2012a).

In this single case study, the observational approach was accepted by foster carers and social workers, was set up with little delay, and was reported to have been helpful by the foster carer and the social work network. The grounded theory methodology I used to analyse the research data involved a line-by-line analysis of the notes that fits well with the detailed note-writing of the therapeutic observation model (Strauss & Corbin, 1990) Grounded theory is oriented to a "context of discovery" rather than a "context of validation" (Glaser and Strauss, 1967; M. J. Rustin, 2001b) and, like infant observation, relies on an attitude of receptive openness to new connections. "Constant comparison" is used in reading through data to uncover recurrent themes and underlying categories that may generate hypotheses and new questions (Anderson, 2006; Holton, 2007). This methodology aims to produce "rich description", conveying something of the depth and detail of interpersonal interactions.

A central theme became apparent during the date analysis: coming together and coming apart. Four ways of coming together and coming apart were prominent in my observations of Rahan and his interactions with Nadira; more or less integrated states were also observable in my own emotional responses to the experiences that I witnessed and in the group dynamics of the professional network. The observational material made it possible to link the different ways of coming together and coming apart with contrasting types of organization and functioning. It seemed that at times of transition, organization was more likely to be driven by the dynamics of trauma, bringing heightened risks of dissociation, fragmentation, panic and depersonalization, in the social care network as well as in the foster-carer–child dyad. I explored the hypothesis that vicious circles of dysfunctional interaction are generated by the escalating impact of undigested psychic pain and result in a loss of contact with the emotional reality of the infant. These findings were linked to discussions in the social care and psychoanalytic literature of "blind spots" created by defences against intolerable anxiety (Boswell & Cudmore, 2014; Cooper, 2010; Ferguson, 2017; Menzies, 1960; M. E. Rustin, 2005).

Three aspects of trauma-driven organization—which I named "tornado", "machine", and "limbo"—fluctuated at different periods in the life of the temporary foster placement. Each involve a loss of contact with emotional reality: in "tornado", as the result of fragmentation; in "machine", through dissociation and the separation of thought from feeling; and in "limbo", through withdrawal and the suspension of time. The research also highlighted a different type of organization, which I called "matrix". This is a developmental type of functioning in which the child's experiences and states of mind are central in the thoughts, preoccupations, and feelings of the responsible adults. This more integrated type of organization and functioning shapes conditions in which emotional contact with painful realities can be sustained and tolerated.

Another finding from the observation project was the crucial role of play in mitigating the impact of experiences of discontinuity, rupture, and provisionality during the infant's time in temporary foster care. In the Observation 5, with Rahan, now 4 months 2 weeks old, his foster carer, Nadira, tells me that she has just remembered the game of peekaboo, noticing that she had previously forgotten about it.

> Rahan lies on his back, draws up his knees, and takes hold of one foot in each hand. He drops the left foot, almost cries, and then again holds a foot in each hand. He repeats this movement several times. He murmurs and makes some repetitive humming sounds. ... His stare moves from my face to my feet and back to my face again. When I then move my feet, he watches with a fascinated expression, and then, as if in answer, moves his own feet.

> When Nadira leaves the room, she carries on talking to Rahan from the kitchen. He mouths the corner of the toy she gave him and looks steadily ahead. When she comes back, I say something about how he watches her when she is there, and when she leaves, he is listening to her voice. She tells me she only just remembered to play peek-a-boo with him, as she did with all her own children when they were babies. She says she had forgotten about it. She says it helps them to be able to wait.

Peekaboo, in all its variants, allows experiences of separation to be experimented with and explored, giving the growing infant a degree of control and agency. The capacity to anticipate and live through a separation is enhanced. Perhaps, for Nadira, preoccupied by the permanent separation to come when her foster baby is adopted, the repeated rehearsal of separation and reunion in the game of peekaboo has felt too raw. When Nadira becomes able to play peekaboo with Rahan, recognizing that it helps him, something has lifted that enables her to hold in mind his current development as well as the imminent separation.

Four months later, when adoptive families were about to be introduced, the three of us—Nadira, Rahan, and I, as the observer—have found a way to be together. Something of this is perhaps reflected in Rahan's interest in the three toys that he holds in his hands.

> Rahan holds three toys between his hands. One is a little doll with waist-length hair like Nadira's and Dina's (the foster family's youngest daughter).
>
> Nadira tells me she held him in her lap all morning before I came. She says she thinks he feels better when I come. I say her lap is a good place for him.

The ease we have found in being together feels encouraging for the prospect of introducing another "third": the adoptive parents. But at a time when every knock at the door startles both Nadira and me with the fantasy that someone has come to take the baby away, this triangulated state of mind feels fragile.

> Nadira sings to Rahan, "One, two, buckle my shoe ..." and breaks off the song.

The next line—"three, four, who's at the door?"—feels like a stage too far. Mourning for the tiny baby who is growing up is accompanied by dread of the absolute separation when he is adopted. Distress and disarray evoked by the impending upheaval are mitigated by the relief and gratification of seeing Rahan's robust development and his zest for life, but awareness of the separation and loss to come can only be taken in small doses.

These were moments during the observation that sensitized me to challenges and inhibitions in temporary care-giving relationships that may subtly impinge on the foster carer's capacity to encompass the child's future development in her mind. These moments also highlighted the potential for play and playful states of mind to mitigate the impact of trauma and disruption.

Service development informed by clinical research

When the research findings from this observational study were disseminated through feedback meetings, workshops, and conversations with social workers, the service began to receive more referrals for babies and young children in care. Social workers began to consult with us more often in relation to family finding and the planning of placement moves for infants and young children. Workshops with a focus on exploring and learning from the experiences of all those involved in transition planning have provided opportunities for continuing learning and the building up of shared knowledge and understanding of the experiences of the youngest children in care.

Subsequent observational interventions have involved children whose early start in life had been overshadowed by drug and alcohol exposure, developmental difficulties, medical interventions, and family tragedy. We have been able to further develop the observer's role in advocating for children's psychological needs, liaising with professional networks and providing pre- and post-adoption support. The new service model identified the need for a brief intervention model that would help to sustain a focus on the emotional experiences of babies and young children who have been exposed to early adversity.

Developing a brief intervention model: "Watch Me Play!"

When 5-year-old Angus, the son of friends, asked me one weekend to "Shut the door and watch me play!", he expressed an intuitive expectation for the kind of attention that may be impaired or less available for children in the care system. In our outreach service, we could not think of a better name for the intervention we were developing than "Watch Me Play!" (WMP). The approach aims to promote child-led play in foster placements by encouraging foster carers to provide children with their undivided attention at regular times during the week.

It consists of three inter-related elements: promoting child-led play, encouraging carers to give their foster child their undivided attention in a quiet environment for regular, short periods during the week, and, together with the foster carer, attending to the quality and atmosphere of the child's play. Developmental guidance leaflets are provided for foster carers and social workers along with regular invitations to training workshops and forums.[1] Sharing the observations of foster carers and clinicians facilitates a child-centred focus in professional meetings and informs care-planning discussions. One social worker commented: "Watch Me Play! is the voice of the child through their play."

"Watch me play!" is not a "brand": the aim is not to market a supposedly new and unique way of intervening but, rather, to focus on core principles that have been common to evidence-based approaches and clinical practice with distressed and troubled young children for decades and are supported by child development research from many perspectives. Recognizing that insight into the emotional lives and the psychological consequences of early trauma and disruption are not at the forefront of legal and social care discourse or in trainings for foster carers, a distinctive feature of Watch Me Play! is the focus on advocacy and on observed play to bring the child's lived emotional experience to the centre of attention.

The developmental value of play that is fundamental in early years' education is often less well understood in social care contexts. Fragmentation of parenting, when children are looked after by a succession of different adults or when different aspects of parenting are divided among many adults, can also result in an erosion of the reflective tenderness that the young infant ordinarily elicits from those around her or him. Busy foster homes can create routines where children's physical needs are met but the fundamental need for individual attention and intimacy is overlooked (Hardy et al., 2013; Meakings & Selwyn, 2016). Foster carers are routinely encouraged by social workers to take children to stay and play in nursery groups to extend their play experiences and interact with other children, but little attention is explicitly given to interaction, play, and physical comfort and interaction in the foster home; trainings that mainly focus on physical care, behaviour management, and protecting carers from allegations rarely address these important topics (Narey & Owers, 2018). The dynamics of child protection work can also impact on adults' awareness of children's emotional experiences: when children have been injured or assaulted or are at risk of significant harm, the necessary focus on physical safety may result in sensitivity to psychological experience becoming blunted.

WMP draws on child psychotherapy training in infant observation and child development, and on child psychotherapy practice in combining direct work with the child–carer dyad and indirect work with professional networks. It is a psychoanalytic approach that relies on the concept of containment, looks for the development of symbolic play in children and reflective attention in caregivers, and draws on Freud's understanding of attention in both its active and passive aspects. This brief intervention also includes reflection on the emotional quality of the child's play and of the child's interactions with the carer during play. Mutual delight may be experienced as child and carer become more attuned, exploration begins, and playfulness affords some relief from the sequelae of trauma.

Child-led play, underpinned by the attention of the primary caregiver for regular short periods, is central to interventions for young children with psychological vulnerability or developmental delay, including Speech & Language therapy, the Solihull Approach, the Webster Stratton Incredible Years and Fostering Changes training programmes, Watch Wait and Wonder, Floor-time, Special Time, as well as psychoanalytic child psychotherapy and parent–infant psychotherapy (Alvarez & Phillips, 1998; Bratton, Landreth, Kellam, & Blackard, 2006; Elliot & Reis, 2003; Pallet, Blackeby, Yule, Weissman, & Scott, 2000). This particular attention to play, in which the caregiver comments on and describes the child's play, has been found to enhance confidence, trust, self-efficacy or agency, imagination, self-esteem, concentration, regulation, and coordination in the child, mutual understanding and communication between child and caregiver, and sensitivity and attunement in the caregiver (Ayling & Stringer, 2013; Panksepp, 2007; Sunderland, 2007). In Africa, studies of children recovering from malnourishment report reduced mortality and increased speed of recovery in children who received intensive feeding together with psychosocial support, in the form of promoting play and attention on the child, compared to children who received intensive feeding only (WHO, 2006). A focus on psychological well-being generated the life-giving emotional connectedness with caregivers is also critical for children in care.

In Watch Me Play! trainings and workshops, core principles from child development research are discussed, and developmental guidance is provided for foster carers and social workers working with babies and young children in care. Foster carers and social workers who are anxious about how a move to adoption may be experienced by a child who is deeply attached to the foster carer and the foster family may find encouragement in the finding from attachment theory that a secure attachment in infancy is the foundation for future relationships. The psychoanalytic concept of the stability that comes with internalizing a good object is intuitively understood by many foster carers and social workers. Understanding that exploratory play comes before formal learning and may involve making a mess or getting things "wrong" is reassuring for foster carers who are zealous about promoting children's learning. This can help to validate and prioritize the time given to free exploratory play. The central principle that "Thinking about meaning helps children of all ages" can be liberating for foster carers and social workers when a child's behavioural difficulties seem to mirror difficulties in the birth family, or when a child who has experienced prolonged neglect is difficult to remember and hold in mind.

The following clinical vignettes illustrate various aspects of the WMP approach.

Children who "cannot play": Kiara and Kyeshawn

Kiara and Kyeshawn entered foster care, aged 2 and 3 years, after receiving hospital treatment for fractures caused by physical abuse in their birth family. They also had feeding and sleeping difficulties following prolonged exposure to domestic violence and force-feeding by their parents. Four months after entering care, they were referred with concerns about their feeding and also about the strain on their foster carer, Susan, as a result of their post-traumatic hyperactivity and dysregulation. She described the children's arrival in the foster home as "like a tornado hitting us". During my first visit, as the two children hurtled around the room, making identical, high-pitched shrieks, it was hard to imagine either child ever dropping their guard enough to make new relationships or to develop the confidence to explore their world in play.

Over time, both children responded well to regular play sessions, for Kyeshawn with Susan, and for Kiara with Susan's daughter, her back-up carer. The television was switched off, and battery-operated toys were replaced with a small number of soft toys, toy animals, cars, and puzzles (Lerner & Barr, 2015). Susan sat on the floor with Kyeshawn and talked quietly to him about what was happening in his play. For some weeks she found herself describing cars being crashed together, over and over again; then the cars were repeatedly pushed under a sofa, and Kyeshawn would ask Susan to find them for him. Susan described the deadening, controlling atmosphere of this repetitive, driven play: ten minutes was as much as could be managed during this period. Drawing on what was known of Kyeshawn's early history, the clinician discussed with Susan the possible links with terrifying experiences of unpredictable adults and with the drastic changes in his young life.

After three months, Kyeshawn began to "find" his cars for himself; Susan spoke of a shared delight in Kyeshawn's newly found sense of his own agency. With Susan sitting on the floor alongside him, Kyeshawn was able to explore other toys, talk to the toy animals, or join in with a nursery rhyme. The feeding difficulties resolved, and it became possible for Kyeshawn to relax a little of his vigilant watching. The siblings started to sleep in separate beds, and Kyeshawn was able to start nursery for a few hours a day.

For the carers of Kiara and Kyeshawn, experiencing and reflecting with the clinician on something that felt driven, controlled or coercive in the play experience, and linking this with the children's experiences of repeated rejection, physical abuse or domestic violence, allowed something to shift over time. Sitting close to the carer with a selection of simple toys in a quiet environment created conditions in which the children's anxieties and high arousal could begin to be contained. Over time, more exploratory play could begin. Observation and child-led play were complementary: observing with warmth and interest helped to facilitate children's play; careful attention to play helped foster carers and clinicians to notice, take in and remember the children's communications.

My involvement continued with play-based sessions in the clinic playroom until adoptive parents came forward for the two children, and I had the opportunity to meet them. They were keen to discuss Kyeshawn and Kiara's differing needs and interests and their observations of the children as they got to know them. In the course of intermittent telephone support that continued for another two years, I had the pleasure of hearing about two children who went on to thrive in their adoptive family.

"Do I matter to her?": Molly

Under the pressure of numerous subtle messages and anxieties, a foster carer may efface herself and, instead of her own physical, individual, living presence, present the infant in her care with wall-to-wall television and a sea of automated toys. Instead of intimacy and responsive interaction, the child experiences a cacophony of recorded voices, fragments of electronic music, and the over-stimulation of randomly flashing lights. The child's signals and cues cannot be noticed or responded to, and both carer and child may increasingly withdraw, leading to a situation where adequate physical care is being provided, but the child is living in an emotional void. The following brief intervention brought it home to me how hard it must have been for Jane, a first-time foster carer, to feel that she could be close to and important for the traumatized infant in her care. From the day after Molly's arrival in the foster home, Jane was obliged to take the 3-month-old baby on a two-hour journey five times a week, for supervised contact with her parents.

Molly was 5 months old when consultation was requested to discuss concerns about her shrill, persistent crying and sudden mood changes. She had been born addicted to heroin and had spent her first two weeks of life in a special care baby unit. When I visited the foster home, Jane told me more about her worries. A large television was on in the bright living room where Molly was surrounded by battery-operated toys making random sounds and flashing lights as she pressed their buttons; a radio could also be heard from the adjoining kitchen. I saw that Molly repeatedly glanced briefly in Jane's direction after a particularly loud noise, then dropped her gaze when Jane was looking elsewhere. As this went on, Molly's face became paler and her arms and legs seemed to stiffen. It seemed to me that Jane may have lacked any belief that her presence and attention were important for Molly. Together with Jane's supervising social worker, we were able to think about the conditions Molly might need to help her to regulate her high levels of arousal and that would help Jane to attune to the infant in her care. Turning the television off for some hours of the day and putting away the mechanical toys created a quieter environment in which Jane could hold Molly in her arms, talk quietly or sing to her, and watch and get to know her rapid, fleeting facial expressions. This helped Jane to see when Molly was ready for play and when she needed to rest. It also helped Molly to send clearer signals and cues to the caregiver whose attention was now on her.

Encouraging Jane to provide Molly with undivided attention for regular periods during the week increased Jane's confidence in attuning and interacting with a foster baby who had seemed worryingly withdrawn and irritable. Repeatedly experiencing familiar responses in the transitional space provided by play created a "rhythm of safety" (Tustin, 1986a). Increasingly, pleasurable interactions began to be described as Molly began to seek Jane's attention, her long gazes giving way to slow smiles as Jane talked to her and waited for her response. Jane reported to the social worker that she felt she was getting to know Molly in a different way. She began to recognize the likely stressors for Molly and felt more able to anticipate her changes of mood and more confident about soothing her when she was upset. The long periods of inconsolable crying lessened.

"She doesn't like me": Ameera

Ameera, aged 2 months 2 weeks, and her foster carer Dulcie both appeared depressed when I met them following concerns that the care being provided in the foster home was "functional". Ameera was a sturdy, thick-set toddler with a sombre expression who glanced at the dolls' house in the clinic playroom without moving towards it or looking to her carer. I sat on the floor with a small selection of toys, which I placed near Ameera. Slowly, with no change of expression, she picked up one animal after another and looked at it. In a loud voice, Dulcie began to tell Ameera the names of the animals and asked her to repeat them. Ameera turned away and stared into space. Dulcie told me that this was Ameera acting like a sulky teenager.

I encouraged Dulcie to sit on the floor and to watch what Ameera chose to do and suggested we could talk afterwards about what we each saw. When Dulcie sat down near her, Ameera put some cushions on the floor and took a blanket and played at going to bed. Dulcie now talked to her in a quieter voice, describing what she was doing. At the end of the session, Dulcie told me she had never seen Ameera play in this way before. In the next two sessions, Ameera repeated this game with increasing delight and began to play peekaboo with Dulcie, hiding behind the blanket. During the third session, Ameera lifted her arms to be held by Dulcie. I felt a deep relief as I saw her relax into Dulcie's lap, her rigid muscle tone softened. Ameera's sombre expression lifted more often into a smile, and she vocalized more freely; Dulcie told me: "the house feels lighter".

I did not have the scope to explore the underlying causes of the alienation that seemed to have come about between Dulcie and Ameera, or the opportunity to follow up this intervention, but it seemed that the transitional space of play and the experience of mutual delight that it afforded had allowed something to become freed up and created more warmth and attunement between carer and child.

Many factors may lead to foster carers becoming distant from the children they are looking after. Burn-out is a professional risk, under the impact of repeated, often unprocessed losses and repeated experiences of rejection by children whose interactive styles appear indifferent or dismissive. Foster carers may feel unvalued in a climate that militates against validating the parenting that they provide.

Becoming a child: George

Foster carers looking after toddlers may find it difficult to allow the kind of free play that provides opportunities for children to express themselves. George, a shy and constrained 3-year-old, had experienced repeated placement breakdowns and sudden moves. He spoke in a whisper, rarely raising his eyes, and avoided any physical comfort from his thoughtful foster carers. A shift was seen after two WMP sessions and telephone support for his foster carer, Simeera. My colleague noticed that as soon as George started to play, Simeera asked many questions and made suggestions about what he could do next. It seemed that Simeera very much wanted to find a way of giving something to George, and in doing so, unwittingly, became intrusive.

The focus on play and attention helped child and carer to find each other. When Simeera was able to take a step back and started to see how George was then able to play more freely, a new side of George began to emerge. Now he could show the toy animals fighting, shout when he was winning at Snap, and ask to be held on Simeera's lap when he was upset. Simeera felt that George had come alive and had become a 3-year-old child instead of a "mini-adult". She began to enjoy looking after George much more, even when the placement became more challenging as George became less compliant.

Evaluation

Service evaluation and feedback suggested that integrating different aspects of a child's life through a focus on observation and play allows professionals to provide more containment for the child. A pilot feasibility study of "Watch Me Play!" found that the intervention was accepted by foster carers and was valued by social workers. Social workers commented on the skills that this approach could help foster carers to develop.

> It's not an area where in my experience foster carers are even aware of how this kind of work could help them, the routines are attended to but play is always a gap.

> It would help the carers to understand the children, because sometimes even the young ones do not get time to play with their foster carers.
>
> This could allow foster carers to get more enjoyment from being with the children. It could help the carers to feel involved and help the children to feel they are wanted.

This study also showed that it was sadly not possible to obtain permission from birth parents during or after care proceedings to recruit children to evaluate the effects of a six-session WMP intervention. Feedback also suggested that in another trial, flexibility would be needed in relation to the number of sessions offered.

A deeper understanding of risk and protective factors for babies and young children in care

A dissemination project following the development of the "Watch Me Play!" approach provided opportunities to share experiences with professionals working with infants and young children in care across the country and to evaluate a half-day training workshop. Data from individual evaluation forms and transcriptions of focus groups discussion were analysed using content analysis, extracting themes by frequency and salience.

The resulting themes highlighted the common experiences of professionals in different parts of the country that the psychological experiences and needs of young children in care tend to become overlooked. One respondent poignantly commented,

> They are this kind of forgotten.

This aspect of the research gave a deeper resonance to concerns about "under-involved" foster care, which has been highlighted as a risk factor for mental health difficulty and adoption breakdown in later childhood (Hardy et al., 2013; Hillen, Gafson, Conlon, & Rosen, 2012; Meakings and Selwyn, 2016; Selwyn, Wijedasa, & Meakings, 2014). Discussions in training workshops and focus groups confirmed earlier findings that under-involved foster care may reflect the wider, systemic under-involvement of organizations in the emotional lives and experiences of young children in care.

The value for young children of free exploratory play was recognized as something that many professionals were aware of in principle, but that quickly becomes lost to sight in social care contexts.

> We often see children who have no idea about play. It's all about the care proceedings and the care planning.
>
> Play is paramount for any child and it is lost by professionals.

The need for preventative intervention was flagged up by many respondents:

> To help children develop resources so they are more able to manage later.
>
> It would save problems in the long term. All the evidence suggests the earlier you intervene the better—rather than waiting for children to act up when they are 7, 8, 9, 11—or 17.

The Watch Me Play approach was felt to be feasible and acceptable, particularly as an introductory way of working:

> Helpful starting point as a way in.
>
> You feel you can do it.
>
> There's not a lot of instructions but there's a lot to gain.

Respondents pointed to other areas of work in which the WMP approach could be applied, including work with children on the edge of care or under child protection arrangements, and in post-adoption support, potentially leading into subsequent video-based interventions.

Focus group discussions identified topics for further training. The recognition that foster carers may feel anxious about what might be expressed in the child's play highlighted the need for reflective discussion to be an intrinsic part of the intervention.

Some respondents felt that the simplicity of the WMP approach might lead parents and carers to think it unimportant, suggesting that trainers draw attention to the child development research underpinning it and the potential benefits for children and caregivers. Others commented that the observing and attending stance in WMP involves a change of gear that might feel challenging until it has become embedded in daily or weekly routines.

The next stage

Social workers, foster carers, contact supervisors, children in care nurses, and paediatricians and legal professionals in the local authority have participated in forums focusing on the needs and experiences of young children in care. Alongside individual case consultations with social workers and therapeutic interventions with foster carers and children's networks, termly "Relationships and Transitions" workshops allow experiences and good practice to be shared among foster carers, social workers, and health professionals. The service continues to offer brief interventions and longer therapeutic observations with infants and young children in care, as resources permit. A manual in preparation for the Watch Me Play! approach is aimed to be a free downloadable resource.

Applications of the WMP approach as a preventative intervention are currently being explored with teenage parents who are in care or leaving care. This work may provide a potential context for a pilot feasibility study exploring the impact of WMP for young parents, their children, and for the parent–child relationship.

Concluding thoughts

The dialogue between clinical research and practice is a fruitful one that has helped to bring new ideas and approaches into work with a group of particularly vulnerable children. A focus on partnership in learning and on learning from experience has helped to facilitate closer working partnerships and to advocate for emotional and psychological dimensions of the lives of young children who are at risk of being overlooked during complex care proceedings and temporary caregiving contexts. At times when hope and hopefulness may be hard to find, a new interest in and focus on the child's experiences can help to generate the life-seeking drive for development that is particularly important for foster carers living with the trauma of young children as well as for professionals working in a beleaguered climate.

Notes

1. Further information on this service, First Step, can be found at: https://tavistockandportman.nhs.uk/care-and-treatment/our-clinical-services/first-step.

I am grateful to the children, foster carers, and social workers who have contributed to this work; to my colleagues in First Step and the local authority for our work together; and to the Tavistock Clinic Foundation for funding the research.

APPENDIX A

Completed doctoral theses in child and adolescent psychotherapy

The following theses in child and adolescent psychotherapy were completed between 2000 and 2018 at the Tavistock Clinic and the University of East London's Professional Doctorate Programme in Child Psychotherapy.

Child psychotherapists within the Professional Doctorate Programme undertook their research at the Tavistock and Portman NHS Trust in London; at the Northern School for Child and Adolescent Psychotherapy in Leeds; at the Birmingham Trust for Psychoanalytic Psychotherapy in Birmingham; and at the Scottish Child Psychotherapy Training in Glasgow and Edinburgh. Research was also undertaken within this programme by child psychiatrists or psychoanalysts working for doctoral awards.

Akhtar, Khuzuma. *Brief psychotherapy with children in a specialist school: An exploration of the underlying issues for children and mainstream schools.*

Allnutt, Louise. *Transitions, boundaries and thresholds: How can child psychotherapy help a child in care find a place of his own?*

Anderson, Janet. *Risk-taking, dangerous behaviour in childhood.*

Baker, Tim. *An exploration of the workings of the staff team in an adolescent psychiatric in-patient unit.*

Ball, Jillian. *An investigation into the impact which a mother's death has on her adolescent daughter's adolescent development.*

Bannerman-Haig, Sara. *Switching a Light On: Can Intensive Psychoanalytic Psychotherapy Enable a Child Diagnosed with Development Delay Become Unstuck?*

Bradley, Marie. *No man's land? Making a map: The contribution of child psychotherapy to decision-making for looked after children in transition.*

Brown, Davina. *"The emerging butterfly": How can a boy considered likely to receive an ADHD diagnosis at age 5 be provided with a different developmental experience?*

Chantrell, Sue. *A study of how a child in foster care and in transition to adoption expressed, explored and developed his internal representations of self and carer in psychoanalytic psychotherapy.*

Cherry-Swaine, Janine. *What is the impact of intermittent strabismus upon the therapeutic relationship?*

Chester, Christine. *What can be learned from comparing a child's psychotherapist's experience of children in a children's psychotherapy group with the narrative accounts of foster carers describing the same children in their care?*

Chinoy, Freni. *Psychotherapeutic work with families with serious parental illness.*

Cohn, Nancy. *A study in the process of consultation under the auspices of UNICEF in former Yugoslavia.*

Coyle, Anne-Marie. *The complex world of hide and seek: Investigations into the use and meaning of hide and seek play and how it is related to processes of change within a looked after boy engaged in psychoanalytic psychotherapy.*

Creaser, Miriam. *A comparison of audio recordings and therapists' process notes in child and adolescent psychoanalytic psychotherapy.*

Crehan, Geraldine. *Issues of transference: Psychotherapy with a severely traumatized child placed for adoption.*

Curen, Valerie. *Exploration of intensive psychotherapy with adolescent patients.*

Dawson, Andrew. *Stuck cases: Understanding the experience of children, families and clinicians in CAMHS when the helping relationship becomes stuck.*

De Rementeria, Alexandra. *Observing the nature and trajectory of infant defences against disturbing mothering on a mother and baby unit.*

Della Rosa, Elena. *An exploration of transference interpretations in short term psychoanalytic psychotherapy (STPP) with adolescents suffering from depression (IMPACT study).*

Douglas, Hazel. *Containment and reciprocity: Integrating psychoanalytic theory and child development research for work with children.*

Elfer, Jane. *To investigate the emotional impact of adolescent sibling bone marrow donation.*

Evans, Angela. *An investigation into the interactions between a child psychotherapist as a consultant/researcher and three primary school SENCOs.*

Fan, Hsueh-Mei. *Imitation in Development and in Developmental Failure: A Case Study Based on a Child's Psychotherapy.*

Fleming, Robert. *New perspectives on the dynamics of the adoption triangle using biographical, literary and psychoanalytic sources.*

Frances, Fionualla. *Problems coming into the therapy room: An investigation into how anxieties entering the transition from waiting room to therapy room are linked with the work of the therapy in intensive work with a 5-year-old girl who has been sexually abused.*

Goldberger, Danny. *The struggle to separate: Psychoanalytic psychotherapy with boys living alone with their mothers.*

Grunbaum, Liselotte (PhD). *Anxieties and dilemmas relating to breaks in the therapeutic relationship.*

Hindle, Debbie. *An intensive assessment of a small sample of siblings placed together in foster care.*

Hodgson, Sarie. *Internal and external home and homelessness: The Emotional Experience of Children Looked After in Residential Care, & Care Staff.*

Ironside, Leslie. *Living in a storm: An examination of the impact of deprivation and abuse on the psychotherapeutic process and the implications for clinical practice.*

Jones, Hilary (PhD). *A study of intensive outpatient psychotherapy with sexually abused children.*

Junor Sheppard, Sean. *An investigation of the transference to determine the usefulness of cross-cultural psychotherapy in the development of the patient's self.*

Keenan, Amanda. *Parental loss in early adolescence and its subsequent impact on adolescent development.*

Klingert-Hall, Julie. *An exploration of a patient's use of her body within the transference relationship in intensive psychotherapy: Towards allowing thoughts to become thinkable.*

Lane, Harriet. *Can a reflective space be established in a Family Assessment Centre and what might such a space provide for the staff observing contact? An exploration into the benefits and challenges of this intervention.*

Langton, Patricia. *Don't shoot the messenger: An exploration of how professional networks struggle to receive, contain and process painful communications from and about adolescents in the care system.*

Lewis, Catherine. *A clinical investigation of impairment in the development of healthy aggression as a result of confusion of destructive and non destructive aggression, with reference to the work of Child Psychoanalyst Henri Parens and his research group.*

Lorenz, Gabrielle. *Play as a bridge to communication: The gains and risks of playing imaginatively in psychotherapy sessions with developmentally delayed and traumatised children.*

Lush, Margaret. *Links between states of mind and drawing: A case study of an adolescent boy.*

Lusher Nikki. *Addressing the negative transference in intensive child psychotherapy.*

Maher, Emmett. *The role of shame and humiliation in relation to the technical difficulties providing child psychotherapy to a 6-year-old boy in care.*

Maxwell, Monique. *What is the nature of the therapeutic encounter in an adolescent psychotherapy group?*

McLatchey, Jo. *Am I the only one? What happens in a parent support group in a Neonatal Intensive Care Unit (NICU)?*

Meehan, Deirdre. *Coming into being": The process of developmental growth in a severely deprived child in intensive psychoanalytic psychotherapy.*

Mees, Peta. *Generic assessments: The contribution of the child psychotherapist.*

Midgen, Melissa. *The child analytic tradition of the Society of Analytical Psychology: Birth, death and beyond.*

Millar, Tennyson. *Race, identity and the transference/countertransference: A mixed-race patient and a mixed-race therapist. A single case study.*

Nesic-Vuckovic, Tanya. *Visual perception in children diagnosed with Asperger's syndrome.*

Nicholson, Joanne. *What developments can be seen in a year's intensive psychotherapy with a 10-year-old adopted boy with mild learning difficulties?*

O'Dwyer, Louise. *"I'm No More Your Mother or Your Father": Parents' Experience of Having a Child Hospitalized for an Eating Disorder.*

O'Shea, Daniel. *An investigation into perinatal psychotherapy as a treatment for first-time mothers with anxiety disorders.*

Philps, Janet. *Applications of child psychotherapy to work with children in temporary foster care.*

Pollard, Laura. *How do members of a multi-disciplinary team involved in running a therapeutic play group understand their role in the work?*

Pozzi, Maria. *A research study into the process of change in under-five's psychoanalytic psychotherapy.*

Quagliata, Emanuela. *A psychoanalytic study of recurrent miscarriage: Brief psychotherapeutic work with pregnant women.*

Reid, Marguerite. *The mother's state of mind following the loss of a baby and the birth of the next infant.*

Russell, Jo. *Dissociative identities in childhood: An exploration of the relationship between adopting these identities and painful states of mind in three young people. Are there implications for psychoanalytic technique?*

Ryan, Emily. *Tracking change: A thematic analysis of change in a deprived boy in long term foster care during intensive psychoanalytic psychotherapy.*

Sanderson, Nicholas. *An attempt to identify distinguishable patterns of projective identification in the child & adolescent psychotherapy setting, produced around the experience of disappointment.*

Scott, Alexandra. *On the effects of trauma experienced in infancy: A single case study.*

Serlin, Mel. *What can we learn from interviews with kinship carers, teachers and therapists about the experiences of children in kinship care?*

Shallcross, Wendy. *Psychoanalytical infant observation and research: What can be learned from a single case study?*

Sharma, Rajni. *An exploration into the effects a Child Psychotherapist's pregnancy has on her clinical work.*

Slater, Peter. *A study of how the experience of a violent father has impacted on a latency boy's development.*

Sloan Donachy, Gillian. *Placement breakdown in foster care with children under-five: A psychoanalytic view of the caregiving relationship under stress.*

Sternberg, Janine. *An examination of the relevance of the study of infant observation to psychoanalytic psychotherapy trainings.*

Sutton, Sarah. *Being taken in: How can psychoanalytic psychotherapy lead to better relationships for an adopted child?*

Sweeney, Lynne. *"A baby mouse in a tiny boat" in psychotherapy treatment: Can the experience of premature birth be considered significant in understanding the internal world of a child?*

Tamm Lessa de Sá, Carlos (PhD). *Autistic functioning and language development.*

Taylor, Georgina. *An investigation into the implementation of CYP-IAPT routine outcome measures in their first year of integration into child psychotherapy practice.*

Taylor, Lynne. *How can a child psychoanalytic psychotherapy assessment contribute to the understanding of the individual experiences of children who are refugees?*

Thomas, Louis. *The suicide attempt of a 7-year-old boy: An exploration of precipitating and protective factors.*

Thomas, Sayi. *Stuck at three: Psychoanalytic psychotherapy treatment for a young boy with obsessive-compulsive disorder.*

Tiltina, Kristine. *Challenges facing long term foster carers: Exploration of the nature of psychoanalytic parent/carer support.*

Trice, Julie. *Investigating links between intimacy and violence in intensive psychotherapy.*

Wakelyn, Jenifer. *What can be learned from a therapeutic observation of an infant or young child in foster care?*

Wakitani, Junko. *From verbal to bodily expression: The nature of and meanings of regression. A single case study of a 7-year-old boy.*

Watt, Ferelyth. *Crossing the threshold: An inquiry into the lived experience of Bangladeshi parents with young children; their worries and sources of support.*

Wedd, Anne-Marie. *How observational material might be used in a collaborative consultation with teachers to further their understanding of their pupils.*

Weir-Jeffrey, Tessa. *An investigation into the process of recovery from an early history of deprivation and trauma through the use of psychoanalytic psychotherapy.*

Wood, Sam. *Finding the order in disorder: Exploring possible links between child & adolescent psychotherapy and chaos theory.*

Wright, Hilary. *Emotional Turbulence: The Development of Symbolic Thinking in the Psychotherapeutic Treatment of an Adolescent Girl.*

Young, Joanne. *The Internal World of Children with Insulin Dependent Diabetes Mellitus (IDDM): The Use of the Winnicott Squiggle Game as an Assessment Tool.*

REFERENCES

Adamo, S. M. G., & Rustin, M. E. (Eds.) (2014). *Young Child Observation: A Development in the Theory and Method of Infant Observation*. London: Karnac.

Akhtar, S. (2009). *A Comprehensive Dictionary of Psychoanalysis*. London: Karnac.

Allawi, A. (2009). *The Crisis of Islamic Civilisation*. New Haven, CT: Yale University Press.

Alvarez, A. (1992). *Live Company: Psychoanalytic Psychotherapy with Autistic, Borderline, Deprived and Abused Children*. London: Routledge.

Alvarez, A. (2006). Some questions concerning states of fragmentation: Unintegration, under-integration, disintegration, and the nature of early integrations. *Journal of Child Psychotherapy, 32* (2): 158–180.

Alvarez, A., & Phillips, A. (1998). The importance of play: A child psychotherapist's view. *Child Psychology and Psychiatry Review, 3* (3): 99–104.

Alvarez, A., & Reid, S. (Eds.) (1999). *Autism and Personality: Findings from the Tavistock Autism Workshop*. London: Routledge.

Anderson, J. (2003). The mythic significance of risk-taking, dangerous, behaviour. *Journal of Child Psychotherapy, 29* (1): 75–91.

Anderson, J. (2006). Well-suited partners: Psychoanalytic research and grounded theory. *Journal of Child Psychotherapy, 32* (3): 329–348.

Appelbaum, S. A. (1973). Psychological-mindedness: Word, concept and essence. *International Journal of Psychoanalysis, 54*: 35–46.

Atkins, K., & Chattoo, S. (2007). The dilemmas of providing welfare in an ethnically diverse state: Seeking reconciliation in the role of a "reflexive practitioner". *Policy & Politics, 35* (3): 377–393.

Avello, J. J. (1998). Metapsychology in Ferenczi: Death instinct or death passion? *International Forum of Psychoanalysis, 7*: 229–234.

Ayling, P., & Stringer, B. (2013). Supporting carer-child relationships through play: A model for teaching carers how to use play skills to strengthen attachment relationships. *Adoption and Fostering, 37* (2): 130–143.

Baginsky, M., Gorin, S., & Sands, C. (2017). *The Fostering System in England: Evidence Review*. London: Department of Education. Available at: https://www.gov.uk/government/publications/the-fostering-system-in-england-review

Bailey, K. (2000). Comparison of verbatim transcripts and psychoanalytic process notes for emotion tone, abstraction, and referential activity using computerized text analysis methods. *Dissertation Abstracts International: Section B: The Sciences and Engineering, 61*: 3269.

Balsam, R. (2003). The vanished pregnancy body in psychoanalytic female developmental theory. *Journal of the American Psychoanalytic Association, 51*: 1153–1179.

Balsam, R. (2012). *Women's Bodies in Psychoanalysis*. London: Routledge.

Baradon, P. (2005). *The Practice of Psychoanalytic Parent–Infant Psychotherapy: Claiming the Baby*. London: Routledge.

Bardyshevsky, M. (1998). The compensation of autistic features during a little boy's second year: Overcoming pain through the development of attachment. *Infant Observation, 2* (1): 40–57.

Bartram, P. (2003). Some oedipal problems in work with adopted children and their parents. *Journal of Child Psychotherapy, 29* (1): 21–36.

Bateman, A., & Fonagy, P. (2010). Mentalization-based treatments for borderline personality disorder. *World Psychiatry, 9* (1): 11–15.

Bateman, A., & Fonagy, P. (2016). *Mentalization-Based Treatments for Personality Disorder*. Oxford: Oxford University Press.

Bateson, M. C. (1971). The interpersonal context of infant vocalization. *Quarterly Progress Report of the Research Laboratory of Electronics, 100*: 170–176.

Bick, E. (1964). Notes on infant observation in psychoanalytic training. *International Journal of Psychoanalysis, 45*: 558–566.

Bick, E. (1968). The experience of the skin in early object relations. *International Journal of Psychoanalysis, 49*: 484–486.

Bick, E. (1986). Further considerations of the function of the skin in early object relations. *British Journal of Psychotherapy, 2*: 292–299.

Bion, W. R. (1959). Attacks on linking. *International Journal of Psychoanalysis, 40*: 308–315. Reprinted in: *Second Thoughts: Selected Papers on Psycho-Analysis* (pp. 93–109). London: Karnac, 1984. Also in: E. Bott Spillius (Ed.), *Melanie Klein Today, Vol. 1: Mainly Theory* (pp. 87–101). London: Routledge, 1988.

Bion, W. R. (1962a). *Learning from Experience*. London: Heinemann.

Bion, W. R. (1962b). A theory of thinking. In: *Second Thoughts: Selected Papers on Psycho-Analysis* (pp. 110–119). London: Karnac, 1984.

Bion, W. R. (1963). *Elements of Psycho-Analysis*. London: Karnac, 1984.

Bion, W. R. (1965). *Transformations*. London: Heinemann.

Bion, W. R. (1967). *Second Thoughts: Selected Papers on Psycho-Analysis*. London: Karnac, 1984.

Bion, W. R. (1970). *Attention and Interpretation*. London: Tavistock.

Bion, W. R. (1977). *Two Papers: The Grid and Caesura*. London: Karnac, 1989.

Bion, W. R. (1991). *A Memoir of the Future*. London: Karnac.

Bion, W. R. (1992). *Cogitations*. London: Karnac.

Birk Irner, T. (2012). Substance exposure in utero and developmental consequences in adolescence: A systematic review. *Child Neuropsychology, 18* (6): 521–549.

Birksted-Breen, D. (1996). Phallus penis and mental space. *International Journal of Psychoanalysis, 77*: 649–657.

Blass, R. B., & Blatt, S. J. (1992). Attachment and separateness: A theoretical context for the integration of object relations theory with self psychology. *Psychoanalytic Study of the Child, 47*: 189–204.

Blatt, S. J., & Luyten, P. (2009). A structural-developmental psychodynamic approach to psychopathology: Two polarities of experience across the life span. *Development and Psychopathology, 21*: 793–814.

Blessing, D. (2007). Hiding in plain sight: The sibling connection in eating disorder. *Journal Child Psychotherapy, 33* (1): 36–50.

Blessing, D., & Block, K. (2014). Sewing on a shadow: Acquiring dimensionality in a participant observation. In S. M. G. Adamo, & M. E. Rustin (Eds.), *Young Child Observation: A Development in the Theory and Method of Infant Observation* (pp. 215–223). London: Karnac.

Blumer, H. (1992). *Symbolic Interactionism: Perspective and Method*. Oakland, CA: University of California Press.

Bonnin, N. (2011). *Therapeutic Memory: A Study of Therapists' Process Notes* Doctoral dissertation, Wright Institute, Graduate School of Psychology, Berkeley, CA.

Boston, M., & Lush, D. (1994). Further considerations of methodology for evaluating psychoanalytic psychotherapy with children: Reflections in the light of research experience. *Journal of Child Psychotherapy, 20* (2): 205–229.

Boston, M., & Szur, R. (Eds.) (1983). *Psychotherapy with Severely Deprived Children*. London: Routledge.

Boswell, S., & Cudmore, L. (2014). "The children were fine": Acknowledging complex feelings in the move from foster care into adoption. *Adoption and Fostering, 38* (1): 5–21.

Bradley, E., & Emanuel, L. (2008). *What Can the Matter Be? Therapeutic Interventions with Parents, Infants and Young Children*. London: Karnac.

Bradley, S. B., Selby, J., & Urwin, C. (2012). Group life in babies: Opening up perceptions and possibilities. In: C. Urwin & J. Sternberg (Eds.), *Infant Observation and Research: Emotional Processes in Everyday Lives* (pp. 137–148). Hove: Routledge.

Bratton, S. C., Landreth, G. L., Kellam, T., & Blackard, S. R. (2006). *Child Parent Relationship Therapy (CPRT) Treatment Manual: A 10-Session Filial Therapy Model for Training Parents*. New York: Routledge/Taylor & Francis Group.

Braun, V., & Clarke, V. (2006). Using thematic analysis in psychology. *Qualitative Research in Psychology, 3*: 77–101.

Brenman, E. (2006). The recovery of the good object relationship: The conflict with the superego. In: G. F. Spoto (Ed.), *Recovery of the Lost Good Object* (pp. 94–106). London: Routledge.

Briggs, A. (Ed.) (2012). *Waiting to Be Found: Papers on Children in Care*. London: Karnac.

Briggs, S. (1997). Observing when infants are at potential risk. In: S. Reid (Ed.), *Developments in Infant Observation: The Tavistock Model* (pp. 207–227). London: Routledge.

Britton, R. (1989). The missing link: Parental sexuality in the Oedipus complex. In: R. Britton, M. Feldman & E. O'Shaughnessy (Eds.), *The Oedipus Complex Today: Clinical Implications* (pp. 83–101). London: Karnac.

Britton, R. (Ed.) (1998). Belief and Imagination. London: Routledge.

Britton, R., & Steiner, J. (1994). Interpretation: Selected fact or overvalued idea? *International Journal of Psychoanalysis, 75*: 1069–1078.

Bruner, J. S. (1978). The role of dialogue in language acquisition. In: A. Sinclair, R. J. Jarvelle & W. J. M. Levelt (Eds.), *The Child's Conception of Language* (pp. 241–256). New York: Springer-Verlag.

Bruschweiler-Stern, N., Harrison, A. M., Lyons-Ruth, D., Morgan, A. C., Nahum, J. P., Sander, L. W., et al. (2002). Explicating the implicit: The local level and the microprocess of change in the analytic situation. *International Journal of Psychoanalysis, 83* (5): 1051–1062.

Bryant, A., & Charmaz, K. (2007). Grounded theory in historical perspective: An epistemological account. In: A. Bryant & K. Charmaz (Eds.), *The Sage Handbook of Grounded Theory* (pp. 31–57). London: Sage.

Burnell, A., Castell, K., & Cousins, G. (2009). *Siblings Together or Apart*. Northampton: Family Futures. Available at: https://www.familyfutures.co.uk/

wp-content/uploads/2015/05/Siblings-Together-or-Apart-Practice-Paper.compressed.pdf

Burstall, S. (2004). *Regaining Equilibrium: Understanding the Process of Sibling Adjustment to Pediatric Acquired Brain Injury*. Unpublished doctoral thesis Griffith University, South East Queensland, Australia.

Canham, H. (1999). The development of the concept of time in fostered and adopted children. *Psychoanalytic Inquiry, 19* (2): 160–172.

Canham, H. (2002). Group and gang states of mind. *Journal of Child Psychotherapy, 28* (2): 113–127.

Canham, H. (2003). The relevance of the Oedipus myth to fostered and adopted children. *Journal of Child Psychotherapy, 29* (1): 5–19.

Canham, H. (2004). Spitting, kicking and stripping: Technical difficulties encountered in the treatment of deprived children. *Journal of Child Psychotherapy, 30*: 143–154.

Canham, H., & Emanuel, L. (2000). Tied together feelings' group psychotherapy with latency children: The process of forming a cohesive group. *Journal of Child Psychotherapy, 26* (2): 281–302.

Cardenal, M. (1999). A psychoanalytically informed approach to clinically ill babies. *Infant Observation, 2* (1): 90–101.

Carlberg, G. (2007). Laughter opens the door: Turning points in child psychotherapy. *Journal of Child Psychotherapy, 23* (3): 331–349.

Carroll, L. (1865). *Alice's Adventures in Wonderland*. Kindle Edition, Wisehouse Classics, 2016.

Charmaz, K. (1995). Grounded theory. In: J. A. Smith, R. Harré, & L. Van Langenhove (Eds.), *Rethinking Methods in Psychology* (pp. 27–50). London: Sage.

Charmaz, K. (2006). *Constructing Grounded Theory: A Practical Guide through Qualitative Analysis*. London: Sage.

Cioffi, F. (1970). Freud and the idea of a pseudoscience. In: F. Borger & F. Cioffi (Eds.), *Explanation in the Behavioural Sciences* (pp. 115–142). London: Cambridge University Press.

Cioffi, F. (1998). *Freud and the Question of Pseudoscience*. London: Open Court.

Cohen, D., Mitchell, J., & Britton, R. (2009). Siblings in development: Towards a metapsychology. In: V. Lewin & B. Sharp (Eds.), *Siblings in Development: A Psychoanalytic View* (pp. 77–100). London: Karnac.

Coles, P. (2003). *The Importance of Sibling Relationships in Psychoanalysis*. London: Karnac.

Conte, H. R., Ratto, R., & Byram Karusa, T. (1996). The Psychological Mindedness Scale: Factor, structure and relationship to outcome of psychotherapy. *Journal of Psychotherapy Practice and Research, 5*: 250–259.

Cooper, A. (2010). *A Short Cultural History of British Child Maltreatment and Protection: Case Studies in Problems of Mourning in the Public Sphere*. Paper presented at Tavistock Centre Scientific Meeting, 8 February.

Corbin, J., & Strauss, A. (2008). *Basics of Qualitative Research: Techniques and Procedures for Developing Grounded Theory* (3rd edition). London: Sage.

Covner, B. J. (1944a). Studies in phonographic recordings of verbal material: III. The completeness and accuracy of counselling interview reports. *Journal of General Psychology, 30*: 181–203.

Covner, B. J. (1944b). Studies in phonographic recordings of verbal material: IV. Written reports of interviews. *Journal of Applied Psychology, 28* (2): 89–98.

Craven, P., & Lee, R. (2006). Therapeutic interventions for foster children: A systematic research synthesis. *Research on Social Work Practice, 16*: 287–304.

Crews, F. (2017). *Freud: The Making of an Illusion*. London: Profile Books.

Crews, F., & Crews, F. (1997). *The Memory Wars: Freud's Legacy in Dispute*. London: Granta Books.

Davidsen, A. S. (2013). Phenomenological approaches in psychology and health sciences. *Qualitative Research in Psychology, 10* (3): 318–339.

Dawson, L. (2005). Local survey. In: *Views on Access to CAMHS Tower Hamlets*. Unpublished.

Dein, S. (2013). Magic and jinn among Bangladeshis in England suffering from physical and mental health problems: Controlling the uncontrollable. *Research in the Social Scientific Study of Religion, 24*: 193–219.

Department of Education and Skills (2006). *Care Matters: Transforming the Lives of Children and Young People in Care*. London: TSO Blackwell.

Diamond, J. (2012). Creating a "third position" to explore oedipal dynamics in the task and organization of a therapeutic school. In: A. Briggs (Ed.), *Waiting to Be Found: Papers on Children in Care*. London: Karnac.

Diem-Wille, G. (2011). *The Early Years of Life: Psychoanalytical Development Theory according to Freud, Klein, and Bion*. London: Karnac.

Douglas, H., & Brennan, A. (2004). Containment, reciprocity and behaviour management: Preliminary evaluation of a brief early intervention (the Solihull Approach) for families with infants and young children. *International Journal of Infant Observation, 7* (1): 89–107.

Eco, T., & Seboek, T. (Eds.) (1988). *The Sign of Three—Dupuin, Holmes, Pierce: Advances in Semiotics*. Bloomington, IN: Indiana University Press.

Edwards, J. (2000). On being dropped and picked up: Adopted children and their internal objects. *Journal of Child Psychotherapy, 26* (3): 349–367.

Edwards, J. (2008). Early splitting and projective identification. *International Journal of Infant Observation and Its Applications, 11* (1): 57–65.

Egelund, T., & Hestbæk, A. (2003). *Anbringelse af børn og unge uden for hjemmet. En forskningsoversigt*. København: Socialforskningsinstituttet.

Elliot, A. J., & Reis, H. T. (2003). Attachment and exploration in adulthood. *Journal of Personality and Social Psychology, 85* (2): 317–331.

Emde, R. (1988a). Development terminable and interminable: I. Innate and motivational factors from infancy. *International Journal of Psychoanalysis, 69* (1): 23–42.

Emde, R. (1988b). Development terminable and interminable: II. Recent psychoanalytic theory and therapeutic considerations. *International Journal of Psychoanalysis, 69* (2): 283–296.

Etchegoyen, A. (1993). The analyst's pregnancy and its consequences on her work. *International Journal of Psychoanalysis, 74*: 141–149.

Eysenck, H. (1973). *The Uses and Abuses of Psychology*. London: Pelican.

Eysenck, H. (2002). *The Decline and Fall of the Freudian Empire*. Piscataway, NJ: Transaction Books.

Fagan, M. (2011). Relational trauma and its impact on late adopted children. *Journal of Child Psychotherapy, 37* (2): 129–146.

Fairbairn, W. R. D. (1952). The repression and the return of bad objects (with special reference to the "war neuroses"). In: *Psychoanalytic Studies of the Personality* (pp. 59–81). London: Routledge & Kegan Paul.

Ferguson, H. (2017). How children become invisible in child protection work: Findings from research into day-to-day social work practice. *British Journal of Social Work, 47* (4): 1007–1023.

Fernald, A. (1985). Four-month-old infants prefer to listen to motherese. *Infant Behavior and Development, 8* (2): 181–195.

Fisher, J. (2011). The emotional experience of K. In: C. Mawson (Ed.), *Bion Today* (pp. 43–63). London: Routledge.

Fonagy, P. (1993). The research agenda: The vital need for empirical research in child psychotherapy. *Journal of Child Psychotherapy, 29* (2): 129–136.

Fonagy, P. (2001). *Attachment Theory and Psychoanalysis*. London: Karnac.

Fonagy, P. (2003). Psychoanalysis today. *World Psychiatry, 2* (2): 73–80.

Fonagy, P., Gergely, G., Jurist, E. J., & Target, M. (2004). *Affect Regulation, Mentalization and the Development of the Self*. London: Routledge.

Fonagy, P., Rost, F., Carlyle, J. A., McPherson, S., Thomas, R., Pasco Fearon, R. M., et al. (2015). Pragmatic randomized controlled trial of long-term psychoanalytic psychotherapy for treatment-resistant depression: The Tavistock Adult Depression Study (TADS). *World Psychiatry, 14*: 312–321.

Ford, T., Vastanis, P., Meltzer, H., & Goodman, R. (2007). Psychiatric disorder among British children looked after by local authorities: Comparison with children living in private households. *British Journal of Psychiatry, 190*: 319–325.

Fraiberg, S. H., Adelson, E., & Shapiro, V. (1985). Ghosts in the nursery: A psychoanalytic approach to the problem of impaired infant–mother relationships. *Journal of the American Academy of Child Psychiatry, 14*: 387–421.

Freud, A. (1936). Identification with the aggressor. In: *The Ego and the Mechanisms of Defence* (pp. 109–121). New York: International Universities Press, 1966.

Freud, A. (1955). Special experiences of young children, particularly in times of social disturbance. In: K. Soddy (Ed.), *Mental Health and Infant Development. Proceedings of the International Seminar held by the World Federation for Mental Health at Chichester, England* (pp. 141–159). London: Routledge & Kegan Paul.

Freud, A. (1978). The principal task of child analysis. In: *The Writings of Anna Freud, Vol. 8*. New York: International Universities Press.

Freud, A., & Dann, S. (1951). An experiment in group upbringing. *Psychoanalytic Study of the Child, 6*: 127–168.

Freud, S. (1901b). The Psychopathology of Everyday Life. *Standard Edition, 6*.

Freud, S. (1905d). Three Essays on the Theory of Sexuality. *Standard Edition, 7*.

Freud, S. (1909b). Analysis of a phobia in a five-year-old boy. *Standard Edition, 10*: 5–149.

Freud, S. (1911b). Formulations on the two principles of mental functioning. *Standard Edition, 12*.

Freud, S. (1912e). Recommendations to physicians practising psycho-analysis. *Standard Edition 12*: 109–120.

Freud, S. (1914g). Remembering, repeating and working-through. *Standard Edition, 12*: 145–156.

Freud, S. (1917a). A difficulty in the path of psychoanalysis. *Standard Edition, 17*: 137–144.

Freud, S. (1918a). The taboo of virginity. *Standard Edition, 11*: 192–208.

Freud, S. (1920g). Beyond the Pleasure Principle. *Standard Edition, 18*: 1–64.

Freud, S. (1921c). Group Psychology and the Analysis of the Ego. *Standard Edition, 18*: 67–143.

Freud, S. (1923a). Two encyclopaedia articles. *Standard Edition, 18*: 235–262.

Freud, S. (1926d). Inhibitions, Symptoms and Anxiety. *Standard Edition, 20*.

Gabbard, G. O. (1997). Case histories and confidentiality. *International Journal of Psychoanalysis*, 78 820–821.

Gabbard, G. O. (2000). Disguise or consent: Problems and recommendations concerning the publication and presentation of clinical material. *International Journal of Psychoanalysis, 81* (6): 1071–1086.

Gaddini, R., & Gaddini, E. (1959). Rumination in infancy. In: L. Jessner & E. Pavenstedt (Eds.), *Dynamic Psychopathology in Childhood* (pp. 166–185). New York: Grune & Stratton.

Gaensbauer, T. J. (1994). Therapeutic work with a traumatized toddler. *Psychoanalytic Study Child, 49*: 412–433.

Gaensbauer, T. J. (1995). Trauma in the preverbal period: Symptoms, memories and developmental impact. *Psychoanalytic Study Child, 50*: 123–149.

Gallie, W. B. (1952). *Peirce and Pragmatism*. Harmondsworth: Pelican.

Garfinkel, H. (1967). *Studies in Ethnomethodology*. Cambridge: Polity Press.

Garland, C. (Ed.) (2002). *Understanding Trauma: A Psychoanalytical Approach* (2nd enlarged edition). London: Karnac.

Geertz, C. (1973). *The Interpretation of Cultures*. London: Basic Books.

Gerhardt, S. (2004). *Why Love Matters: How Affection Shapes a Baby's Brain*. London: Routledge.

Gilbert, R., Widom, C., Browne, K., Fergusson, D., Webb, E., & Janson, S. (2009). Burden and consequences of child maltreatment in high-income countries. *The Lancet, 373* (9657): 68–81.

Glaser, B. G., & Strauss, A. (1965). *Awareness of Dying*. New York: Aldine, 2009.

Glaser, B. G., & Strauss, A. (1967). *The Discovery of Grounded Theory: Strategies for Qualitative Research*. Chicago, IL: Aldine.

Glaser, D. (2000). Child abuse and neglect and the brain: A review. *Journal of Child Psychology and Psychiatry, 41* (8): 1076.

Glasser, M. (1992). Problems in the psychoanalysis of certain narcissistic disorders. *International Journal of Psychoanalysis, 73*: 493–503.

Goffman, E. (1968). *Asylums: Essays on the Social Situation of Mental Patients and Other Inmates*. London: Penguin.

Golse, B. (1999). Le development du language. In: *Au début de la vie psychique. Le dévelopment du petit enfant*. Paris: Editions Odile Jacob.

Goodyer, I. M., Reynolds, S., Barrett, B., Byford, S., Dubicka, B., Hill, J., et al. (2017). Cognitive behavioural therapy and short-term psychoanalytical psychotherapy versus a brief psychosocial intervention in adolescents with unipolar major depressive disorder (IMPACT): A multicentre, pragmatic, observer-blind, randomised controlled superiority trial. *The Lancet, 4* (2): 109–119.

Goodyer, I. M., Tsancheval, S., Byford, S., Dubicka, B., Hill, J., Kelvin, R., et al. (2011). Improving mood with psychoanalytic and cognitive therapies (IMPACT): A pragmatic effectiveness superiority trial to investigate whether specialised psychological treatment reduces the risk for relapse in adolescents with moderate to severe unipolar depression: Study protocol for a randomised controlled trial. *Trials, 12*, 175. Available at: www.trialsjournal.com/content/12/1/175

Grandin, T. (1992). Calming effects of deep touch pressure in patients with autistic disorder, college students, and animals. *Journal of Child and Adolescent Psychopharmacology, 2* (1): 63–72.

Green, A. (1975). The analyst, symbolization and absence in the analytical setting. In: *On Private Madness* (pp. 30–59). London: Hogarth Press & The Institute of Psycho-Analysis, 1986.

Green, A. (1977). The borderline concept. In: *On Private Madness* (pp. 60–83). London: Hogarth Press & The Institute of Psycho-Analysis, 1986.

Greenson, R. (1967). *The Technique and Practice of Psychoanalysis, Vol. 1.* London: Routledge, 2016.

Gretton, A. (2006). An account of a year's work with a mother and her 18-month-old son. *International Journal of Infant Observation, 9*: 21–34.

Griffith, L. (2009). Motherhood, ethnicity and experience: A narrative analysis of the debates concerning culture in the provision of health services for Bangladeshi mothers in East London. *Anthropology & Medicine, 17* (3) 2010: 289–299.

Groarke, S. (2008). Psychoanalytical infant observation: A critical assessment. *European Journal of Psychotherapy and Counselling, 10* (4): 299–321.

Grünbaum, L. (2014). *Anxieties and Dilemmas Relating to Breaks in the Therapeutic Relationship with Children Whose Relationships in Early Infancy Were Reported to Have Been Emotionally Unstable and Traumatised: A Systematic Study of Child Psychotherapy with a Young Child Who Had Suffered Early Abuse and Neglect.* Doctoral dissertation, University of East London/ Tavistock and Portman NHS Foundation Trust.

Grünbaum, L., & Mortensen, K. V. (2017). *Psychodynamic Child and Adolescent Psychotherapy: Theories and Methods.* London: Karnac.

Gunnar, M. R. (2010). A commentary on deprivation-specific psychological patterns: Effects of institutional deprivation. *Monographs of the Society for Research in Child Development, 75* (1): 232–247.

Hannett, F. (1949) Transference reactions to an event in the life of the analyst. *Psychoanalytic Review, 36*: 69–81.

Hardy, C., Hackett, E., Murphy, E., Cooper, B., Ford, T., & Conroy, S. (2013). Mental health screening and early intervention: Clinical research study for under 5-year-old children in care in an inner London borough. *Clinical Child Psychology and Psychiatry, 20*: 261–275.

Harré, R., & Madden, E. H. (1975). *Causal Powers: A Theory of Natural Necessity.* Oxford: Blackwell.

Harris, M., & Bick, E. (2011). *The Tavistock Model: Papers on Child Development and Psychoanalytic Training* (2nd revised edition). London: Karnac.

Harris, M., & Carr, H. (1966). Therapeutic consultations. *Journal of Child Psychotherapy, 1*: 13–19. Reprinted in: M. Harris & E. Bick, *The Tavistock*

Model: Papers on Child Development and Psychoanalytic Training (2nd revised edition, pp. 304–311). London: Karnac, 2011.

Heimann, P. (1950). On counter-transference. *International Journal of Psycho-analysis, 31*: 81–84.

Heritage, J. (1984). *Garfinkel and Ethnomethodology*. Cambridge: Polity Press.

Hillen, T., Gafson, L., Conlon, L., & Rosen, L. (2012). Assessing the prevalence of mental health disorders and needs among preschool children in care in England: An unmet need for greater care. *Infant Mental Health Journal, 33* (4): 411–420.

Hindle, D. (2007). Clinical research: A psychotherapeutic assessment model for siblings in care. *Journal of Child Psychotherapy, 33* (1): 70–93.

Hindle, D. (2014). Clinical research: A psychotherapeutic assessment model for siblings in care. In D. Hindle & S. Sherwin-White (Eds.), *Sibling Matters: A Psychoanalytic, Developmental, and Systemic Approach* (pp. 225–250). London: Karnac.

Hinshelwood, R. D. (1991). Psychodynamic formulation in assessment for psychotherapy. *British Journal of Psychotherapy, 8* (2): 166–174.

Hinshelwood, R. D. (1994). *Clinical Klein*. London: Free Association Books.

Hobson, P. (2002). *The Cradle of Thought: Exploring the Origins of Thinking*. London: Macmillan.

Hobson, P. R., Patrick, M. P. H., & Valentine, J. D. (1998). Objectivity in psychoanalytic judgements. *British Journal of Psychiatry, 173*: 172–177.

Hodges, J., & Tizard, B. (1989). Social and family relationships of ex-institutional adolescents. *Journal of Child Psychology, Psychiatry, and Allied Disciplines, 30*: 77–97.

Hollway, W. (2011). In between external and internal worlds: Imagination in transitional space. *Methodological Innovations, 6* (3): 50–60.

Hollway, W. (2012). Infant observation: Opportunities, challenges, threats. *International Journal of Infant Observation, 15* (1): 21–32.

Hollway, W., & Jefferson, T. (2000). *Doing Qualitative Research Differently: Free Association, Narrative and the Interview Method*. London: Sage.

Hollway, W., Phoenix, A., Elliott, H., Urwin, C., & Gunaratnam, Y. (2008). *Identities in Process: Becoming Bangladeshi, African Caribbean and White Mothers*. Swindon: ESRC.

Holton, J. A. (2007). The coding process and its challenges. In: A. Bryant & K. Charmaz (Eds.), *The Sage Handbook of Grounded Theory* (pp. 265–281). London: Sage.

Hopkins, J. (2004). Conscience and conflict: Darwin, Freud and the origins of human aggression. In: D. Evans & P. Cruse (Eds.), *Emotions, Evolution and Rationality* (pp. 225–248). Oxford: Oxford University Press.

Houzel, D. (1999). A therapeutic application of infant observation in child psychiatry. *Infant Observation, 2* (3): 42–53.

Houzel, D. (2001). The "nest of babies" fantasy. *Journal of Child Psychotherapy, 27* (2): 125–138.

Houzel, D. (2004). The psychoanalysis of infantile autism. *Journal of Child Psychotherapy, 30* (2): 225–237.

Houzel, D. (2008). The creation of psychic space, the "nest of babies" fantasy and the emergence of the Oedipus complex. In: K. Barrows (Ed.), *Autism in Childhood and Autistic Features in Adults: A Psychoanalytic Perspective* (pp. 119–145). London: Karnac.

Houzel, D. (2010). Infant observation and the receptive mind. *Infant Observation, 13* (2): 119–133.

Hoxter, S. (1983). Some feelings aroused in working with severely deprived children. In: M. Boston, & R. Szur (Eds.), *Psychotherapy with Severely Deprived Children* (pp. 125–132). London: Karnac, 1990.

Hoyningen-Huene, P. (1987). Context of discovery and context of jusification. *Studies in History and Philosophy of Science, 18* (4): 501–515.

Hughes, A. (1988). The use of manic defence in the psychoanalysis of a 10-year-old girl. *International Review Psycho-Analysis, 15*: 157–164.

Hughes, J. (2004). *From Obstacle to Ally: The Evolution of Psychoanalytic Practice*. London: Brunner-Routledge.

Hunter, M. (2002). *Psychotherapy with Young People in Care*. Hove: Brunner-Routledge.

Hurry, A. (1998). *Psychoanalysis and Developmental Therapy*. London: Karnac.

Jones, C. (2016). Sibling relationships in adoptive and fostering families: A review of the international research literature. *Children and Society, 30*: 324–334.

Joseph, B. (1985). Transference: The total situation. *International Journal of Psychoanalysis, 66*: 447–454. Reprinted in: M. Feldman & E. B. Spillius (Eds.), *Psychic Equilibrium and Psychic Change: Selected Papers of Betty Joseph*. London: Routledge, 1989.

Joseph, B. (1986). *Psychic Equilibrium and Psychic Change: Selected Papers of Betty Joseph*. London: Routledge.

Kanner, L. (1943). Autistic disturbances of affective contact. *Nervous Child, 2*: 217–225.

Kearney, R. (2004). Emmanuel Levinas: Ethics of the infinite. In: *Debates in Continental Philosophy: Conversations with Contemporary Thinkers*. Manchester: Manchester University Press.

Kenrick, J. (2010). "Be a kid": The traumatic impact of repeated separations on children who are fostered or adopted. *Journal of Child Psychotherapy, 26* (3): 393–412.

Klein, M. (1926). Psychological principles of early analysis. In: *Love, Guilt and Reparation and Other Works 1921*–1945 (pp. 128–138). London: Hogarth Press, 1975.

Klein, M. (1927a). Symposium on child-analysis. In: *Love, Guilt and Reparation and Other Works 1921–1945* (pp. 139–169). London: Hogarth, 1975.

Klein, M. (1927b). Criminal tendencies in normal children. In: *Love, Guilt and Reparation and Other Works 1921–1945* (pp. 170–185). London: Hogarth Press, 1975.

Klein, M. (1930). The importance of symbol-formation in the development of the ego. *International Journal of Psychoanalysis, 11*: 24–39.

Klein, M. (1931). A contribution to the theory of intellectual inhibition. In: *Love, Guilt and Reparation and Other Works 1921–1945* (pp. 236–247). London: Hogarth Press, 1975.

Klein, M. (1932). *The Psychoanalysis of Children*. London: Virago, 1994.

Klein, M. (1935). A contribution to the psychogenesis of manic-depressive states. *International Journal of Psychoanalysis, 16*: 145–174.

Klein, M. (1936a). Weaning. In: *Love, Guilt and Reparation and Other Works 1921–1945* (pp. 290–305). London: Hogarth Press, 1975.

Klein, M. (1936b). Weaning. In: *Love, Guilt and Reparation and Other Works 1921–1945* (pp. 290–305). London: Hogarth Press, 1975.

Klein, M. (1940). Mourning and its relation to manic-depressive states. *International Journal of Psychoanalysis, 21*: 125–153.

Klein, M. (1945). The Oedipus complex in the light of early anxieties. In: *Love, Guilt and Reparation and Other Works 1921*–1945 (pp. 370–419). London: Hogarth Press, 1975.

Klein, M. (1946). Notes on some schizoid mechanisms. In: *Envy and Gratitude and Other Works 1946–1963* (pp. 1–24). London: Hogarth Press, 1975.

Klein, M. (1952). The origins of transference. In: *Envy and Gratitude and Other Works 1946–1963* (pp. 48–56). London: Hogarth Press, 1975.

Klein, M. (1955). On identification. In: *Envy and Gratitude and Other Works 1946–1963* (pp. 141–175). London: Hogarth Press, 1975.

Klein, M. (1961). *Narrative of a Child Analysis: The Conduct of the Psycho-Analysis of Children as Seen in the Treatment of a Ten-Year-Old Boy*. New York: Delta Book, 1975.

Klein, S. (1980). Autistic phenomena in neurotic patients. *International Journal of Psychoanalysis, 61*: 395–402.

Knapp, P. H., Mushatt, C., & Nemetz, S. J. (1966). Collection and utilization of data in a psychoanalytic psychosomatic study. In: L. A. Gottshalk & A. A. Auerbach (Eds.), *Methods of Research in Psychotherapy* (pp. 401–422). New York: Appleton-Century-Crofts.

Knorr-Cetina, K. (1999). *Epistemic Cultures: How the Sciences Make Knowledge*. Cambridge, MA: Harvard University Press.

Korbivcher, C. F. (1995). Supervisão com Frances Tustin. *Ide, 27*.

Kronengold, H. (2010). Hey Toy Man. *Journal of Infant, Child, and Adolescent Psychotherapy, 9*: 3–17.

Kuhn, T. S. (1962). *The Structure of Scientific Revolutions*. Chicago, IL: Chicago University Press.

Labastida, A. T. (1976). Ansiedades de separation y reunion en la transferencia en quatro ninos [Separation and reunion anxieties in the transference of four children]. *Neurología, Neurocirugía, Psiquiatría, 17* (2): 95–101.

Laplanche, J., & Pontalis, J.-B. (1973). *The Language of Psychoanalysis*. London: Hogarth Press. reprinted London: Karnac, 1988.

Latour, B., & Woolgar, S. (1979). *Laboratory Life: The Construction of Scientific Facts*. London: Sage.

Lawson, K., & Cann, R. (2018). *State of the Nation's Foster Care 2016: Impact Report*. London: The Fostering Network.

Lax, R. (1969). Some considerations about transference and countertransference manifestations evoked by the analyst's pregnancy. *International Journal of Psychoanalysis, 30*: 363–372.

Layard, R., & Clarke, D. (2015). *Thrive: The Power of Psychological Therapy*. London: Penguin.

Lerner, C., & Barr, R. (2015). Screen Sense: Setting the record straight. Research-based guidelines for screen use for children under 3 years old. *Zero To Three, 35* (4): 1–10.

Loftus, E. (1979). *Eyewitness Testimony*. Cambridge, MA: Harvard University Press.

Løpez-Corvo, R. E. (2003). *The Dictionary of the Work of W. R. Bion*. London: Karnac.

Lord, C., Rutter, M., Goode, S., Heemsbergen, J., Jordan, H., Mawhood, L., et al. (1989). Autism diagnostic observation schedule: A standardized observation of communicative and social behavior. *Journal of Autism and Developmental Disorders, 19* (2): 185–212.

Lord, C., Rutter, M., & Le Couteur, A. (1994). Autism Diagnostic Interview–Revised: A revised version of a diagnostic interview for caregivers of individuals with possible pervasive developmental disorders. *Journal of Autism and Developmental Disorders, 24* (5): 659–685.

Lord, J., & Borthwick, S. (2008). *Together or Apart: Assessing Siblings for Permanent Placement*. London: BAAF. Available at: https://www.familyfutures.co.uk/wp-content/uploads/2015/05/Siblings-Together-or-Apart-Practice-Paper.compressed.pdf

Loshak, R. (Ed.) (2012). *Out of the Mainstream: Helping the Children of Parents with a Mental Illness*. London: Routledge.

Loxterkamp, L. (2009). Contact and truth: The unfolding predicament in adoption and fostering. *Clinical Child Psychology and Psychiatry, 14*: 423–435.

Luborsky, L. (1997). The core conflictual relationship theme (CCRT): A basic case formulation method. In: T. Eels (Ed.), *Handbook of Psychotherapy Case Formulation* (pp. 58–83). New York: Guilford Press.

Luborsky, L., & Luborsky, E. (2006). *Research and Psychotherapy: The Vital Link*. Lanham, MA: Jason Aronson.

Lush, D., Boston, M., Morgan, J., & Kolvin, I. (1998). Psychoanalytic psychotherapy with disturbed adopted and foster children: A single case follow-up study. *Clinical Child Psychology and Psychiatry, 3* (1): 51–69.

Magagna, J. (2007). Transformation: From twin to individual. *Journal Child Psychotherapy, 33* (1): 51–69.

Magagna, J. (2014). Envy, jealousy, love, and generosity in sibling relations: The impact of sibling relations on future family relations. In: K. Skrzypek, B. Maciejewska-Sobczak, & Z. Stadnicka-Dmitriew (Eds.), *Siblings: Envy and Rivalry: Coexistence and Concern* (pp. 195–217). London: Karnac.

Maiello, S. (1995). The sound-object. *Journal of Child Psychotherapy, 21* (1): 23–41. [First published as: "Loggetto sonoro". In: *Richard e Piggle*, Vol. 1, No. 1, pp. 31–47. Roma: Il Pensiero Scientifico, 1993].

Maiello, S. (1997). Interplay: Sound aspects in mother–infant observation. In: S. Reid (Ed.), *Developments in Infant Observation: The Tavistock Model*. London: Routledge.

McDougall, J. (1986). *Theatres of the Mind: Illusion and Truth on the Psychoanalytic Stage*. London: Free Association Books.

McFadyen, A. (1994). *Special Care Babies and Their Developing Relationships*. London: Routledge.

Meakings, S., & Selwyn, J. (2016). She was a foster mother who said she didn't give cuddles": The adverse early foster care experiences of children who later struggle with adoptive family life. *Clinical Child Psychology and Psychiatry, 21* (4): 509–519.

Mehlbye, J., Bonfils, I. S., & Andersen, K. R. (2011). *Netværksanbringelser. Praksis og erfaringer i tre nordiske lande*. Købmagergade: AKF, Anvendt Kommunal Forskning.

Meltzer, D. (1967). *The Psycho-Analytical Process*. London: Heinemann.

Meltzer, D. (1975a). Adhesive identification. *Contemporary Psychoanalysis, 11*: 289–310.

Meltzer, D. (1975b). Dimensionality in mental functioning. In: *Explorations in Autism: A Psycho-Analytical Study*. Strath Tay: Clunie Press.

Meltzer, D. (1975c). Mutism in infantile autism, schizophrenic and manic-depressive states: The correlation of clinical psycho-pathology and linguistics. In: *Explorations in Autism.* London: Karnac.

Meltzer, D., Bremner, J., Hoxter, S., Weddell, D., & Wittenberg, I. (1975d). *Explorations in Autism.* London: Karnac.

Meltzer, D., & Harris, M. (1976). A psychoanalytic model of the child-in-the-family-in-the-community. In: A. Hahn (Ed.), *Sincerity and Other Works: Collected Papers of Donald Meltzer* (pp. 387–454). London: Karnac, 1995.

Meltzer, D., & Harris Williams, M. (1973). The apprehension of beauty. In: D. Meltzer & M. Harris Williams (Eds.), *The Role of Aesthetic Conflict in Development, Art and Violence* (pp. 1–6). Strath Tay: Clunie Press.

Meltzer, D., & Harris Williams, M. (1988). Aesthetic conflict: Its place in development. In: D. Meltzer & M. Harris Williams (Eds.), *The Apprehension of Beauty: The Role of Aesthetic Conflict in Development, Art and Violence* (pp. 7–33). Strath Tay: Clunie Press.

Mendelsohn, A. (2005). Recovering reverie: Using infant observation in interventions with traumatised mothers and their premature babies. *Infant Observation, 8* (3): 195–205.

Menzies, I. E. P. (1960). A case study in the functioning of social systems as defence against anxiety. A report on a study of the nursing service of a general hospital. *Human Relations, 13*: 95–121. Reprinted in: *Containing Anxiety in Institutions. Selected Essays, Vol. 1.* London: Free Association Books, 1990.

Menzies Lyth, I. (1988). *Containing Anxiety in Institutions.* London: Free Association Books.

Midgley, N. (2006). The "inseparable bond between cure and research": Clinical case study as a method of psychoanalytic inquiry. *Journal of Child Psychotherapy, 32* (2): 122–147.

Midgley, N. (2009). *Child Psychotherapy and Research.* London: Routledge.

Midgley, N., Anderson, J., Grainger, E., Nesic-Vuckovic, T., & Urwin, C. (2009). *Child Psychotherapy and Research: New Approaches, Emerging Findings* (pp. 56–71). London: Routledge.

Midgley, N., & Kennedy, E. (2011). Psychodynamic psychotherapy for children and adolescents: A critical review of the evidence base. *Journal of Child Psychotherapy, 37* (3): 232–260.

Miller, L., Rustin, M. E., Rustin, M. J., & Shuttleworth, J. (1989). *Closely Observed Infants.* London: Bloomsbury.

Mitchell, J. (2003). *Siblings, Sex and Violence.* Cambridge: Polity Press/Blackwell Publishing, 2004.

Money-Kyrle, R. (1956). Normal counter-transference and some of its deviations. *International Journal of Psychoanalysis, 37*: 360–366.

Morgan, D. L. (1997). *Focus Groups as Qualitative Research*. London: Sage.

Morgan, R. (2012). *Adoption with Siblings: Contact with Parents*. London: Ofsted.

Music, G. (2011). *Nurturing Natures: Attachment and Children's Emotional, Socio-Cultural and Brain Development*. Hove: Psychology Press.

Narey, M., & Owers, M. (2018). *Foster Care in England: A Review for the Department for Education*. London Department for Education. Available at: https://assets.publishing.service.gov.uk/government/uploads/system/uploads/attachment_data/file/679320/Foster_Care_in_England_ Review.pdf

Needell, B., & Booth, R. P. (1998). Infants entering foster care compared to other infants using birth status indicators. *Child Abuse and Neglect, 22* (12): 1179–1189.

Negri, R. (1994). *The Newborn in the Intensive Care Unit: A Neuropsychoanalytic Prevention Model*. London: Karnac.

O'Callaghan, P., Storey, L., & Rafferty, H. (2012). Narrative analysis of former child soldiers' traumatic experiences. *Educational & Child Psychology, 29*: 87–97.

Ogden, T. H. (1989). *The Primitive Edge of Experience*. Lanham, MA: Jason Aronson.

Ogden, T. H. (1999) *Reverie and Interpretation: Sensing Something Human*. London: Karnac.

Olden, C. (1953). On adult empathy with children. *Psychoanalytic Study of the Child, 8* (1): 111–126.

Ornstein, P. H., & Ornstein, A. (1994). On the conceptualisation of clinical facts in psychoanalysis. *International Journal of Psychoanalysis, 75*: 977–994.

O'Shaughnessy, E. (1964). The absent object. In: P. S. Barrows (Ed.), *Key Papers from the Journal of Child Psychotherapy* (pp. 13–23). Hove: Brunner-Routledge, 2004.

O'Shaughnessy, E. (1981). A commemorative essay on W. R. Bion's theory of thinking. *Journal of Child Psychotherapy, 7* (2): 181–192. Reprinted as: W. R. Bion's theory of thinking and new techniques in child analysis. In: E. B. Spillius (Ed.), *Melanie Klein Today: Developments in Theory and Practice. Vol. 2: Mainly Practice* (pp. 177–190). London: Routledge, 1988.

O'Shaughnessy, E. (1989). The invisible Oedipus complex. In: R. Britton, M. Feldman & E. O'Shaughnessy (Eds.), *The Oedipus Complex Today: Clinical Implications* (pp. 129–150). London: Karnac.

O'Shaughnessy, E. (1994). What is a clinical fact? *International Journal of Psychoanalysis, 75*: 939–947.

Pallet, C., Blackeby, K., Yule, W., Weissman, R., & Scott, S. (2000). *Fostering Changes: How to Improve Relationships and Manage Difficult Behaviour. A Training Programme for Foster Carers*. London: BAAF.

Pally, R. (2000). *The Mind–Brain Relationship*. International Journal of Psychoanalysis Key Papers Series. London: Karnac.

Palmer, M., Larkin, M., De Visser, R., & Fadden, G. (2010). Developing an interpretative phenomenological approach to focus group data. *Qualitative Research in Psychology, 7* (2): 99–121.

Panksepp, J. (2007). Can PLAY Diminish ADHD and facilitate the construction of the social brain? *Journal of the Canadian Academy of Child and Adolescent Psychiatry, 16* (2): 57–66.

Phillips, A., Wellman, H. M., & Spelke, E. S. (2002). Infants' ability to connect gaze and emotional expression to intentional action. *Cognition, 85* (1): 53–78.

Philps, J. F. (2003). *Applications of Child Psychotherapy to Work with Children in Temporary Foster Care*. Doctoral dissertation, University of East London, London.

Philps, J. F. (2009). Mapping process in child psychotherapy: Steps towards drafting a new method for evaluating psychoanalytic case studies. In: N. Midgley, J. Anderson, E. Grainger, T. Nesic-Vuckovic, & C. Urwin (Eds.), *Child Psychotherapy and Research: New Approaches, Emerging Findings* (pp. 56–71). London: Routledge.

Piontelli, A. (1992). *From Foetus to Child: An Observational and Psychoanalytic Study*. London: Routledge.

Popper, K. R. (1963). *Conjectures and Refutations*. London: Routledge & Kegan Paul.

Raphael-Leff, J. (Ed.) (2003). *Parent–Infant Psychodynamics: Wild Things, Mirrors and Ghosts*. London: Whurr.

Reicherz, J. (2007). Abduction: The logic of discovery in grounded theory. In: A. Bryan, & K. Charmaz (Eds.), *The Sage Handbook of Grounded Theory* (pp. 214–228). London: Sage.

Reid, M. (2007). The loss of a baby and the birth of the next infant. *Journal of Child Psychotherapy, 33* (2): 181–201.

Rey, H. (1986). The schizoid mode of being and the space-time continuum (beyond metaphor). *Journal of the Melanie Klein Society, 4*: 12–52.

Rey, H. (1994). *Universals of Psychoanalysis in the Treatment of Psychotic and Borderline States: Factors of Space–Time and Language*. London: Free Association Books.

Rhode, M. (2003). Sensory aspects of language development in relation to primitive anxieties. *International Journal of Infant Observation and Its Applications, 6* (2): 12–32.

Rhode, M. (2007). Infant observation as an early intervention. In: S. Acquarone (Ed.), *Signs of Autism in Infants: Recognition and Early Intervention*. London: Karnac.

Rhode, M. (2011). The "autistic" level of the Oedipus complex. *Psychoanalytic Psychotherapy, 25* (3): 262–276.

Rosenbluth, D. (1970). Transference in child psychotherapy. *Journal of Child Psychotherapy, 2* (4): 72–87. Reprinted in: P. S. Barrows (Ed.), *Key Papers from the Journal of Child Psychotherapy* (pp. 44–61). Hove: Brunner-Routledge, 2004.

Rosenfeld, H. (1964). On the psychopathology of narcissism: A clinical approach. In: *Psychotic States: A Psychoanalytic Approach*. London: Hogarth Press, 1965.

Rosenfeld, H. (1971). A clinical approach to the psychoanalytic theory of the life and death instincts: An investigation into the aggressive aspects of narcissism. *International Journal of Psychoanalysis, 52*: 169–178.

Rosenfeld, H. (2008). *Impasse and Interpretation: Therapeutic and Anti-Therapeutic Factors in the Psychoanalytic Treatment of Psychotic, Borderline, and Neurotic Patients*. London: Routledge.

Roth, A., & Fonagy, P. (1998). *What Works for Whom? A Critical View of Psychotherapy Research* (2nd edition). New York: Guilford Press, 2005.

Rowe, J., Cain, H., Hundleby, M., & Keane, A. (Eds.) (1984). *Long-Term Foster Care*. London: Batsford Academic and Educational, in association with the BAFF.

Rushton, A., Dance, C., Quinton, D., & Mayes, D. (2001). *Siblings in Late Permanent Placement*. London: BAFF.

Rustin, M. E. (1989). Identity: Fragmentation and recovery in psychoanalytic psychotherapy. *Social Discourse, 2*: 311–319.

Rustin, M. E. (1998). Observation, understanding and interpretation: The story of a supervision. *Journal of Child Psychotherapy, 24* (3): 433–448.

Rustin, M. E. (1999). Work with parents. In: M. Lanyado & A. Home (Eds.), *The Handbook of Child and Adolescent Psychotherapy: Psychoanalytic Approaches* (pp. 206–219). London: Routledge.

Rustin, M. E. (2001). The therapist with her back against the wall. *Journal of Child Psychotherapy, 27* (3): 273–284.

Rustin, M. E. (2005). A conceptual analysis of critical moments in Victoria Climbiés life. *Child and Family Social Work, 10* (1): 11–19.

Rustin, M. E. (2006). Where I belong: Dilemmas for children and adolescents who have been adopted or brought up in long-term foster care. In: J. Kenrick, C. Lindsey, & L. Tollemache (Eds.), *Creating New Families: Therapeutic Approaches to Fostering, Adoption and Kinship Care* (pp. 107–125). London: Karnac.

Rustin, M. E. (2007). Taking account of siblings: A view from child psychotherapy. *Journal of Child Psychotherapy, 33* (1): 21–35.

Rustin, M. E. (2008). Multiple families in mind. In: D. Hindle, & G. Shulman (Eds.), *The Emotional Experience of Adoption* (pp. 77–89). London: Routledge.

Rustin, M. E. (2014). The relevance of infant observation for early intervention: Containment in theory and practice. *Infant Observation, 17* (2): 97–114.

Rustin, M. E., & Rustin, M. J. (2017). *Reading Klein.* London: Routledge.

Rustin, M. J. (1997). The generation of psychoanalytic knowledge: Sociology and clinical perspectives. Part one: Give me a consulting room. *British Journal of Psychotherapy, 13* (4): 527–541.

Rustin, M. J. (2001a). Give me a consulting room … the generation of psychoanalytic knowledge. In: M. J. Rustin (Eds.), *Reason and Unreason: Psychoanalysis, Science, Politics* (pp. 30–51). London: Continuum.

Rustin, M. J. (2001b). Research, evidence and psychotherapy. In: C. Mace, S. Moorey & B. Roberts (Eds.), *Evidence in the Psychological Therapies: A Critical Guide for Practitioners* (pp. 27–45). London: Brunner-Routledge.

Rustin, M. J. (2009). What do child psychotherapists know? In: N. Midgley, J. Anderson, E. Grainger, N. Anderson, J. Grainger & T. Nesic-Vuckovic (Eds.), *Child Psychotherapy and Research: New Approaches, Emerging Findings* (pp. 35–49). London: Routledge.

Rustin, M. J. (2012). Infant observation as a method of research. In: C. Urwin & J. Sternberg (Eds.), *Infant Observation and Research Emotional Processes in Everyday Lives* (pp. 13–22). London: Routledge.

Rustin, M. J. (2019). *Researching the Unconscious: Principles of Psychoanalytic Method.* London: Routledge.

Salomonsson, B. (2004). Some psychoanalytic viewpoints on neuropsychiatric disorders in children. *International Journal of Psychoanalysis, 85* (1): 117–135.

Sanderson, N. (2014). Frustration and disappointment. *Journal of Child Psychotherapy, 40* (1): 36–57.

Sandler, J., & Freud, A. (1985). *The Analysis of Defenses: The Ego and the Mechanisms of Defense Revisited.* New York: International Universities Press.

Sandler, P. C. (2005). *The Language of Bion: A Dictionary of Concepts.* London: Karnac.

Schacter, D. L. (1996). *Searching for Memory: The Brain, the Mind and the Past.* New York: Basic Books.

Schore, A. (2001). The effects of early relational trauma on right brain development, affect regulation and infant mental health. *Infant Mental Health Journal, 22* (1–2): 201–269.

Segal, H. (1957). Notes on symbol formation. *International Journal of Psycho-analysis, 39*: 391–397.

Segal, H. (1997). The uses and abuses of counter-transference. In: H. Segal (Ed.), *Psychoanalysis, Literature and War, Papers 1972–1995* (pp. 111–119). London: Routledge.

Selwyn, J., Wijedasa, D., & Meakings, S. (2014). *Beyond the Adoption Order: Challenges, Interventions and Adoption Disruption. Research Report*. London: Department for Education.

Shallcross, W. (2012). What can be learned from a single case of psychoanalytic infant observation? In: C. Urwin & J. Sternberg (Eds.), *Infant Observation and Research: Emotional Processes in Everyday Lives* (pp. 69–80). London: Routledge.

Sharpe, S. A., & Rosenblatt, A. D. (1994). Oedipal sibling triangles. *Journal of the American Psychoanalytic Association, 42* (2): 491–523.

Silverstone, J. (2006). Siblings. In: P. Coles (Ed.), *Sibling Relationships*. London: Karnac.

Sklar, J. (2017). *Balint Matters: Psychosomatics and the Art of Assessment*. London: Karnac.

Smith, J. A. (1996). Beyond the divide between cognition and discourse: Using interpretative phenomenological analysis in health psychology. *Psychology & Health, 11*: 261–271.

Smith, J. A. (2004). Reflecting on the development of interpretative phenomenological analysis and its contribution to qualitative research in psychology. *Qualitative Research in Psychology, 1*: 39–54.

Smith, J. A., Flowers, P., & Larkin, M. (2009). *Interpretative Phenomenological Analysis: Theory, Method and Research*. London: Sage.

Smith, J. A., Harré, R., & Van Langenhove, L. V. (Eds.) (1995a). *Rethinking Psychology*. London: Sage.

Smith, J. A., Harré, R., & Van Langenhove, L. V. (Eds.) (1995b). *Rethinking Methods in Psychology*. London: Sage.

Smith, J. A., & Osborn, M. (2008). Interpretative phenomenological analysis. In: J. A. Smith (Ed.), *Qualitative Psychology: A Practical Guide to Methods* (pp. 53–80). London: Sage.

Solms, M. (2015). *The Feeling Brain: Selected Papers on Neuropsychoanalysis*. London: Karnac.

Spence, D. P. (1982). Narrative truth and theoretical truth. *Psychoanalytic Quarterly, 51*: 43–69.

Spence, D. P. (1984). *Narrative Truth and Historical Truth: Meaning and Interpretation in Psychoanalysis*. New York: Norton.

Spence, D. P. (1993). Traditional case studies and prescriptions for improving them. In: N. E. Miller, L. Luborsky, J. P. Barber & J. P. Docherty (Eds.), *Psychodynamic Treatment Research* (pp. 37–52). New York: Basic Books.

Spence, D. P. (1994). The special nature of clinical facts. *International Journal of Clinical Psychoanalysis, 75* (5/6): 915–926.

Spence, D. P. (1998). Rainforest or mud field? *International Journal of Psychoanalysis, 79*: 643–647.

Spence, D. P. (2000). Remembrance of things past. *Journal of Clinical Psychoanalysis, 9* (1): 149–162.

Spence, D. P. (2002). The virtual case report. *Psychoanalytic Quarterly, 71*: 679–698.

Spence, D. P. (2007). Perils and pitfalls of memory-based reporting: How case histories can become more evidenced-based. *Psychoanalytic Inquiry, 27* (5): 602–616.

Spillius, E. B. (Ed.) (1988a). *Melanie Klein Today: Developments in Theory and Practice. Vol. 1: Mainly Theory*. London: Routledge.

Spillius, E. B. (Ed.) (1988b). *Melanie Klein Today: Developments in Theory and Practice. Vol. 2: Mainly Practice*. London: Routledge.

Steiner, J. (1993). *Psychic Retreats: Pathological Organizations in Psychotic, Neurotic, and Borderline Patients*. London: Routledge.

Stern, D. (1985). *The Interpersonal World of the Infant*. New York: Basic Books.

Strachey, J. (1934). The nature of the therapeutic action in psychoanalysis. *International Journal of Psychoanalysis, 15*: 127–159.

Strauss, A., & Corbin, J. A. (1990). *Basics of Qualitative Research: Grounded Theory, Procedures and Techniques*. Thousand Oaks, CA: Sage.

Sunderland, M. (2007). *What Every Parent Needs to Know: The Incredible Effects of Love, Nurture and Play on Your Childs Development*. London: Dorling Kindersley.

Swedberg, R. (2012). Theorising in sociology and social science: Turning to the context of discovery. *Theory and Society, 41*: 1–40.

Tagore, R. (1913). *The Crescent Moon*. London & New York: Macmillan & Co.

Tarsoly, E. (1998). The relationship between failures in containment and early feeding difficulties: A participant observational study in a Hungarian residential nursery. *Infant Observation, 2* (1): 58–78.

Tizard, B., & Hodges, J. (1978). The effect of early institutional rearing on the development of eight-year-old children. *Journal Child Psychology and Psychiatry, 19*: 99–118.

Tomkins, L., & Eatough, V. (2010). Reflecting on the use of IPA with focus groups: Pitfalls and potentials. *Qualitative Research in Psychology, 7* (3): 244–262.

Trevarthen, C. (1974). Conversations with a two-month-old. *New Scientist*, 6 June, pp. 3–6.

Trevarthen, C. (2010). Communication and cooperation in early infancy: A description of primary intersubjectity. In: M. Bullowa (Ed.), *Before Speech: The Beginning of Interpersonal Communication* (pp. 321–349). Cambridge: Cambridge University Press.

Trevarthen, C., Aitken, K., Papoudi, D., & Robarts, J. (1998). *Children with Autism: Diagnosis and Interventions to Meet Their Needs* (2nd edition). London: Jessica Kingsley.

Trowell, J. (Ed.) (2011). *Childhood Depression: A Place for Psychotherapy*. London: Karnac.

Tuckett, D. (1994). Developing a grounded hypothesis to understand clinical process: The role of conceptualization in validation. *International Journal of Psychoanalysis, 75* (5/6): 1159–1180.

Tustin, F. (1966). A significant element in the development of autism. *Journal of Child Psychology and Psychiatry, 7*: 53–67.

Tustin, F. (1972). *Autism and Childhood Psychosis*. London: Hogarth Press reprinted London: Karnac, 1995.

Tustin, F. (1984). Autistic shapes. *International Review of Psycho-Analysis, 11*: 279–290.

Tustin, F. (1986a). *Autistic Barriers in Neurotic Patients*. London: Karnac.

Tustin, F. (1986b). A significant element in the development of psychogenic autism. In: K. Barrows (Ed.), *Autism in Childhood and Autistic Features in Adults: A Psychoanalytic Perspective* (pp. 39–62). London: Karnac, 2008.

Tustin, F. (1990a). Autistic encapsulation in neurotic patients. In: L. Bryce-Boyer & P. Giovacchini (Eds.), *Master Clinicians on Treating the Regressed Patient*. Northvale, NJ: Jason Aronson.

Tustin, F. (1990b). *The Protective Shell in Children and Adults*. London: Karnac.

Tustin, F. (1994). The perpetuation of an error. *Journal of Child Psychotherapy, 20*: 3–23.

Urwin, C. (2003). Breaking ground. Hitting ground: A sure start rapid response service for parents and their under fours. *Journal of Child Psychotherapy, 29* (3): 375–392.

Urwin, C., & Sternberg, J. (Eds.) (2012). *Infant Observation and Research: Emotional Processes in Everyday Lives*. London: Routledge.

Waddell, M., & Williams, G. (1991). Reflections on perverse states of mind. *Free Associations, 2*: 203–213.

Wade, J., Biehal, N., Farrelly, N., & Sinclair, I. (2010). *Maltreated Children in the Looked After System: A Comparison of Outcomes for Those Who Go Home and Those Who Do Not*. London: Department for Education.

Wakelyn, J. (2007). Entangled bonds. Psychodynamic assessments of sibling relationships for the family courts. In: C. Thorpe & J. Trowell (Eds.), *Re-Rooted Lives. Interdisciplinary Work within the Family Justice System*. Bristol: Jordan Publishing.

Wakelyn, J. (2008). Transitional psychotherapy for looked-after children in short-term foster care. *Journal of Social Work Practice, 22* (1): 27–36.

Wakelyn, J. (2011). Therapeutic observation of an infant in foster care. *Journal of Child Psychotherapy, 37* (3): 280–310.

Wakelyn, J. (2012a). Observation as a therapeutic intervention for infants and young children in care. *Infant Observation, 15* (1): 49–66.

Wakelyn, J. (2012b). A study of therapeutic observation of an infant in foster care. In: C. Urwin. & J. Sternberg (Eds.), *Infant Observation and Research Emotional Processes in Everyday Lives* (pp. 81–92). London: Routledge.

Wallerstein, R. S. (1988). One psychoanalysis or many? *International Journal of Psychoanalysis, 69*: 5–21.

Wallerstein, R. S. (2005). Will psychoanalytic pluralism be the enduring state of our discipline? *International Journal of Psychoanalysis, 86*: 623–626.

Wallerstein, R. S., & Fonagy, P. (1999). Psychoanalytic research and the IPA: History, present status and future potential. *International Journal of Psychoanalysis, 80* (1): 91–110.

Wallerstein, R. S., & Sampson, H. (1971). Issues in research in the psychoanalytic process. *International Journal of Psychoanalysis, 52*: 11–50.

Ward, H., Munro, E., & Dearden, C. (2006). *Babies and Young Children in Care: Life Pathways, Decision-Making and Practice*. London: Jessica Kingsley.

White, N. (2004). Review of literature. *Psychoanalytic Psychotherapy, 18* (1): 15–26.

WHO (2006). *Mental Health and Psychosocial Well-Being among Children in Severe Food Shortage Situations*. Department of Mental Health and Substance Abuse (MSD). Geneva: World Health Organization.

Williams, G. (1997). *Internal Landscapes and Foreign Bodies: Eating Disorders and Other Pathologies*. London: Duckworth.

Willig, C. (2001). *Introducing Qualitative Research in Psychology: Adventures in Theory*. Buckingham: Open University Press.

Wilson, A., & Malatesta, C. (1989). Affect and the compulsion to repeat: Freud's repetition compulsion revisited. *Psychoanalysis and Cotemporary Thought, 12*: 265–312.

Winnicott, D. (1949a). Birth memories, birth trauma, and anxiety. In: *Through Paediatrics to Psychoanalysis* (pp. 174–193). London: Karnac, 1984.

Winnicott, D. W. (1949b). Hate in the counter-transference. *International Journal of Psychoanalysis, 30*: 69–74.

Winnicott, D. W. (1952). Anxiety associated with insecurity. In: *Through Paediatrics to Psychoanalysis* (pp. 97–100). London: Karnac, 1984.

Winnicott, D. W. (1956). The antisocial tendency. In: *Through Paediatrics to Psychoanalysis* (pp. 306–315). London: Karnac, 1984.

Winnicott, D. W. (1960). The theory of the parent–infant relationship. In: *The Maturational Processes and the Facilitating Environment* (pp. 37–55). London: Karnac, 1990.

Winnicott, D. W. (1967). Mirror-role of mother and family in child development. In: *Playing and Reality*. London: Tavistock, 1971.

Winnicott, D. W. (1974). The fear of breakdown. *International Review of Psycho-Analysis, 1*: 103–107.

Winnicott, D. W. (1990). *The Maturational Processes and the Facilitating Environment*. London: Karnac.

Wittgenstein, L. (1953). *Philosophical Investigations* (2nd edition). Oxford: Blackwell, 1997.

Wolfson, A., & Sampson, H. (1976). A comparison of process notes and tape recordings: Implications for therapy research. *Archives of General Psychiatry, 33* (5): 558–563.

Yakeley, J. (2013). Seeing, mirroring, desiring: The impact of the analysts pregnancy body on the patient's body image. *International Journal of Psychoanalysis, 94*: 667–688.

Zeanah, C. H., & Boris, N. W. (2000). Disturbances and disorders of attachment in early childhood. In: C. H. Zeanah (Ed.), *Handbook of Infant Mental Health, Second Edition* (pp. 353–368). New York: Guilford Press.

Žižek, S. (1990). East Europe's Republics of Gilead, *New Left Review 183* (Sept.–Oct): 50–62.

Žižek, S. (1993). Enjoy your nation as yourself. In: *Tarrying with the Negative: Kant, Hegel and the Critique of Ideology* (pp. 200–238). Durham, NC: Duke University Press.

INDEX

For Product Safety Concerns and Information please contact our EU representative GPSR@taylorandfrancis.com Taylor & Francis Verlag GmbH, Kaufingerstraße 24, 80331 München, Germany

Batch number: 10725793

Printed by Printforce, the Netherlands